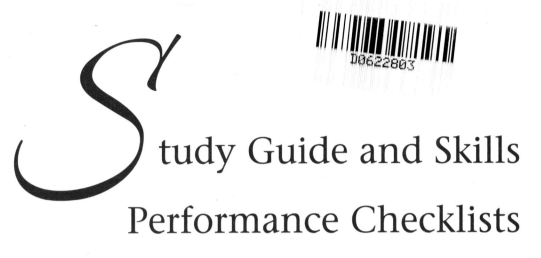

# Study Guide and Skills Performance Checklists

to Accompany

## POTTER/PERRY
### *Canadian Fundamentals of Nursing*
#### 5th edition

**Geralyn Ochs, RN, MSN, BC-ACNP, ANP**
Assistant Professor of Nursing
St. Louis University School of Nursing
St. Louis, Missouri

**Kyla C. Janzen, RN, BScN, MSN**
Trinity Western University
Langley, British Columbia

*Skills Performance Checklists by*
**Jerilee LaMar, PhD, RN, BC**
Assistant Professor of Nursing
University of Evansville
Evansville, Indiana

**Linda Turchin, RN, MSN**
Assistant Professor
Fairmont State University
Fairmont, West Virginia

ELSEVIER

**ELSEVIER**
MOSBY

---

**NOTICE**

Knowledge and best practice in this field are constantly changing. As new research and expertise broaden our knowledge, changes in practice, treatment, and drug therapy may become necessary or appropriate. Readers are advised to check the most current information provided (i) on procedures featured or (ii) by the manufacturer of each product to be administered, to verify the recommended dose or formula, the method and duration of administration, and contraindications. It is the responsibility of the practitioner, relying on their own experience and knowledge of the patient, to make diagnoses, to determine dosages and the best treatment for each individual patient, and to take all appropriate safety precautions. To the fullest extent of the law, neither the Publisher nor the Authors assumes any liability for any injury and/or damage to persons or property arising out of or related to any use of the material contained in this book.

The Publisher

---

**Library and Archives Canada Cataloguing in Publication**

Ochs, Geralyn
Study guide and skills performance checklists to accompany Potter/Perry Canadian fundamentals of nursing, 5th edition / Geralyn Ochs, Kyla C. Janzen; skills performance checklists by Jerilee LaMar, Linda Turchin.

ISBN 978-1-926648-52-1

1. Nursing—Problems, exercises, etc.  2. Nursing—Handbooks, manuals, etc.
I. Janzen, Kyla C  II. LaMar, Jerilee  III. Turchin, Linda  IV. Potter, Patricia Ann. Canadian fundamentals of nursing.  V. Title.

RT41.P68 2013 Suppl.                    610.73                    C2012-906675-3

*Vice President, Publishing:* Ann Millar
*Developmental Editor:* Christine Langone
*Managing Developmental Editor:* Martina van de Velde
*Project Manager:* Siva Raman Krishna Moorthy
*Copy Editor:* Judy Jamison
*Typesetting and Assembly:* GW Tech, India
*Printing and Binding:* Edward Brothers, MI, USA

Elsevier Canada
905 King Street West, 4th Floor,
Toronto, ON, Canada M6K 3G9
Phone: 1-866-896-3331
Fax: 1-866-359-9534

1   2   3   4   5   14   13

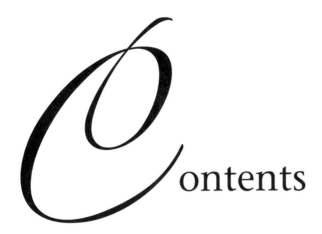

# ontents

# Unit IV - Working With Patients and Families

# Unit V - Caring Throughout the Lifespan

# Unit VI - Psychosocial Considerations

# Unit VII - Scientific Basis for Nursing Practice

# Unit VIII - Basic Physiological Needs

## Unit IX - Patients With Special Needs

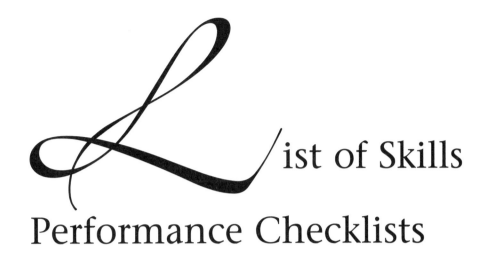

# List of Skills

# Performance Checklists

# Introduction

The *Study Guide and Skills Performance Checklists to accompany Canadian Fundamentals of Nursing*, Fifth Edition, has been developed to encourage independent learning for beginning nursing students. As you begin to read the text, you may note a difference in style and format from other books you've used in the past. The terms are new, and the focus of the content is different. You may be wondering, "How will I possibly learn all of the material in this chapter?" The essential objective of this study guide is to assist you in this endeavour—to help you learn what you need to know and then self-test with hundreds of review questions.

This study guide follows the text chapter for chapter. Whatever chapter your instructor assigns, you will use the same chapter number in this study guide. The outline format was designed to help you learn to read nursing content more effectively and with greater understanding. Each chapter of this study guide has the following sections to assist you to comprehend and recall.

The *Preliminary Reading* section is designed to teach pre-reading strategies. You need to become familiar with the chapter by first reading the chapter title, the key concepts and key terms, and all headings, as well as review all photographs, drawings, tables, and boxes. This can be done rather quickly and will give you an overall idea of the content of the chapter.

The *Comprehensive Understanding* section is next and is in outline format. This will prove to be a very valuable tool, not only as you first read the chapter but also as you review for tests. This outline identifies the topics and main ideas of each chapter as an aid to concentration, comprehension, and retaining textbook information. By completing this outline, you will learn to "pull-out" key information in the chapter. As you write the answers in the study guide, you will be reinforcing that content. Once completed, this outline will serve as a review tool for exams.

The *Review Questions* in each chapter provide a valuable means of testing and reinforcing your knowledge of the material read and the answers written in the outline. Each question is multiple choice. As a further aid for independent learning, each answer requires a rationale (the reason why the option you selected is correct). After you have completed the review questions, you can check the answers in the back of the study guide.

Chapters 25 to 29 and 35 to 48 include exercises based on the care plans found in the text. These exercises provide practice in synthesizing the nursing process and critical thinking as you, the nurse, care for patients. Taking one aspect of the nursing process, you will be asked to imagine you are the nurse in the case study and to think about what knowledge, experiences, standards, and attitudes might be used in caring for the patient. Write your answers in the appropriate boxes and check them against the answer key.

When you finish answering the review questions and synthesis exercises, take a few minutes for self-evaluation. If you answered a question incorrectly, begin to analyze the thoughts that led you to the wrong answer:

- Did you miss the key word or phrase?
- Did you read into something that wasn't stated?
- Did you not understand the subject matter?
- Did you use an incorrect rationale for selecting your response?

Each incorrect response is an opportunity to learn. Go back to the text and re-read any content that is still unclear. In the long run, it will be a time-saving activity.

A performance checklist is provided for each of the skills presented in the text. The checklists may be used by instructors to evaluate your competence in performing the techniques. You may need to adapt these skills in order to meet a patient's special needs or follow the particular policy of an institution.

The learning activities presented in this study guide will assist you in completing the semester with a firm understanding of nursing concepts and processes that you can rely on for all of your professional career.

# 1

# Health and Wellness

## *Preliminary Reading*

Chapter 1, pages 1–14

## *Comprehensive Understanding*

### Conceptualizations of Health

**Classifications of Health Conceptualizations**

1. Compare three different conceptualizations of health.

   a. _____

   b. _____

   c. _____

### Historical Approaches to Health in Canada

2. Historically, the three different approaches to health in Canada have been medical, behavioural, and socioenvironmental. Identify the distinguishing features of each of these approaches.

   a. Medical:

   _____

   _____

   b. Behavioural:

   _____

   _____

   c. Socioenvironmental:

   _____

   _____

3. Identify the contributions of the following Canadian documents to the understanding of health and health determinants.

   a. *Lalonde Report*:

   _____

   _____

   b. *Ottawa Charter*:

   _____

   _____

   c. *Epp Report*:

   _____

   _____

   d. *Strategies for Population Health*:

   _____

   _____

   e. *Toronto Charter*:

   _____

   _____

## Determinants of Health

4. Identify 12 major determinants of health, as outlined by Health Canada, the *Ottawa Charter*, and the *Toronto Charter*.

_____  _____
_____  _____
_____  _____
_____  _____
_____  _____
_____  _____

5. Why is it important for nurses to understand the concept of health determinants?

_____
_____
_____

## Strategies to Influence Health Determinants

6. The concepts of *health promotion* and *disease prevention* are distinct yet interrelated. Briefly explain each one.

   a. Health promotion:

   _____
   _____

   b. Disease prevention:

   _____
   _____

7. Define the three levels of prevention, and give an example of each.

   a. *Primary prevention*:

   _____
   _____

   b. *Secondary prevention*:

   _____
   _____

   c. *Tertiary prevention*:

   _____
   _____

## Health Promotion Strategies

8. Define the five health promotion strategies contained in the *Ottawa Charter*, and give examples of activities in each strategy.

   a. *Build healthy public policy*:

   _____
   _____

   b. *Create supportive environments*:

   _____
   _____

   c. *Strengthen community action*:

   _____
   _____

   d. *Develop personal skills*:

   _____
   _____

   e. *Reorient health services*:

   _____
   _____

## Population Health Promotion Model: Putting It All Together

9. What are the four major elements of the Population Health Promotion Model?

   a. _____
   b. _____
   c. _____
   d. _____

10. Provide an example of how you might use this model in your practice.

_____
_____
_____

## Review Questions

Select the appropriate answer, and cite the rationale for choosing that particular answer.

1. The "watershed" document that marked the shift from a lifestyle to a socioenvironmental approach to health was the
   a. *Lalonde Report*
   b. National Forum on Health
   c. *Toronto Charter*
   d. *Ottawa Charter*

   Answer: _____ Rationale: _____

   _____

   _____

2. The major determinants of health in a socioenvironmental view of health are
   a. Psychosocial risk factors and socioenvironmental risk conditions
   b. Physiological risk factors and behavioural risk factors
   c. Behavioural and psychosocial risk factors
   d. Behavioural and socioenvironmental risk factors

   Answer: _____ Rationale: _____

   _____

   _____

3. The main reason that intersectoral collaboration is a necessary strategy to reach the goal of "Health for All" is
   a. The determinants of health are broad
   b. Intersectoral collaboration is cost-effective
   c. Intersectoral collaboration encourages problem solving at a local level
   d. Intersectoral collaboration is less likely to result in conflict

   Answer: _____ Rationale: _____

   _____

   _____

4. Providing immunizations against measles is an example of
   a. Health promotion
   b. Primary prevention
   c. Secondary prevention
   d. Tertiary prevention

   Answer: _____ Rationale: _____

   _____

   _____

5. Which of the following statements does *not* accurately characterize health promotion?
   a. Health promotion addresses health issues within the context of the social, economic, and political environment.
   b. Health promotion emphasizes empowerment.
   c. Health promotion strategies focus primarily on helping people develop healthy behaviours.
   d. Health promotion is political.

   Answer: _____ Rationale: _____

   _____

   _____

6. The belief that health is primarily an individual responsibility is most congruent with which approach to health?
   a. Medical
   b. Behavioural
   c. Socioenvironmental
   d. Public health

   Answer: _____ Rationale: _____

   _____

   _____

7. All of the following statements accurately describe the Population Health Promotion Model, *except*
   a. The model suggests that action can address the full range of health determinants
   b. The model incorporates the health promotion strategies of the *Ottawa Charter*
   c. The model focuses primarily on interventions at the society level
   d. The model attempts to integrate the concepts of population health and health promotion

   Answer: _____ Rationale: _____

   _____

   _____

8. Which of the following is the most influential health determinant?
   a. Personal health practices
   b. Income and social status
   c. Health care services
   d. Physical environment

   Answer: _____ Rationale: _____

   _____

   _____

9. A medical approach to health is to health services as a behavioural approach is to
   a. Income and social status
   b. Employment and working conditions
   c. Physical environments
   d. Personal health practices

Answer:_____ Rationale: _____
_____
_____

10. Understanding the context in which health behaviours occur most accurately reflects which approach to health?
   a. Behavioural
   b. Medical
   c. Socioenvironmental
   d. Primary prevention

Answer:_____ Rationale: _____
_____
_____

# 2

# The Canadian Health Care Delivery System

## *Preliminary Reading*

Chapter 2, pages 15–28

## *Comprehensive Understanding*

### Evolution of the Canadian Health Care System

1. Canada has constructed a social safety net for the protection of its citizens. Medicare is an important part of this safety net. Briefly explain the role of the following in the development of medicare.

   a. *British North America Act:*

     _____

     _____

   b. Great Depression:

     _____

     _____

   c. Tommy Douglas:

     _____

     _____

   d. *Medical Care Act* (1966):

     _____

     _____

   e. *Canada Health Act* (1984):

     _____

     _____

### The Organization and Governance of Health Care

2. Under the *Canadian Constitution Act*, administration and delivery of health care services are primarily provincial or territorial responsibilities. However, the federal government continues to have a role. Briefly explain the following.

   a. The four areas of federal jurisdiction for health care in Canada:

     _____

     _____

     _____

     _____

   b. The role of the provincial and territorial governments in the organization and delivery of health care:

     _____

     _____

     _____

     _____

   c. The five principles enshrined in the *Canada Health Act:*

     _____

     _____

     _____

     _____

## Health Care Spending

3. In 2009, a Conference Board of Canada study stated that despite our significant increase in health care spending, Canada ranked

   _____ in a comparison of 16 industrialized countries on quality indicators such as life expectancy.

## Trends and Reforms in Canada's Health Care System

4. Describe the main recommendations of the *Romanow* and *Kirby* reports.

   _____
   _____
   _____
   _____

## Right to Health Care

5. Explain the role and influence of the *Canada Health Act* in establishing health care as a right for all Canadians.

   _____
   _____
   _____
   _____

## Primary Health Care

6. Explain the difference between primary care (PC) and primary health care (PHC).

   _____
   _____
   _____
   _____

7. Explain the four pillars of PHC.
   a. _____
   b. _____
   c. _____
   d. _____

8. Describe the benefits and potential drawbacks involved with increasing funding to PHC and home care services.

   _____
   _____
   _____
   _____

## Settings for Health Care Delivery

9. Explain the role of each of the following institutions in delivering health care.

   a. Hospitals:

      _____
      _____

   b. Long-term care facilities:

      _____
      _____

   c. Psychiatric facilities:

      _____
      _____

   d. Rehabilitation centres:

      _____
      _____

10. Explain the role of each of the following in delivering health care in the community.

   a. Public health:

      _____
      _____

   b. Physician offices:

      _____
      _____

   c. Community health centres and clinics:

      _____
      _____

   d. Assisted living:

      _____
      _____

e. Home care:

_____

_____

f. Adult day support programs:

_____

_____

g. Community and voluntary agencies:

_____

_____

h. Occupational health:

_____

_____

i. Hospice and palliative care:

_____

_____

j. Parish nursing:

_____

_____

## Levels of Care

11. List and briefly describe the five levels of health care.

a. _____

b. _____

c. _____

d. _____

e. _____

12. Explain primary care, secondary care, and tertiary care.

_____

_____

_____

## Challenges to the Health Care System

13. Describe three cost accelerators in the Canadian health care system.

a. _____

_____

b. _____

_____

c. _____

_____

## *Review Questions*

Select the appropriate answer, and cite the rationale for choosing that particular answer.

1. When the *Canada Health Act* of 1984 amalgamated the previous acts of 1957 and 1966, it added which principle to the existing four?
   a. Accessibility
   b. Comprehensiveness
   c. Portability
   d. Public administration

Answer:_____ Rationale: _____

_____

_____

2. The amount of money (public and private) Canada spent on health care per capita in 2010 was approximately:
   a. $1870
   b. $3839
   c. $5614
   d. $2440

Answer:_____ Rationale: _____

_____

_____

3. A 16-year-old student sees a physician at a walk-in clinic to find out if she is pregnant. This service can be best described as an example of
   a. Primary care
   b. Primary health care
   c. Tertiary care
   d. Secondary care

Answer:_____ Rationale: _____
_____
_____

4. The 16-year-old student attends a community program on prenatal health for teenage mothers. The program is taught by a nurse, a nutritionist, and a social worker. This service can best be described as an example of
   a. Primary care
   b. Primary health care
   c. Tertiary care
   d. Secondary care

Answer:_____ Rationale: _____
_____
_____

5. Which of the following is a *false* statement?
   a. Most nurses work in institutional settings in Canada.
   b. Most nursing graduates are degree prepared.
   c. Most nurses are over age 40.
   d. The ratio of nurses in Canada is one registered nurse for every 127 persons.

Answer:_____ Rationale: _____
_____
_____

# 3

# The Development of Nursing in Canada

## *Preliminary Reading*

Chapter 3, pages 29–41

## *Comprehensive Understanding*

1. Define *nursing* (according to the International Council of Nurses [ICN]).

   _____

   _____

   _____

### Highlights of World Nursing History

2. All of the following statements are true *except*
   a. The Egyptians understood that a good diet was important in maintaining health
   b. The Romans focused on public health and sanitation
   c. The Hebrews believed in the spiritual basis of illness
   d. After the Protestant Reformation, new hospitals were staffed by trained and suitable individuals

### Early History of Nursing in Canada

#### The First Nurses and Hospitals in New France

3. What was the contribution of Mme Hébert to health care in the new colony?

   _____

   _____

   _____

4. List five important milestones in the development of nursing in Canada.

   a. _____

      _____

   b. _____

      _____

   c. _____

      _____

   d. _____

      _____

   e. _____

      _____

#### The Birth of Home Visiting and the Grey Nuns

5. Describe the beginnings and mission of the Grey Nuns.

   _____

   _____

   _____

#### Nursing During the British Regime

6. How did British nursing compare with French nursing during the eighteenth century?

   _____

   _____

   _____

7. _____ carried by _____ and _____ spread rapidly in the British colonies. Established French Canadian orders expanded their services, and new English-speaking orders were founded to help the sick and the poor.

**Health Care in the West and the Grey Nuns**

8. The Grey Nuns travelled from Montreal and cared for the sick in these parts of Canada:

a. _____

b. _____

c. _____

d. _____

**The Nineteenth Century and Florence Nightingale**

9. Nightingale became an advocate for

_____, _____, and

_____.

# Globalization and the Emergence of Modern Nursing

The history of modern nursing, at its heart, is a story of globalization. Nursing history is strewn with examples of nurses travelling across geographic and national boundaries to bring nursing service and training to communities in need.

**Missionary Nursing**

10. Discuss the sociopolitical developments that allowed Canadian missionary nurses into China in the 1880s.

_____

_____

_____

_____

_____

**Nursing in Remote Regions of Canada**

11. The _____ of the _____ brought an onset of resource development in northern regions of Canada, including health care.

**Gender and Diversity in Nursing**

12. Since the 1960s and 1970s, the nursing profession has become increasingly aware of the

need for _____ _____,

and _____, _____, and

_____ _____.

# Nursing Education in Canada

13. What was the main reason for establishing the first Canadian nursing schools?

_____

_____

_____

14. Describe the growth of hospital nursing schools in the late nineteenth century.

_____

_____

_____

**The Impact of Nursing Organizations on Nursing Education**

15. How did the ICN influence the development of nursing organizations worldwide?

_____

_____

_____

_____

16. The Canadian Nurses Association (CNA) became a federation of provincial associations in:
a. 1924
b. 1907
c. 1930
d. 1899

17. Licensure laws are designed to protect the public against unqualified and incompetent practitioners. Highlight the differences between *permissive* and *mandatory* legislation.

_____

_____

_____

18. How did the struggle for women's rights influence nursing?

_____

_____

_____

**The First University Programs**

19. When and where was the first university program in nursing established?

_____

_____

_____

## Health Care and Educational Reform

20. Describe the following reports:
    a. *Weir Report*
    b. The report of the Royal Commission on Health Services of 1964
    c. CNA reports
    d. Baccalaureate entry-to-practice report

## Influence of Periods of Social Upheaval on Nursing

21. In the first quarter of the twentieth century, women in western Canada became seriously involved in commenting on needs in health and education, and developed organizations to put forward their ideas. These five Albertan women petitioned the Supreme Court of Canada for women's rights:
    a. _____
    b. _____
    c. _____
    d. _____
    e. _____

22. Describe the relationship between the Canadian Red Cross and university programs in nursing.

    _____
    _____
    _____

### From the Depression to the Post–World War II Years

23. The Great Depression brought _____ and _____ to nurses.

24. How did World War II affect health education?

    _____
    _____
    _____

### Emerging from Economic and Military Crises

25. Describe the development of graduate programs during the years following World War II.

    _____
    _____
    _____

### Nursing Education Today

26. Where does the responsibility for monitoring standards of nursing education lie?

    _____
    _____

27. A master's degree in nursing is necessary for

    _____.

28. Nurses with doctorates can _____

    _____.

29. _____, a hallmark of any profession, remains an important characteristic of the nursing profession despite vast differences between the health care settings of the early days and those of today.

## *Review Questions*

Select the appropriate answer, and cite the rationale for choosing that particular answer.

1. Hippocrates is considered the father of scientific medicine because
   a. He was the first to make observations of patients and develop treatments on the basis of symptoms
   b. He recognized the importance of fresh water and hygiene for public health
   c. He believed in a spiritual basis of illness
   d. He recognized the importance of nutrition in maintaining health

   Answer: _____ Rationale: _____
   _____
   _____

2. The first visiting nurses in Canada were
   a. Led by Jeanne Mance in 1642
   b. The first three Augustinian nuns in 1639
   c. Marie Rollet Hébert and her surgeon-apothecary husband in 1617
   d. The Grey Nuns under Marguerite d'Youville in 1737

   Answer: _____ Rationale: _____
   _____
   _____

3. Which of the following is *not* attributed to Florence Nightingale?
   a. Dramatically reduced morbidity and mortality rates among the wounded
   b. Developed nursing as a profession independent from medicine
   c. Introduced nursing to the British army during the Crimean War
   d. Made nursing an acceptable field of work for middle- and upper-class women outside the home

Answer: _____ Rationale: _____
_____
_____

4. The first undergraduate degree program in nursing in Canada was developed at
   a. St. Francis Xavier University
   b. University of Toronto
   c. University of Alberta
   d. University of British Columbia

Answer: _____ Rationale: _____
_____
_____

5. This struggle helped nurses secure laws to regulate their profession in Canada:
   a. Public health
   b. Crimean War
   c. Women's rights
   d. University education

# 4

# Community Health Nursing Practice

## *Preliminary Reading*

Chapter 4, pages 42–53

## *Comprehensive Understanding*

1. Community health nursing care focuses on

   _____

   _____

   _____

### Promoting the Health of Populations and Community Groups

2. Distinguish between a *population* and a *community*, and give an example of each.

   _____

   _____

   _____

3. Compare the characteristics of a *healthy population* and a *healthy community*.

   _____

   _____

   _____

   _____

### Community Health Nursing Practice

4. Describe the scope of *community health nursing practice*.

   _____

   _____

   _____

5. Define *social justice*.

   _____

   _____

   _____

6. Briefly explain the nursing focus in *primary health care* (PHC).

   _____

   _____

   _____

7. Briefly explain the nursing focus on *empowerment* in community health nursing guided by PHC.

   _____

   _____

   _____

8. Briefly describe the contributions of public health and population health to *public health nursing*.

   _____

   _____

   _____

   _____

9. Give an example of each of the strategies identified in the framework for public health programs.

   a. Promote individual and family action:

      _____

      _____

   b. Provide direct care:

      _____

      _____

c. Influence the environment:

_____

_____

d. Build partnerships:

_____

_____

10. A strong theoretical foundation for *home health nursing* is provided by

_____

_____.

11. Briefly describe key distinctions between public health nursing and home health nursing.

a. Public health nursing:

_____

_____

b. Home health nursing:

_____

_____

## The Changing Focus of Community Health Nursing Practice
### Vulnerable Populations

12. *Vulnerable populations* of patients are those who are

_____

_____

_____.

13. Explain how a nurse approaches diversity to provide culturally sensitive, competent, and safe care.

_____

_____

_____

_____

14. List some of the reasons why vulnerable populations typically experience poorer health outcomes.

_____

_____

_____

_____

15. Briefly describe the following vulnerable groups, and identify the circumstances that contribute to their vulnerability.

a. Poor and homeless people:

_____

_____

b. People in precarious circumstances:

_____

_____

c. People with chronic conditions and disabilities:

_____

_____

d. People who engage in stigmatizing risk behaviours:

_____

_____

### Standards, Competencies, Roles, and Activities in Community Health Nursing

16. A nurse in a community health practice must have a variety of skills and knowledge to assist individuals and families within the community, as well as communities broadly. Briefly explain the competencies the community nurse needs to develop.

a. Communication:

_____

_____

b. Facilitation:

_____

_____

c. Leadership:

_____

_____

d. Advocacy:

_____

_____

e. Consultation:

_____

_____

f. Team building and collaboration:

_____

_____

g. Building capacity:

_____

_____

h. Building coalitions and networks:

_____

_____

i. Outreach:

_____

_____

j. Resource management, planning, coordination:

_____

_____

k. Case management:

_____

_____

l. Care/counselling:

_____

_____

m. Referral and follow-up:

_____

_____

n. Screening:

_____

_____

o. Surveillance:

_____

_____

p. Health threat response:

_____

_____

q. Health education:

_____

_____

r. Community development:

_____

_____

s. Policy development and implementation:

_____

_____

t. Research and evaluation:

_____

_____

## Community Assessment

17. The community is viewed as having three components. Briefly explain each one.

a. Locale or structure:

_____

_____

b. Social systems:

_____

_____

c. People:

_____

_____

18. Briefly describe each of the following strategies to assess the locale or structure of a community.

a. Windshield or walking survey:

_____

_____

b. Observation of activities:

_____

_____

c. Key informant interviews:

_____

_____

d. Population data review:

_____

_____

e. Focus group interviews:

_____

_____

## Promoting Patients' Health

19. The challenge is how to promote and protect the patient's health, whether within the context of the community or with the community as the focus. The most important theme to consider, to be an effective community health nurse, is to _____.

20. Identify some factors that nurses must consider in community nursing practice.

_____
_____
_____
_____

## *Review Questions*

Select the appropriate answer, and cite the rationale for choosing that particular answer.

1. Which of the following would *not* typically be considered an example of PHC?
   a. Lunchtime nutrition and activity program in an inner-city school run by nurses, nutritionists, social workers, and teachers
   b. A rehabilitation program in a hospital provided by physiotherapists, physicians, nurses, and social workers for patients and families recovering from a stroke
   c. Activities provided by child care workers in a day care centre at a corporation
   d. A well-baby clinic conducted by nurses and nutritionists for new mothers at a neighbourhood health centre

Answer:_____ Rationale: _____
_____
_____

2. Among the communication skills needed to provide nursing care to community patients is the ability to
   a. Clarify patient values and care expectations
   b. Follow medical prescriptions in many settings
   c. Manage generational interfamilial conflict
   d. Speak the patient's language or dialects

Answer:_____ Rationale: _____
_____
_____

3. Poor and homeless people
   a. Have a high incidence of mental illness and substance abuse
   b. Have more resources than low-income people
   c. Eat nutritious food
   d. Have great trust in health and social services

4. When the community health nurse refers patients to appropriate resources, and monitors and coordinates the extent and adequacy of services to meet family health care needs, the nurse is functioning in the role of:
   a. Collaborator
   b. Educator
   c. Consultant
   d. Coordinator

Answer:_____ Rationale: _____
_____
_____

5. Which of the following is *not* identified as a challenge in community health nursing?
   a. Increased task orientation, specialization, and working in silos
   b. Staying current on health information
   c. Limited demand for acute care in the community
   d. Conflict between prescribed programs and community partnership activities

Answer:_____ Rationale: _____
_____
_____

# 5

# Theoretical Foundations of Nursing Practice

## *Preliminary Reading*

Chapter 5, pages 54–64

## *Comprehensive Understanding*

1. Define the terms *theory* and *nursing theory*, and explain why knowledge of nursing theory can help nurses become better practitioners.

   _____

   _____

   _____

   _____

### Early Nursing Practice and the Emergence of Theory

2. Briefly describe how developments in science and technology affected the development of nursing as a science.

   _____

   _____

   _____

   _____

3. Explain the relationship between the development of nursing theory and the challenge of building curriculum for nursing education.

   _____

   _____

   _____

   _____

   _____

### Nursing Process

4. Describe the four basic steps of the *nursing process*.

   a. Assessment:

   _____

   _____

   b. Planning:

   _____

   _____

   c. Intervention:

   _____

   _____

   d. Evaluation:

   _____

   _____

5. The relationship between clinical judgement and nursing process is

   _____.

## Conceptual Frameworks

6. Briefly describe how systematic thinking using conceptual nursing models differs from linear reasoning processes.

_____

_____

_____

_____

## Metaparadigm Concepts

7. Explain the importance of each *metaparadigm* concept for the clinical reasoning process in nursing.

   a. Person:

   _____

   _____

   b. Environment:

   _____

   _____

   c. Health:

   _____

   _____

   d. Nursing:

   _____

   _____

8. For each metaparadigm concept, identify at least two possible ways it might be defined for the purpose of guiding nursing practice.

   a. Person:

   _____

   _____

   b. Environment:

   _____

   _____

   c. Health:

   _____

   _____

   d. Nursing:

   _____

   _____

## Philosophy of Nursing Science

9. Thomas S. Kuhn's ideas about paradigms helped nurses understand the scientific basis of nursing not simply as theoretical propositions but as

   _____

   _____.

10. Chaos theory provided nurses with a new way to think about

   _____.

## Ways of Knowing in Nursing Practice

11. List four forms of knowledge identified by Carper that have contributed to excellent nursing practice.

   a. _____

   b. _____

   c. _____

   d. _____

## Paradigm Debates Within Nursing

12. The two distinct paradigms that have been associated with debates surrounding nursing's theoretical development are _____ and _____.

## Nursing Diagnosis

13. Identify advantages and disadvantages of adopting a fixed list of diagnostic categories for nursing care.

   a. Advantages:

   _____

   _____

   _____

   b. Disadvantages:

   _____

   _____

   _____

## Reflections on Conceptualizing Nursing

Instead of arguing the advantages of one nursing theory over another, nursing scholars of today appreciate the creativity of their predecessors within the constrained conceptual contexts in which they were expected to operate.

## Major Theoretical Models

14. Identify one characteristic of each of the following categories of theoretical models.

    a. Practice-based theories:

    _____

    _____

    b. Needs theories:

    _____

    _____

    c. Interactionist theories:

    _____

    _____

    d. Systems theories:

    _____

    _____

    e. Simultaneity theories:

    _____

    _____

15. Name one theory or theorist as an example for each of the categories listed in question 14.

    a. _____

    b. _____

    c. _____

    d. _____

    e. _____

16. *Praxis* is a dialogue representing the dynamic interaction between theorizing and clinical practice. This newer form of theorizing does not

    seek _____ truths about nursing

    practice as _____.

## *Review Questions*

Select the appropriate answer, and cite the rationale for choosing that particular answer.

1. Which of the following is *not* an intended outcome of a *grand theory*?
   a. To provide guidance for specific nursing interventions
   b. To provide a framework for broad ideas about nursing
   c. To provide a structural framework within which smaller range theories can be developed
   d. To stimulate critical thinking about nursing ideas

   Answer: _____ Rationale: _____

   _____

   _____

2. Which of the following is *not* an intended outcome of a *prescriptive theory*?
   a. To provide insight into general and broad phenomena
   b. To be action oriented
   c. To test validity
   d. To predict the consequence of a specific intervention

   Answer: _____ Rationale: _____

   _____

   _____

3. Which nursing theorist's model conceptualizes the person as an adaptive system?
   a. Virginia Henderson
   b. Rosemary Parse
   c. Hildegard Peplau
   d. Sister Callista Roy

   Answer: _____ Rationale: _____

   _____

   _____

4. Which nursing theorist's model conceptualizes the person as an irreducible energy field, coextensive with the universe?
   a. Adam's interactionist theory
   b. Orem's self-care theory
   c. Rogers's simultaneity theory
   d. Watson's transpersonal theory

Answer: _____ Rationale: _____
_____
_____

5. Which of the following levels of abstraction is *not* part of Liaschenko's ideas about nursing knowledge?
   a. Knowing the case
   b. Knowing the patient
   c. Knowing the disease
   d. Knowing the person

Answer: _____ Rationale: _____
_____
_____

# 6

# Research as a Basis for Practice

## Preliminary Reading

Chapter 6, pages 65–79

## Comprehensive Understanding

### Why Evidence?

1. Define *evidence-informed practice*.

_____

_____

_____

2. Briefly describe the relationship between research and practice.

_____

_____

_____

3. What are the sources of evidence used to inform practice?

_____

_____

_____

### Researching the Evidence

#### Ask the Clinical Question

4. Describe a PICO question.

_____

_____

_____

_____

#### Collect the Best Evidence

5. Describe where and how to find research studies in nursing.

_____

_____

_____

### Critique the Evidence

6. How is research evidence assessed for applicability in practice?

_____

_____

_____

7. The typical research article has the following parts. Briefly explain each section.

a. Introduction: _____

_____

b. Methods: _____

_____

c. Results: _____

_____

d. Discussion (Clinical Implications): _____

_____

e. References: _____

_____

#### Integrate the Evidence

8. Using an evidence-informed practice approach helps you improve_____.

### Evaluate the Practice Decision or Change

9. Two questions must be asked to evaluate the effect of an intervention:

a. _____

b. _____

## Support for Evidence-Informed Practice

10. Differentiate *research-based practice* from *evidence-informed practice*.

_____

_____

_____

## Knowledge Development in Nursing

11. Briefly describe the fundamental patterns of knowing in nursing.

_____

_____

_____

_____

_____

## The Development of Research in Nursing

12. Nursing research involves

_____

_____

_____.

13. Briefly describe the relationship between research and theory.

_____

_____

_____

## The History of Nursing Research in Canada

14. Briefly explain the significance of each of the following.

a. Florence Nightingale:

_____

_____

_____

b. Development of master's and doctoral degree programs in nursing:

_____

_____

_____

c. Establishment of nursing research journals:

_____

_____

_____

## Nursing Research

### The Scientific Paradigm

15. The scientific paradigm gave rise to *the scientific method*, which involves posing _____, and _____ and _____ data to find answers to those questions.

16. The dominant paradigm for most of the nineteenth and twentieth centuries has been

_____.

17. *Positivism* emphasizes _____ and _____ experience, rather than speculation, and focuses on the search for _____ and _____ relationships to explain phenomena.

Wood and Ross-Kerr (2011) described the research process as beginning with a researchable question, reviewing the literature to determine what is already known about the topic of the question, and then designing a study to answer the question. A goal of scientific research is to understand phenomena so that the knowledge can be applied generally, not just to isolated cases. Researchers conduct studies that contribute to the testing or development of theories, thereby advancing knowledge that can be applied in practice.

### The Qualitative (Interpretive) Paradigm

18. _____ is an alternative to positivism and promotes the idea that many truths exist depending on the perceptions of people in the situation. This philosophy leads to _____, which strives to understand the situation from the perspective of the participant, not the researcher.

## Research Designs

19. The two broad approaches to research are
_____ and _____.

### Quantitative Nursing Research

20. Briefly describe the three requirements of a true experiment.

_____
_____
_____

21. A quasi experiment is one in which groups are formed and the conditions are controlled, but

_____
_____
_____.

22. Surveys are designed to

_____
_____.

Exploratory descriptive designs provide in-depth descriptions of populations or variables not previously studied.

### Qualitative Nursing Research

Qualitative studies stem from questions that cannot be quantified and measured.

23. Define the following designs that are used with qualitative research.

   a. Ethnography:

   _____

   b. Phenomenology:

   _____

   c. Grounded theory:

   _____

### Conducting Nursing Research

24. Who should conduct nursing research?

_____
_____

## Ethical Issues in Research

25. Describe the purpose and responsibilities of a research ethics board.

_____
_____
_____

26. *Informed consent* means that research subjects

_____
_____
_____.

27. Briefly describe the five guiding ethical principles for research in Canada.

   a. _____
   b. _____
   c. _____
   d. _____
   e. _____

## Applying Research Findings to Nursing Practice

28. To use findings in clinical practice, nurses must

_____
_____, and
_____.

## *Review Questions*

Select the appropriate answer, and cite the rationale for choosing that particular answer.

1. The researcher's refusal to disclose the names of subjects is
   a. Respect for privacy and confidentiality
   b. Minimizing harm
   c. Informed consent
   d. Balancing harms and benefits

Answer: _____ Rationale: _____
_____
_____

2. The purpose of a research ethics board is to
   a. Ensure that federal funds are equitably appropriated
   b. Conduct research benefiting the public
   c. Determine the risk status of patients in research projects
   d. Ensure that ethical principles are being upheld

Answer: _____ Rationale: _____
_____
_____

3. Research studies can most easily be identified by
   a. Looking for the word "research" in the title of the report
   b. Looking for the study only in research journals
   c. Examining the contents of the report
   d. Reading the abstract of the report

Answer: _____ Rationale: _____
_____
_____

4. Which statement concerning research articles is accurate?
   a. Nursing textbooks are current sources of information.
   b. Systematic reviews and meta-analysis of randomized controlled trials (RCTs) provide the best evidence.
   c. RCTs do not provide scientific evidence.
   d. Peer-reviewed articles have been reviewed by a panel of nurses before publication.

Answer: _____ Rationale: _____
_____
_____

5. A research article includes all of the following *except*
   a. A summary of literature used to identify the research problem
   b. The researcher's interpretation of the study results
   c. A summary of other research studies with the same results
   d. A description of methods used to conduct the study

Answer: _____ Rationale: _____
_____
_____

# 7

# Nursing Values and Ethics

## Preliminary Reading

Chapter 7, pages 80–93

## Comprehensive Understanding

1. A value is a

_____

_____.

2. Ethics is the study of

_____

_____.

### Values

3. Values formation is

_____

_____.

4. Value conflict occurs when

_____

_____.

5. Values clarification is

_____

_____.

6. Identify three values clarification questions.

a. _____

b. _____

c. _____

### Ethics

7. Define *ethics* or *morality*.

_____

_____

_____

_____

**Nursing and Ethics**

8. A *code of ethics* serves

_____

_____.

9. Identify and briefly describe the seven values that must be upheld by Canadian nurses according to the Canadian Nurses Association.

a. _____

b. _____

c. _____

d. _____

e. _____

f. _____

g. _____

10. Define the following terms, and explain how they apply to the role of the nurse.

a. *Responsibility*:

_____

_____

b. *Accountability*:

_____

_____

c. *Advocacy*:

_____

_____

**Ethical Theory**

11. Define the following terms.

a. *Deontology*:

_____

_____

b. *Utilitarianism*:

_____

_____

c. *Bioethics*:

_____

_____

d. *Autonomy*:

_____

_____

e. *Beneficence*:

_____

_____

f. *Nonmaleficence*:

_____

_____

g. *Justice*:

_____

_____

h. *Social justice*:

_____

_____

i. *Feminist ethics*:

_____

_____

j. *Relational ethics*:

_____

_____

k. *Environment*:

_____

_____

l. *Embodiment*:

_____

_____

m. *Mutuality*:

_____

_____

n. *Engagement*:

_____

_____

## Ethical Analysis and Nursing

12. An ethical dilemma is

_____

_____.

13. Briefly describe each of the seven steps in the processing of an ethical dilemma.

a. Step 1:

_____

_____

b. Step 2:

_____

_____

c. Step 3:

_____

_____

d. Step 4:

_____

_____

e. Step 5:

_____

_____

f. Step 6:

_____

_____

g. Step 7:

_____

_____

### Ethical Issues in Nursing Practice

**Patient Care Issues**

14. Explain the following patient care issues and how they apply to nursing.

    a. Informed consent:

    _____

    _____

    b. Futile care:

    _____

    _____

    c. Advance directives:

    _____

    _____

    d. Withdrawal of food and hydration:

    _____

    _____

## *Review Questions*

Select the appropriate answer, and cite the rationale for choosing that particular answer.

1. Nursing codes of ethics fulfill which of the following purposes?
    a. They help nurses and the public understand professional nursing conduct.
    b. They outline actions to be implemented in specific nursing care situations.
    c. They define the scope of nursing practice on a national level.
    d. They define the roles of the nurse, the patient, other health care providers, and society.

    Answer: _____ Rationale: _____

    _____

    _____

2. Identify the statement below that is *not* accurate regarding advance directives.
    a. Advance directives offer direction of care goals to health care providers.
    b. Two broad categories exist within an advance directive: proxy and interactive.
    c. The instructive directive is commonly called a durable power of attorney.

    d. Proxy directives permit patients to name a surrogate decision maker on their behalf.

    Answer: _____ Rationale: _____

    _____

    _____

3. With regard to ethical situations in patient care, the most important nursing responsibility is to
    a. Remain neutral in clinical decisions
    b. Realize that the professional health care team collectively must be responsible for deciding ethical questions
    c. Be accountable for the morality of one's own actions
    d. Act only when absolutely certain that the action is ethically correct

    Answer: _____ Rationale: _____

    _____

    _____

4. You are working with the parents of a seriously ill newborn. Surgery has been proposed for the infant, but the chances of success are unclear. In helping the parents resolve this ethical conflict, you know that the next step is
    a. Exploring reasonable courses of action
    b. Collecting all available information about the situation
    c. Clarifying values related to the cause of the dilemma
    d. Identifying people who can solve the difficulty

    Answer: _____ Rationale: _____

    _____

    _____

5. The goal of informed consent is to protect the patient's right to
    a. Autonomy
    b. Beneficence
    c. Ethic of care
    d. Advocacy

    Answer: _____ Rationale: _____

    _____

    _____

b. *Battery*:

_____

_____

c. *Invasion of privacy*:

_____

_____

d. *False imprisonment*:

_____

_____

8. Discuss the concerns surrounding nurses and the use of social media.

_____

_____

_____

## Unintentional Torts

### Negligence

9. Define *negligence*.

_____

_____

10. Briefly explain how a nurse can avoid being liable for negligence.

_____

_____

_____

## Criminal Liability

11. Describe the difference between the tort of negligence and criminal negligence charges.

_____

_____

_____

_____

## Consent

12. The following factors must be verified for consent to be legally valid.

a. _____

b. _____

c. _____

A signed consent form is required for all routine treatment, hazardous procedures, some treatment programs such as chemotherapy, and research involving patients.

### Informed Consent

13. *Informed consent* is a person's agreement to

_____

_____.

14. The following factors provide adequate information for the patient to formulate a decision and are required to have met the standard of *informed consent*.

a. _____

b. _____

c. _____

d. _____

15. The nurse's signature witnessing the consent means

_____

_____

_____.

## Nursing Students and Legal Liability

16. If a patient is harmed as a direct result of a nursing student's actions or lack of action, who is liable?

_____

_____

_____

17. When students are employed as nursing assistants or nurses' aides when not attending classes, which tasks should they not perform?

_____

_____

_____

## Abandonment, Assignment, and Contract Issues

### Short Staffing

18. Briefly explain the process that a nurse needs to follow when a staffing assignment is unreasonable.

_____

_____

_____

### Floating

19. Identify what the nurse's responsibility is when he or she "floats" to another nursing unit.

_____

_____

_____

## Ethical Issues in Nursing Practice

**Patient Care Issues**

14. Explain the following patient care issues and how they apply to nursing.

    a. Informed consent:

    _____
    _____

    b. Futile care:

    _____
    _____

    c. Advance directives:

    _____
    _____

    d. Withdrawal of food and hydration:

    _____
    _____

## *Review Questions*

Select the appropriate answer, and cite the rationale for choosing that particular answer.

1. Nursing codes of ethics fulfill which of the following purposes?
   a. They help nurses and the public understand professional nursing conduct.
   b. They outline actions to be implemented in specific nursing care situations.
   c. They define the scope of nursing practice on a national level.
   d. They define the roles of the nurse, the patient, other health care providers, and society.

   Answer: _____ Rationale: _____
   _____
   _____

2. Identify the statement below that is *not* accurate regarding advance directives.
   a. Advance directives offer direction of care goals to health care providers.
   b. Two broad categories exist within an advance directive: proxy and interactive.
   c. The instructive directive is commonly called a durable power of attorney.

   d. Proxy directives permit patients to name a surrogate decision maker on their behalf.

   Answer: _____ Rationale: _____
   _____
   _____

3. With regard to ethical situations in patient care, the most important nursing responsibility is to
   a. Remain neutral in clinical decisions
   b. Realize that the professional health care team collectively must be responsible for deciding ethical questions
   c. Be accountable for the morality of one's own actions
   d. Act only when absolutely certain that the action is ethically correct

   Answer: _____ Rationale: _____
   _____
   _____

4. You are working with the parents of a seriously ill newborn. Surgery has been proposed for the infant, but the chances of success are unclear. In helping the parents resolve this ethical conflict, you know that the next step is
   a. Exploring reasonable courses of action
   b. Collecting all available information about the situation
   c. Clarifying values related to the cause of the dilemma
   d. Identifying people who can solve the difficulty

   Answer: _____ Rationale: _____
   _____
   _____

5. The goal of informed consent is to protect the patient's right to
   a. Autonomy
   b. Beneficence
   c. Ethic of care
   d. Advocacy

   Answer: _____ Rationale: _____
   _____
   _____

# 8

# Legal Implications in Nursing Practice

## Preliminary Reading

Chapter 8, pages 94–106

## Comprehensive Understanding

### Legal Limits of Nursing

1. The legal guidelines that nurses must follow are derived from the following. Briefly explain each one.

   a. Statute law:

   _____

   _____

   b. Nursing practice acts:

   _____

   _____

   c. Standards of care:

   _____

   _____

   d. Common law:

   _____

   _____

2. Define the following terms.

   a. *Criminal law*:

   _____

   _____

   b. *Civil law*:

   _____

   _____

3. Standards of care are the legal guidelines for nursing practice and are defined by the

   _____

   _____

   _____.

4. Nursing practice acts establish

   _____

   _____.

5. In a negligence lawsuit, these standards are used to determine

   _____

   _____.

### Legal Liability Issues in Nursing Practice

#### Torts

6. Define *tort*.

   _____

   _____

#### Intentional Torts

7. Define the following.

   a. *Assault*:

   _____

   _____

b. *Battery*:

_____

_____

c. *Invasion of privacy*:

_____

_____

d. *False imprisonment*:

_____

_____

8. Discuss the concerns surrounding nurses and the use of social media.

_____

_____

_____

## Unintentional Torts

### Negligence

9. Define *negligence*.

_____

_____

10. Briefly explain how a nurse can avoid being liable for negligence.

_____

_____

_____

### Criminal Liability

11. Describe the difference between the tort of negligence and criminal negligence charges.

_____

_____

_____

_____

### Consent

12. The following factors must be verified for consent to be legally valid.

a. _____

b. _____

c. _____

A signed consent form is required for all routine treatment, hazardous procedures, some treatment programs such as chemotherapy, and research involving patients.

### Informed Consent

13. *Informed consent* is a person's agreement to

_____

_____.

14. The following factors provide adequate information for the patient to formulate a decision and are required to have met the standard of *informed consent*.

a. _____

b. _____

c. _____

d. _____

15. The nurse's signature witnessing the consent means

_____

_____

_____.

## Nursing Students and Legal Liability

16. If a patient is harmed as a direct result of a nursing student's actions or lack of action, who is liable?

_____

_____

_____

17. When students are employed as nursing assistants or nurses' aides when not attending classes, which tasks should they not perform?

_____

_____

_____

## Abandonment, Assignment, and Contract Issues

### Short Staffing

18. Briefly explain the process that a nurse needs to follow when a staffing assignment is unreasonable.

_____

_____

_____

### Floating

19. Identify what the nurse's responsibility is when he or she "floats" to another nursing unit.

_____

_____

_____

**Physicians' Orders**

The physician is responsible for directing the medical treatment.

20. What is the nurse's responsibility with physicians' orders?

_____

_____

_____

21. One of the most frequently litigated issues is whether the nurse

_____

_____

_____.

22. If a verbal order is necessary, it should be written out and _____ by the physician within _____ hours.

## Legal Issues in Nursing Practice

**Abortion**

23. Summarize the legal rights of women in Canada relative to abortion in Canada.

_____

_____

_____

**Drug Regulations and Nurses**

24. Describe the two federal acts that control the manufacture, distribution, and sale of food, medications, and therapeutic devices in Canada.

a. _____

_____

b. _____

_____

**Communicable Diseases**

25. If nurses become aware of communicable diseases in their jurisdiction, what must they do?

_____

_____

26. What must a nurse do whenever confidential health care information is requested by a third party?

_____

_____

**Death and Dying**

27. Explain the legal definition of *death* that is used as standard medical practice across Canada.

_____

_____

_____

28. Define the following terms, and explain their legal status in Canada.

a. *Euthanasia*:

_____

_____

b. *Assisted suicide*:

_____

_____

c. *Withdrawing or withholding treatment*:

_____

_____

**Advance Directives and Health Care Surrogates**

29. Describe the function of an advance directive for health care.

_____

_____

_____

30. Differentiate an advance directive from a living will.

_____

_____

_____

If the existence of an advance directive for health care is known, the instructions must be followed.

31. Describe the two forms that an advance directive assumes.

a. _____

b. _____

**Organ Donation**

32. Every province and territory has human tissue legislation that provides for both _____ and _____ of tissues and organs.

**Mental Health Issues**

33. What is true about the rights of patients admitted to a psychiatric unit on a voluntary basis?

_____

_____

34. What special consideration must be kept in mind for a patient who has a history and medical records that indicate suicidal tendencies?

_____

_____

Documentation of precautions against suicide is essential.

**Public Health Issues**

35. Briefly explain the purpose of public health legislation.

_____

_____

_____

36. Describe nurses' obligation when child abuse or neglect is witnessed or suspected.

_____

_____

_____

## Risk Management

37. Risk management is

_____

_____.

38. The steps involved in risk management include

a. _____

b. _____

c. _____

d. _____

39. Name a tool used by risk managers and discuss its purpose.

_____

_____

40. Risk management includes documentation. It should be

a. _____

b. _____

c. _____

## Review Questions

Select the appropriate answer and cite the rationale for choosing that particular answer.

1. Nursing practice acts are an example of
   a. Statute law
   b. Common law
   c. Public law
   d. Criminal law

   Answer: _____ Rationale: _____

   _____

   _____

2. An example of an *unintentional tort* is
   a. Assault
   b. Battery
   c. Invasion of privacy
   d. Negligence

   Answer: _____ Rationale: _____

   _____

   _____

3. What should you do if you doubt a patient's capacity to give informed consent?
   a. Do not be concerned if the consent is already signed.
   b. Notify the physician, and document your concerns.
   c. Send the patient for the procedure, and discuss it afterward.
   d. Ask a family member to give consent.

   Answer: _____ Rationale: _____

   _____

   _____

4. When a patient is harmed as a result of a nursing student's actions or lack of action, the liability is generally held by
   a. The student
   b. The student's instructor or preceptor
   c. The hospital or health care facility
   d. All of the above

   Answer: _____ Rationale: _____

   _____

   _____

# 9

# Global Health, Culture, and Diversity

## Preliminary Reading

Chapter 9, pages 107–124

## Comprehensive Understanding

### Global Health

1. Briefly define *global health*.

   _____

   _____

### Health Equity

2. Compare *health inequities* and *health equity*.

   _____

   _____

### Global Citizenship

3. Global citizenship is *not*
   a. A responsibility as citizens to engage in our local, national, and international community
   b. Acting upon social injustices and inequities
   c. Disempowering individuals to participate in decision making
   d. Interconnectedness

## Cultural Diversity

4. Canada has always been a multicultural nation. _____ continues to play a pivotal role in shaping Canada's ethnocultural profile.

5. The three largest visible minority groups in Canada are _____, _____, and _____.

### Understanding Cultural Concepts

6. To provide culturally competent care, you must understand cultural concepts. Briefly explain each of the following.

   a. Culture:

   _____

   _____

   b. Ethnicity:

   _____

   _____

   c. Race:

   _____

   _____

   d. Cultural pluralism:

   _____

   _____

   e. Cultural relativism:

   _____

   _____

   f. Enculturation:

   _____

   _____

   g. Acculturation:

   _____

   _____

h. Assimilation:

_____

_____

i. Multiculturalism:

_____

_____

**Cultural Conflicts**

7. Define the following terms.

a. *Cultural imposition*:

_____

_____

b. *Ethnocentrism*:

_____

_____

c. *Stereotypes*:

_____

_____

d. *Discrimination*:

_____

_____

e. *Racism*:

_____

_____

## Historical Development of the Concept of Culture

8. Define *transcultural nursing*.

_____

_____

9. Define *culturally congruent care*.

_____

_____

10. Define *culturally competent care*.

_____

_____

11. Cultural competence has five interlocking components. Briefly explain each one.

a. _____

b. _____

c. _____

d. _____

e. _____

12. Define *cultural awareness*.

_____

_____

13. Briefly describe two strategies a nurse can use to achieve cultural self-awareness.

_____

_____

14. Define *cultural safety*.

_____

_____

Culture is the context in which groups interpret and define their experiences relevant to life transitions.
   Culture is the framework used in defining social phenomena.

## Cultural Assessment

15. The goal of a *cultural assessment* is

_____

_____.

16. Briefly explain how using a cultural assessment model or tool as a guide with a patient can assist with providing culturally competent care.

_____

_____

_____

_____

17. Briefly describe the challenges of using one specific cultural assessment model or tool with every patient.

_____

_____

_____

_____

## Selected Components of Cultural Assessment

18. Describe the following components of cultural assessment:

    a. *Ethnohistory*:

    _____

    _____

    b. *Social organization*:

    _____

    _____

    c. *Socioeconomic status, biocultural ecology, and health risks*:

    _____

    _____

    d. *Language and communication*:

    _____

    _____

    e. *Religion and spirituality*:

    _____

    _____

    f. *Caring beliefs and practices*:

    _____

    _____

    g. *Experience with professional health care*:

    _____

    _____

## Application of Cultural Assessment Components to Aboriginal Peoples of Canada

19. Aboriginal peoples represent an important and growing group within Canada. The three Aboriginal groups in Canada are the _____, _____, and _____. They have their own unique _____, _____, _____, and _____.

20. Discuss the reasons many Aboriginal people find the term *Indian* offensive and outdated.

    _____

    _____

    _____

    _____

### Ethnohistory

21. Discuss the history of the Aboriginals during the following:

    a. Pre–European contact:

    _____

    _____

    b. European contact:

    _____

    _____

    c. Post–European contact:

    _____

    _____

### Social Organization

22. Discuss Aboriginal social organization.

    _____

    _____

    _____

    _____

### Socioeconomic Status

23. All of the following statements are true *except*
    a. Large numbers of Aboriginals live in remote communities
    b. Aboriginals' access to health care is similar to that of other rural Canadians
    c. Aboriginals are marginalized from mainstream society
    d. Colonization disorganized Aboriginal culture

### Biocultural Ecology and Health Risks

24. Identify seven health-related challenges of the Aboriginal people.

    _____

    _____

    _____

    _____

### Language and Communication

25. Approximately _____ Aboriginal languages exist, with Algonquian being the largest and most widespread language family in Canada. Interpreters who can speak the various dialects within a language are invaluable, but _____.

**Religious and Spiritual Practices**

26. The spiritual approaches of Aboriginal peoples incorporate a mind–body–spirit connection that is harmonious with nature. The presence of all components together enables the person to _____.

**Caring Beliefs and Practices**

Aboriginal health and healing incorporates many aspects within the circle of life that includes, for instance, being human, stewarding the land, hunting wild animals, eating traditional foods, and practising herbal medicine.

**Experience With Professional Health Care**

27. Discuss the conceptual links between nursing, Aboriginal peoples, and cultural safety.

_____
_____
_____
_____

**Implications for Nursing Practice**

A deep consideration of **relational practice** and nursing obligations offers you the means to understand experience and to imagine how you might incorporate reflexivity, intentionality, and openness into practice, education, and research.

28. Discuss how to become an exemplary relational practitioner.

a. _____
b. _____
c. _____

## Review Questions

Select the appropriate answer, and cite the rationale for choosing that particular answer.

1. When providing care to patients with diverse cultural backgrounds, it is imperative for you to recognize that
   a. Cultural consideration must be put aside if basic needs are in jeopardy
   b. Generalizations about the behaviour of a particular group may be inaccurate
   c. Current health standards should determine the acceptability of cultural practices
   d. Similar reactions to stress will occur when individuals have the same cultural background

   Answer:_____ Rationale: _____
   _____
   _____

2. To be effective in meeting various ethnic needs, you should
   a. Treat all patients alike
   b. Be aware of patients' cultural differences
   c. Act as if you are comfortable with the patient's behaviour
   d. Avoid asking questions about the patient's cultural background

   Answer:_____ Rationale: _____
   _____
   _____

3. To provide culturally competent nursing care, you should
   a. Identify the patient's values, attitudes, beliefs, and practices
   b. Make decisions based solely on your own assessment of the patient
   c. Not be overly concerned with using knowledge from conceptual or theoretical models
   d. Acknowledge that a patient's response to his or her health is similar among various ethnic groups

   Answer:_____ Rationale: _____
   _____
   _____

4. To respect a patient's personal space, you
   a. Avoid the use of touch
   b. Explain nursing care and procedures
   c. Keep the curtains pulled around the patient's bed
   d. Stand 2.5 m away from the bed, if possible

   Answer:_____ Rationale: _____
   _____
   _____

5. Which of the following is *not* included in providing culturally competent care to a patient?
   a. Being sensitive and open to a patient's cultural beliefs
   b. Providing opportunities for a patient to discuss his or her views with you
   c. Ensuring that a patient's traditional health care practice is handled separately from current health approaches
   d. Working collaboratively with a patient in making health care decisions

Answer:_____ Rationale: _____

_____

_____

# 10

# Nursing Leadership, Management, and Collaborative Practice

## *Preliminary Reading*

Chapter 10, pages 125–139

## *Comprehensive Understanding*

1. Define *collaborative practice*.

_____

_____

_____

### Management and Leadership Roles for Nurses

Building a nursing team and developing a quality work environment begin with the leadership of the nurse executive.

2. Describe the leadership roles and responsibilities of nurses.

_____

_____

_____

### Nursing Care Delivery Models, Collaborative Practice, and Nursing Teams

A nursing care delivery model is a system for organizing and delivering nursing care to patients and their families, and it represents structural and contextual elements of nursing practice. Ideally, the vision for patient care should drive the selection of a care delivery model.

3. Define *continuity of care*.

_____

_____

4. Briefly explain the following delivery systems.

a. *Functional nursing*:

_____

_____

_____

b. *Team nursing*:

_____

_____

_____

c. *Primary nursing*:

_____

_____

_____

d. *Case management*:

_____

_____

_____

e. *Collaborative practice*:

_____

_____

_____

**Decision Making**

5. Briefly explain the following management structures.

   a. Centralized management:

   _____
   _____
   _____

   b. Decentralized management:

   _____
   _____
   _____

   c. Matrix:

   _____
   _____
   _____

6. Identify the responsibilities of a nurse manager in a decentralized management structure.

   _____
   _____
   _____

7. The following are key elements in establishing decentralized decision making. Briefly explain each one.

   a. *Responsibility*:

   _____
   _____

   b. *Autonomy*:

   _____
   _____

   c. *Authority*:

   _____
   _____

   d. *Accountability*:

   _____
   _____

**Supporting Staff Involvement**

8. The nurse manager nurtures and supports staff involvement through the following approaches. Briefly explain each.

   a. Nursing practice or professional shared governance councils:

   _____
   _____

   b. Interprofessional collaboration:

   _____
   _____

   c. Staff communication:

   _____
   _____

   d. Learning organization:

   _____
   _____

9. Give an example of how a student nurse may be involved as a member of a learning organization in a practice setting.

   _____
   _____

**Clinical Care Coordination**

10. Summarize each of the following leadership and management competencies a student nurse may develop for entry into registered nurse (RN) practice.

    a. Clinical decisions:

    _____
    _____

    b. Priority setting:

    _____
    _____

    c. Time management:

    _____
    _____

    d. Evaluation:

    _____
    _____

11. Give an example of how a student nurse may be involved in nursing team development.

_____

_____

_____

12. Define *delegation*.

_____

_____

_____

13. Identify the five rights of delegation.

a. _____

b. _____

c. _____

d. _____

e. _____

14. Identify the purpose of delegation.

_____

_____

_____

_____

15. Summarize the requirements for appropriate delegation.

a. _____

b. _____

c. _____

d. _____

e. _____

## Quality Care and Patient Safety

16. Define *quality improvement*.

_____

_____

_____

### Quality in Nursing Practice

17. Define each of the elements of quality nursing practice.

a. Professional standards:

_____

_____

b. Care and best practice guidelines:

_____

_____

c. Nurse-sensitive outcomes:

_____

_____

18. Give an example of a *nurse-sensitive outcome*.

_____

_____

### Building a Culture of Safety

19. Define *culture of safety for patient care*.

_____

_____

_____

20. Discuss how nurses and other health care providers can contribute to a culture of safe practice.

_____

_____

_____

## Leadership Skills for Nursing Students

Leadership development is ongoing throughout a career, and individual leadership styles are influenced from a variety of sources including theories, best practices, mentors, role models, and experiences.

### Career Development and Mentoring for Nursing Students

21. Discuss the role of a transformational leader in health care.

_____

_____

_____

## *Review Questions*

Select the appropriate answer, and cite the rationale for choosing that particular answer.

1. Primary nursing refers to
   a. Nurses who work with physicians in primary care
   b. Nurses who hold management positions
   c. Placing RNs in a continuous, direct-care role with patients in health care organizations
   d. Nursing carried out in primary health care

Answer:_____ Rationale: _____
_____
_____

2. A student nurse practising in a collaborative-practice model would demonstrate all of the following *except*
   a. Understanding the patient and family perspective
   b. Recognizing other team members for their contribution
   c. Assuming primary responsibility for planning, implementation, follow-up, and evaluation
   d. Developing listening skills and being aware of personal motivation

Answer:_____ Rationale: _____
_____
_____

3. Decentralized management is best described as
   a. Care decisions being made by a manager in another location
   b. Situations in which there is a lack of coordination of care
   c. Situations in which staff overrule the decisions made by managers
   d. Situations in which decision making occurs at the staff level

Answer:_____ Rationale: _____
_____
_____

4. Autonomy is best described as
   a. The duties and activities that an individual is employed to perform
   b. The right to act in areas where an individual has been given and accepts responsibility
   c. The freedom to decide and act
   d. Being answerable for one's actions

Answer:_____ Rationale: _____
_____
_____

5. Which of the following is *not* a purpose for delegation?
   a. Improves efficiency
   b. Provides job enrichment
   c. Transfers accountability for patient care
   d. Improves utilization of health care providers

Answer:_____ Rationale: _____
_____
_____

# 11

# Critical Thinking in Nursing Practice

## Preliminary Reading

Chapter 11, pages 140–152

## Comprehensive Understanding

Critical decision making separates professional nurses from technical or ancillary personnel.

### Critical Thinking Defined

1. Define *critical thinking*.

   _____

   _____

   _____

2. To think critically, you must be able to examine the following within the context of the situation:

   a. _____

   b. _____

   c. _____

   d. _____

   e. _____

3. Identify the core critical thinking skills that apply to nursing.

   a. _____

   b. _____

   c. _____

   d. _____

   e. _____

   f. _____

Learning to think critically helps a nurse to care for patients as their advocate and to assist them in making better informed choices about their care.

### A Critical Thinking Model for Clinical Decision Making

4. Summarize the critical thinking model and list its five components.

   _____

   _____

   _____

   _____

### Levels of Critical Thinking in Nursing

5. Three levels of critical thinking in nursing have been identified. Briefly describe each.

   a. Basic:

   _____

   _____

   b. Complex:

   _____

   _____

   c. Commitment:

   _____

   _____

## Components of Critical Thinking in Nursing

### Specific Knowledge Base

6. Identify what constitutes a nurse's knowledge base.

   _____

   _____

   _____

### Experience

7. Identify the ways in which critical thinking is developed through experience.

   _____

   _____

   _____

## Critical Thinking Competencies

Critical thinking competencies are the cognitive processes a nurse uses to make judgements.

### General Critical Thinking Competencies

#### Scientific Method

8. Define *scientific method*.

   _____

   _____

   _____

9. List the steps of the scientific method.

   a. _____

   b. _____

   c. _____

   d. _____

   e. _____

#### Problem Solving

10. Define *problem solving*.

    _____

    _____

Solving a problem in one situation allows you to apply the knowledge to future patient situations.

#### Decision Making

11. Define *decision making*.

    _____

    _____

12. Explain the process that an individual needs to go through to make a decision.

    _____

    _____

    _____

### Specific Critical Thinking Competencies in Clinical Situations

#### Diagnostic Reasoning and Inference

13. Explain the process of *diagnostic reasoning*.

    _____

    _____

    _____

#### Clinical Decision Making

14. The clinical judgement process requires

    _____

    _____

    _____.

After determining a patient's priorities, a nurse selects therapies most likely to solve each problem.

15. Cite some examples of how nurses make decisions about their patients.

    _____

    _____

    _____

#### Nursing Process as a Critical Thinking Competency

16. The nursing process is a systematic and comprehensive approach for nursing care. List the five steps of the nursing process.

    a. _____

    b. _____

    c. _____

    d. _____

    e. _____

## Developing Critical Thinking Skills

### Reflective Journal Writing

17. Define *reflection*.

    _____

    _____

18. Provide some examples of how a nurse can use reflection.

_____

_____

_____

19. Identify a common approach to reflection that the student nurse may use.

_____

_____

_____

To become a critical thinker, a nurse must be able to use language precisely and clearly. It is important not only to communicate clearly with patients and families but also to be able to communicate findings clearly to other health care providers.

## Critical Thinking Synthesis

Critical thinking is a reasoning process by which you use knowledge, reflect on previous experience, and integrate professional practice standards to provide competent and ethical nursing care to patients.

The nursing process is the traditional critical thinking competency that allows nurses to make clinical judgements and take actions based on reason.

20. Briefly explain how the nursing process and the critical thinking model work together.

_____

_____

_____

## *Review Questions*

Select the appropriate answer, and cite the rationale for choosing that particular answer.

1. Clinical decision making requires you to
   a. Improve a patient's health
   b. Establish and weigh criteria in deciding the best choice of therapy for a patient
   c. Follow the physician's orders for patient care
   d. Standardize care for the patient

Answer: _____ Rationale: _____

_____

_____

2. Which of the following is *not* one of the five steps of the nursing process?
   a. Planning
   b. Evaluation
   c. Hypothesis testing
   d. Assessment

Answer: _____ Rationale: _____

_____

_____

3. Gathering, verifying, and communicating data about the patient to establish a database is an example of which component of the nursing process?
   a. Assessment
   b. Planning
   c. Evaluation
   d. Nursing diagnosis
   e. Implementation

Answer: _____ Rationale: _____

_____

_____

4. Completing nursing actions necessary for accomplishing a care plan is an example of which component of the nursing process?
   a. Assessment
   b. Planning
   c. Evaluation
   d. Nursing diagnosis
   e. Implementation

Answer: _____ Rationale: _____

_____

_____

# 12

# Nursing Assessment and Diagnosis

## Preliminary Reading

Chapter 12, pages 153–172

## Comprehensive Understanding

1. The nursing process comprises the following five steps: _____, _____, _____, _____, and _____.

The nursing process is a dynamic, interactive process; in the clinical setting, practitioners move back and forth within the steps.

### Critical Thinking Approach to Assessment

2. Nursing assessment is the systematic process of _____, _____, and _____.

3. Identify the purpose of the assessment.

_____

_____

As you initiate the assessment component for a specific patient, you are also synthesizing critical knowledge, experience, standards, and attitudes simultaneously.

Accurate assessment makes it possible to develop appropriate nursing diagnoses and to devise appropriate goals and strategies.

### Data Collection

4. Identify some nonverbal behaviours that you may observe during an assessment.

_____

_____

_____

5. A comprehensive nursing health history includes

_____

_____

_____.

6. It is important for the nurse's assessment to first consider the _____, _____, and _____.

7. Assessment data must be _____, _____, and _____.

The collection of inaccurate, incomplete, or inappropriate data leads to incorrect identification of the patient's health care needs and subsequent inaccurate, incomplete, or inappropriate nursing diagnoses.

Whichever approach is used, you must cluster cues of information and identify emerging patterns and potential problems.

## Types of Data

8. Define each of the following.

   a. *Subjective data*:

   _____

   _____

   b. *Objective data*:

   _____

   _____

## Sources of Data

Each source provides information about the patient's level of wellness, anticipated prognosis, risk factors, health practices and goals, and patterns of health and illness.

### Patient

9. Identify the types of information a patient can provide.

   a. _____

   b. _____

   c. _____

   d. _____

   e. _____

### Family and Significant Others

10. Families can be an important secondary source of information about the patient's health status. Give an example.

   _____

   _____

   _____

### Health Care Team

11. Identify the ways that health care team members identify data.

   a. _____

   b. _____

   c. _____

### Medical Records

12. By reviewing medical records, you can find information about a patient's _____, as well as _____ and _____ test results, current physical findings, and _____ plan.

### Literature

Reviewing nursing, medical, and pharmacological literature about an illness helps the nurse complete the database.

### Nurse's Experience

13. A nurse's ability to make an assessment will develop as he or she _____ and _____ propositions, questions, and principle- or standard-based expectations.

## Methods of Data Collection

### Interview

14. During an interview, nurses have the opportunity to

   a. _____

   b. _____

   c. _____

   d. _____

   e. _____

15. Describe the phases of the interview.

   a. _____

   _____

   b. _____

   _____

   c. _____

   _____

16. The nurse uses various types of interview techniques. Describe some of the information obtained in an interview.

   _____

   _____

   _____

## Cultural Considerations in Assessment

It is important that a professional nurse conduct any assessment with cultural competence and cultural safety.

## Nursing Health History

17. The nursing health history is data collected about

   a. _____

   b. _____

   c. _____

d. _____

e. _____

**Family History**

18. The purpose of collecting the family history is to _____. These objectives are to determine whether _____.

**Physical Examination**

19. The physical examination involves the use of _____, _____, _____, _____, and smell.

**Observation of Patient Behaviour**

Throughout an interview and physical examination, it is important for you to observe a patient's verbal and nonverbal behaviour closely. The information enhances your objective database.

**Diagnostic and Laboratory Data**

The results of diagnostic and laboratory tests reveal or clarify alterations questioned or identified during the nursing health history and physical examination.

**Interpreting Assessment Data and Making Nursing Judgements**

Through a process of inferential reasoning and judgement, the nurse decides what information has meaning in relation to the patient's health status.

**Data Validation**

20. Discuss the importance of validation.

_____

**Analysis and Interpretation**

21. After collecting and validating subjective and objective data and interpreting the data, the nurse organizes the information into meaningful clusters. Data analysis involves recognizing

_____.

**Data Documentation**

22. Identify the two essential reasons for thoroughness in data documentation.

a. _____

b. _____

# Nursing Diagnosis

23. Define *nursing diagnosis*.

_____

_____

24. Define *medical diagnosis*.

_____

_____

25. Briefly summarize the evolution of nursing diagnosis.

_____

_____

_____

26. Explain the purpose of NANDA International.

_____

_____

_____

27. Explain the purpose of using nursing diagnoses.

_____

_____

_____

# Critical Thinking and the Nursing Diagnostic Process

28. The diagnostic process includes

_____

_____.

29. Defining characteristics of the nursing diagnostic process are

_____.

Defining characteristics that are beyond healthy norms form the basis for problem identification.

**Formulation of the Nursing Diagnosis**

30. Briefly explain the four types of nursing diagnoses identified by NANDA International.

a. Actual nursing diagnosis:

_____

_____

b. Risk nursing diagnosis:

_____

_____

c. Health promotion nursing diagnosis:

_____

_____

d. Wellness nursing diagnosis:

_____

_____

**Components of a Nursing Diagnosis**

31. Nursing diagnoses are stated in a two-part format: the _____ followed by a _____.

32. The diagnostic label of the nursing diagnosis is

_____

_____

_____.

33. The related factors of the nursing diagnosis are

_____

_____

_____.

NANDA International approves a definition for each diagnosis following clinical use and testing.

34. Risk factors are

_____

_____

_____.

Nursing assessment data must support the diagnostic label.

## Sources of Diagnostic Errors

35. Identify 11 ways nurses can avoid making common diagnostic errors.

a. _____

b. _____

c. _____

d. _____

e. _____

f. _____

g. _____

h. _____

i. _____

j. _____

k. _____

## Review Questions

Select the appropriate answer, and cite the rationale for choosing that particular answer.

1. In most circumstances, the best source of information for nursing assessment of the adult patient is the
   a. Nursing literature
   b. Physician
   c. Patient
   d. Medical record

Answer:_____ Rationale: _____

_____

_____

2. Reviewing the patient's medical record to obtain baseline data about the patient's response to illness occurs during which phase of the nursing process?
   a. Planning
   b. Nursing diagnosis
   c. Evaluation
   d. Assessment

Answer:_____ Rationale: _____

_____

_____

3. A nursing diagnosis
   a. Is a statement of a patient response to a health problem that requires nursing intervention
   b. Identifies health problems within the domain of nursing
   c. Is derived from the physician's history and physical examination
   d. Is not changed during the course of a patient's hospitalization

Answer:_____ Rationale: _____

_____

_____

4. Mr. Margauz, a 52-year-old business executive, is admitted to the coronary care unit. During his admission interview, he denies chest pain or shortness of breath. His pulse and blood pressure are normal. He appears tense and does not want you to leave his bedside. When questioned, he states that he is very nervous. At this moment, which nursing diagnosis is the most appropriate?
   a. Alteration in comfort, chest pain
   b. Alteration in bowel elimination related to restricted mobility
   c. High risk for altered cardiac output related to heart attack
   d. Anxiety related to critical care unit admission

Answer:_____ Rationale: _____
_____
_____

# 13

# Planning and Implementing Nursing Care

## Preliminary Reading

Chapter 13, pages 173–192

## Comprehensive Understanding

### Planning Nursing Care

1. Explain how *planning* is utilized in nursing.

   _____
   _____

### Establishing Priorities

Priority setting involves ranking nursing diagnoses in order of importance.

2. Priorities are classified as high, intermediate, or low. Give an example of each.

   High: _____
   Intermediate: _____
   Low: _____

### Critical Thinking in Establishing Goals and Expected Outcomes

Once a nursing diagnosis is identified for a patient, the nursing process consists of finding the best approach to address and resolve the problem.

Goals and expected outcomes are specific statements of the patient or the nurse to achieve problem resolution.

3. Identify the two purposes for writing goals and expected outcomes.

   a. _____
   b. _____

### Goals of Care

4. Define the following.

   a. *Patient-centred goal*:

      _____
      _____

   b. *Short-term goal*:

      _____
      _____

   c. *Long-term goal*:

      _____
      _____

### Expected Outcomes

5. Define *expected outcomes*.

   _____
   _____
   _____

The expected outcomes should be written in measurable behavioural terms sequentially, with time frames.

**Guidelines for Writing Goals and Expected Outcomes**

6. Define and give an example of each of the seven guidelines to follow when writing goals and expected outcomes.

   a. *Patient-centred*:

   _____

   _____

   b. *Singular*:

   _____

   _____

   c. *Observable*:

   _____

   _____

   d. *Measurable*:

   _____

   _____

   e. *Time-limited*:

   _____

   _____

   f. *Mutual*:

   _____

   _____

   g. *Realistic*:

   _____

   _____

Nursing interventions are those actions designed to assist the patient in moving from the present level of health to that described in the expected outcome.

## Types of Interventions

7. Interventions are based on patients' needs. Define and give an example of each of the three categories of interventions.

   a. *Nurse initiated*:

   _____

   _____

   b. *Physician initiated*:

   _____

   _____

   c. *Collaborative*:

   _____

   _____

## Selection of Interventions

8. Identify the six factors nurses use to select nursing interventions for a specific patient.

   a. _____

   b. _____

   c. _____

   d. _____

   e. _____

   f. _____

**Nursing Interventions Classification**

9. The advantages of the taxonomy of nursing interventions are

   a. _____

   b. _____

   c. _____

   d. _____

## Planning Nursing Care

10. Define *nursing care plan*.

   _____

   _____

   _____

The complete care plan is the blueprint for nursing action. It provides direction for implementation of the plan and a framework for evaluation of the patient's response to nursing actions.

11. A written nursing care plan makes possible

   _____ and _____ of nursing care and consultation by a number of health providers. Written care plans

   _____ information exchanged by

   nurses in _____.

12. Briefly explain each of the following:

a. Institutional care plans:

_____

_____

b. Computerized care plans:

_____

_____

c. Care plans for community-based settings:

_____

_____

d. Critical pathways:

_____

_____

e. Concept maps:

_____

_____

## Consulting Other Health Care Professionals

13. Consultation occurs most often during

_____.

Consulting involves _____ to iden-

tify ways of _____.

Consultation is based on the problem-solving approach, and the consultant is the stimulus for change.

The need to consult occurs when you have identified a problem that cannot be solved using personal knowledge, skills, and resources.

### Implementing Nursing Care

14. Define *implementation*.

_____

_____

15. A nursing intervention is

_____

_____.

16. Define each of the following.

a. Direct care interventions:

_____

_____

b. Indirect care interventions:

_____

_____

## Critical Thinking in Implementation

17. When making decisions about implementing care, you need to consider the following:

a. _____

b. _____

c. _____

d. _____

## Standard Nursing Interventions

18. Nursing interventions can be based on protocols and standing orders. Briefly explain each, and provide an example of where they are commonly used.

a. *Protocols*:

_____

_____

_____

b. *Standing orders*:

_____

_____

_____

## Implementation Process

### Reviewing and Revising the Existing Nursing Care Plan

If the patient's status has changed and the nursing diagnosis and related nursing interventions are no longer appropriate, the nursing care plan must be modified.

19. Identify the steps in modifying the existing care plan.

a. _____

b. _____

c. _____

d. _____

**Organizing Resources and Care Delivery**

Before implementing care, evaluate the plan to determine the need for assistance and the type of assistance required.

20. Describe how each of the following contributes to the preparation of care delivered.

    a. *Equipment*:

    _____

    _____

    b. *Personnel*:

    _____

    _____

    c. *Environment*:

    _____

    _____

    d. *Patient*:

    _____

    _____

**Anticipating and Preventing Complications**

Risks to patients arise from illness, conditions, and treatment.

**Identifying Areas of Assistance**

Certain nursing situations require you to obtain assistance by seeking additional knowledge, nursing skills, unregulated care providers, or a combination of these.

## Direct Care

**Activities of Daily Living**

21. Define *activities of daily living (ADLs)*.

    _____

    _____

Conditions that result in the need for assistance with ADLs can be temporary, permanent, or rehabilitative.

**Instrumental Activities of Daily Living**

22. Instrumental ADLs include such skills as

    _____

    _____.

**Life-Saving Measures**

23. A life-saving measure is

    _____

    _____.

**Counselling**

24. Define *counselling*.

    _____

    _____

25. Identify some areas in which patients or families may need counselling.

    a. _____

    b. _____

    c. _____

**Teaching**

26. Define the following.

    a. *Teaching*:

    _____

    _____

    b. *Teaching–learning process*:

    _____

    _____

**Controlling for Adverse Reactions**

27. What is an *adverse reaction*?

    _____

    _____

    _____

28. How do nurses control for adverse reactions?

    _____

    _____

    _____

## Indirect Care

**Communicating Nursing Interventions**

Nursing interventions are written (via the nursing care plan and medical record) or communicated orally (one nurse to another or to another health care provider).

**Delegating, Supervising, and Evaluating the Work of Other Staff Members**

29. Give examples of tasks you could delegate to another member of the health care team.

    _____

    _____

    _____

## *Review Questions*

Select the appropriate answer, and cite the rationale for choosing that particular answer.

1. The following statement appears on the nursing care plan for an immunosuppressed patient: "The patient will remain free from infection throughout hospitalization." This statement is an example of a (an)
   a. Long-term goal
   b. Short-term goal
   c. Nursing diagnosis
   d. Expected outcome

   Answer:_____ Rationale: _____
   _____
   _____

2. The planning step of the nursing process includes which of the following activities?
   a. Assessing and diagnosing
   b. Evaluating goal achievement
   c. Setting goals and selecting interventions
   d. Performing nursing actions and documenting them

   Answer:_____ Rationale: _____
   _____
   _____

3. The nursing care plan calls for the patient, a 136-kg woman, to be turned every 2 hours. The patient is unable to assist with turning. You know that you may hurt your back if you attempt to turn the patient by yourself. You should
   a. Rewrite the care plan to eliminate the need for turning
   b. Ignore the intervention related to turning in the care plan
   c. Turn the patient by yourself
   d. Ask another nurse to help you turn the patient

   Answer:_____ Rationale: _____
   _____
   _____

4. Ms. Benoit is a patient who recently received a diagnosis of diabetes. You show Mary how to administer an injection. This intervention activity is
   a. Counselling
   b. Communicating
   c. Teaching
   d. Managing

   Answer:_____ Rationale: _____
   _____
   _____

# 14

# Evaluation of Nursing Care

## *Preliminary Reading*

Chapter 14, pages 193–201

## *Comprehensive Understanding*

1. Evaluation involves two components: _____ and then _____.

You conduct evaluative measures to determine whether expected outcomes were attained, not whether nursing interventions were completed.

## Critical Thinking and Evaluation

2. Once an intervention has been performed, what types of data would you collect to see if the intervention has been successful?

_____

_____

_____

Evaluation of care requires you to reflect on the patient's responses to nursing interventions and to determine their effectiveness in promoting the patient's well-being.

Evaluation is the step in the nursing process whereby the nurse continually redirects nursing care to meet patient needs.

## The Evaluation Process

3. Identify the five elements of the evaluation process.

a. _____

b. _____

c. _____

d. _____

e. _____

**Identifying Criteria and Standards**

**Goals**

4. A goal specifies _____

_____.

**Expected Outcomes**

5. Expected outcomes are _____.

6. The purposes of the Nursing Outcomes Classification are

a. _____

b. _____

c. _____

**Collecting Evaluative Data**

7. Identify the two aspects of care that must be addressed.

a. _____

b. _____

8. The primary source of data for evaluation is

_____

**Interpreting and Summarizing Findings**

9. To objectively evaluate the success in achieving a goal, you should use the following steps.

    a. _____

    b. _____

    c. _____

    d. _____

    e. _____

**Documenting Findings**

When documenting the patient's response to interventions, always include the same evaluative measures gathered during assessment.

**Care Plan Revision**

Accurate evaluation leads to the appropriate revision of ineffective care plans and discontinuation of therapy that has been successful.

**Discontinuing a Care Plan**

After determining that expected outcomes and goals have been achieved, confirm this evaluation with the patient and discontinue that care plan.

**Modifying a Care Plan**

When goals are not met, identify the factors that interfered with goal achievement.

Lack of goal achievement may also result from an error in nursing judgement or failure to follow each step of the nursing process.

When a goal is not achieved, repeat the entire sequence to discover changes that must be made to the plan or changes that have occurred in the patient's condition.

10. A complete reassessment of all patient factors relating to the nursing diagnosis and etiology is the first step in re-evaluating the nursing process. Briefly explain the following in relation to modifying a care plan.

    a. Reassessment:

       _____

       _____

    b. Nursing diagnosis:

       _____

       _____

    c. Goals and expected outcomes:

       _____

       _____

    d. Interventions:

       _____

       _____

    e. Evaluation:

       _____

       _____

    f. Patient outcomes:

       _____

       _____

## Review Questions

Select the appropriate answer, and cite the rationale for choosing that particular answer.

1. Evaluation is
   a. Begun immediately before the patient's discharge
   b. Necessary only if the physician orders it
   c. An integrated, ongoing nursing care activity
   d. Performed primarily by nurses in the quality-assurance department

   Answer:_____ Rationale: _____

   _____

   _____

2. Measuring the patient's response to nursing interventions and his or her progress toward achieving goals occurs during which phase of the nursing process?
   a. Planning
   b. Nursing diagnosis
   c. Evaluation
   d. Assessment

   Answer:_____ Rationale: _____

   _____

   _____

# 15

# Documenting and Reporting

*Preliminary Reading*

Chapter 15, pages 202–227

*Comprehensive Understanding*

1. What is *documentation*?

   _____

   _____

   _____

## Confidentiality

2. Explain two reasons why nurses are obligated to keep information about patients confidential.

   a. _____

   b. _____

## Multidisciplinary Communication Within the Health Care Team

3. Caregivers use a variety of ways to exchange information about patients. Briefly explain the following.

   a. Patient record or chart:

   _____

   _____

   _____

   b. Reports:

   _____

   _____

   _____

## Purposes of Records

4. Briefly explain the following purposes of a record.

   a. Communication and care planning:

   _____

   _____

   b. Legal documentation:

   _____

   _____

   c. Education:

   _____

   _____

   d. Funding and resource management:

   _____

   _____

   e. Research:

   _____

   _____

   f. Auditing–monitoring:

   _____

   _____

## Guidelines for Quality Documentation and Reporting

5. High-quality documentation and reporting have six important characteristics: they are factual, accurate, complete, current, and organized, and they comply with standards set by Accreditation Canada and by provincial or territorial regulatory bodies. Explain each one.

   a. Factual:

   b. Accurate:

   c. Complete:

   d. Current:

   e. Organized:

   f. Compliant with standards:

## Common Documentation Systems

### Narrative Documentation

6. Narrative documentation is a storylike format that documents information specific to patient conditions and nursing care. The disadvantages of this style are

   a. _____

   b. _____

   c. _____

### Problem-Oriented Medical Records or Health Care Records

7. *Problem-oriented medical records* place emphasis on the patient's problems. The method corresponds to the nursing process and facilitates communication of patient needs. Explain the following major sections of the problem-oriented medical record.

   a. Database:

   b. Problem list:

   c. Care plan:

   d. Progress notes:

8. Define the acronyms, and briefly explain the forms of documentation of the problem-oriented medical record.

   a. *SOAP or SOAPIE notes*:

   b. *PIE format*:

   c. *Focus charting or DAR*:

9. Briefly explain the following forms of documentation.

   a. *Source records*:

b. *Charting by exception*:

_____

_____

c. *Critical pathways* or *care maps*:

_____

_____

## Common Record-Keeping Forms

10. Briefly explain the following formats used for record keeping.

a. Admission nursing history forms:

_____

_____

b. Flow sheets and graphic records:

_____

_____

c. Patient care summary or Kardex:

_____

_____

d. Acuity records or workload measurement systems:

_____

_____

e. Standardized care plans:

_____

_____

f. Discharge summary forms:

_____

_____

## Home Health Care Documentation

11. Documentation in the home health care system has implications different from those it has in other areas of nursing. List two primary differences.

_____

_____

_____

_____

The nurse is the pivotal person in the documentation of home health care delivery.

## Long-Term Health Care Documentation

12. Because residents are stable, documentation is done using _____, and assessment may be done only _____.

## Computerized Documentation

13. Explain the many benefits of computerized documentation.

_____

_____

_____

### Nursing Information Systems

14. The two basic designs of nursing information systems are

a. _____

b. _____

While there are advantages of nursing information systems, protection of privacy of information in computer systems is a top priority.

15. All _____ containing _____ must be _____ if they are not part of the patient's health record.

## The Electronic Health Record

16. What is an electronic health record?

_____

_____

## Reporting

Nurses communicate information about patients so that all members of the health care team can make appropriate decisions about the patient and his or her care.

**Change-of-Shift Reports**

17. Identify the eight major areas to include in a change-of-shift report.

    a. _____

    b. _____

    c. _____

    d. _____

    e. _____

    f. _____

    g. _____

    h. _____

**Telephone Reports**

It is important that information in a telephone report be clear, accurate, and concise.

**Telephone or Verbal Orders**

18. List the guidelines the nurse should follow when receiving telephone orders from physicians.

    a. _____

    b. _____

    c. _____

    d. _____

    e. _____

    f. _____

**Transfer Reports**

19. List the nine major information areas in a *transfer report*.

    a. _____

    b. _____

    c. _____

    d. _____

    e. _____

    f. _____

    g. _____

    h. _____

    i. _____

**Incident Reports**

20. Describe the purpose of an *incident report*.

    _____

    _____

    _____

## Review Questions

Select the appropriate answer, and cite the rationale for choosing that particular answer.

1. What is the primary purpose of a patient's medical record?
    a. To satisfy the requirements of accreditation agencies
    b. To communicate accurate, timely information about the patient
    c. To provide validation for hospital charges
    d. To provide the nurse with a defence against malpractice

    Answer:_____ Rationale: _____

    _____

    _____

2. Which of the following is charted according to the six guidelines for quality recording?
    a. "Respirations rapid; lung sounds clear."
    b. "Was depressed today."
    c. "Crying. States she doesn't want visitors to see her like this."
    d. "Had a good day. Up and about in room."

    Answer:_____ Rationale: _____

    _____

    _____

3. Which of the following best describes a *change-of-shift report*?
    a. Two or more nurses always visit all patients to review their plan of care.
    b. Nurses should exchange judgements they have made about patient attitudes.
    c. The nurse should identify nursing diagnoses and clarify patient priorities.
    d. Patient information is communicated from a nurse on a sending unit to a nurse on a receiving unit.

    Answer:_____ Rationale: _____

    _____

    _____

4. What is an *incident report*?
   a. A legal claim against a nurse for negligent nursing care
   b. A summary report of all falls occurring on a nursing unit
   c. A report of an event inconsistent with the routine care of a patient
   d. A report of a nurse's behaviour submitted to the hospital administration

Answer:_____ Rationale: _____
_____
_____

5. If an error is made while recording, what should you do?
   a. Erase it or scratch it out.
   b. Obtain a new nurse's note and rewrite the entries.
   c. Leave a blank space in the note.
   d. Draw a single line through the error, and initial it.

Answer:_____ Rationale: _____
_____
_____

# 16

# Nursing Informatics and Canadian Nursing Practice

## Preliminary Reading

Chapter 16, pages 228–241

## Comprehensive Understanding

In an increasingly complex technological environment, long-standing routines and tools in health care are being superseded by strategic, evidence-informed practices that demand high-quality, timely health information.

1. Define *nursing informatics (NI)*.

_____

_____

## Nursing Informatics and the Canadian Health Care System

2. Describe the purpose of the *electronic health record.*

_____

_____

_____

In the 1980s, NI emerged as a new nursing specialty in health information management (IM).

### Defining Nursing Informatics

3. Define the most current definition of NI with the following focuses.

a. *Information technology (IT)*:

_____

_____

b. *Conceptual*:

_____

_____

c. *Role-centred*:

_____

_____

### Evolution of Informatics in the Canadian Health Care System

As defined by the Canadian Organization for Advancement of Computers in Health (COACH), health informatics encompasses all health care disciplines and is the "intersection of clinical, [information management/information technology (IM/IT)] and management practices to achieve better health."

4. Define the acronym and describe the evolution of what is now known as CIHI.

_____

_____

_____

_____

_____

_____

5. Describe the function of the Standards Collaborative Working Groups as part of the Canada Health Infoway.

_____

_____

_____

_____

The events over the last 30 years have culminated in national attention to the need for timely, secure, and appropriate health information access.

Multiple organizations and standards development organizations operate to coordinate documentation of health information and monitoring of the Canadian health care system.

## Standards in Health Informatics

6. Standards in health care data management refer to the established and formally endorsed coding protocols for all health information, including coding of what aspects of health care delivery?

a. _____

b. _____

c. _____

d. _____

Standardization of data management also refers to standardizing forms of technology, information, or business processes.

7. List two benefits of standards in health care data management for each of the following stakeholder groups.

a. Patients:

_____

_____

b. Providers:

_____

_____

c. Service delivery organizations:

_____

_____

d. Educators:

_____

_____

e. Researchers:

_____

_____

Standards play a role in shaping health care data in numerous ways, such as patient registry standards, provider registry standards, diagnostic imaging standards, and pharmacy and laboratory standards, all of which influence how clinical practice is documented.

### Standards Development in Canada

Canada is unique in providing a centralized access point for health information standards development, use, and maintenance.

8. Describe the following two types of needs that can stimulate the need for a data management standard.

a. Technical needs:

_____

_____

b. Business needs:

_____

_____

Canada Health Infoway has standards for adopting, adapting, and developing a new standard that includes testing, evaluation, and retesting before full implementation.

9. Internationally, various standards form the basis for pan-Canadian standards. Define *SNOMED CT*:

_____

_____

### Standardizing Nursing Language

In the 1990s, nursing scholars began to advocate for a standardized nursing language using the following two arguments:

". . . if we cannot name it, we cannot control it, finance it, teach it, research it, or put it into public policy" (Clark & Lang, 1992, p. 109).

". . . without a language to express our concepts we cannot know whether our understanding of their meaning is the same, so we cannot communicate them with any precision to other people" (Clark, 1999, p. 42).

**Health Information: Nursing Components**

10. Describe what is meant by a nursing minimum data set.

    _____

    _____

    _____

11. The majority of Canadian nurses agree that the nursing components of health information known as Health Information: Nursing Components (HI:NC) are composed of five categories of elements. List and describe the five categories.

    a. _____

       _____

    b. _____

       _____

    c. _____

       _____

    d. _____

       _____

    e. _____

       _____

**International Classification for Nursing Practice®**

12. Describe the role of the International Council of Nurses in developing the International Classification for Nursing Practice (ICNP®).

    _____

    _____

    _____

    _____

13. What is the ICNP®, and what is its use?

    _____

    _____

    _____

    _____

The Canadian Nurses Association (CNA) endorses ICNP® as the terminology of choice for documenting professional nursing practice in Canada.

14. ICNP® uses seven axes to capture the core details of nursing practice for coding key nursing data in the electronic health record. Give an example of each of the seven axes.

    a. Focus:

       _____

       _____

    b. Judgement:

       _____

       _____

    c. Means:

       _____

       _____

    d. Action:

       _____

       _____

    e. Time:

       _____

       _____

    f. Location:

       _____

       _____

    g. Patient:

       _____

       _____

## Canadian Privacy Legislation

Although provincial standards of practice and the CNA *Code of Ethics* both address confidentiality, you also need to be aware of Canadian privacy legislation that protects patient data.

Canadians recognize the risk of privacy violation, and many believe that personal health information is one of the most important areas in need of protection under privacy laws.

15. What are the names of the two federal legislative acts that address the privacy of personal information?

    a. _____

    b. _____

16. Describe three examples of personal health information that is protected specifically by the *Personal Information Protection and Electronic Documents Act (PIPEDA)*.

    a. _____

    b. _____

    c. _____

## National E-Nursing Strategy

CNA released the *E-Nursing Strategy for Canada* (2006) to direct the coordinated integration of technology into Canadian nursing practice. The strategy is intended to completely integrate information and communication technologies in nursing.

17. CNA identified seven key outcomes that are projected to emerge from the *E-Nursing Strategy for Canada* (2006). Describe three of these outcomes and how you have seen evidence of each in your practice to date.

   a. _____

   b. _____

   c. _____

The Canadian Nurses Portal known as NurseONE is a key component of the *E-Nursing Strategy* and provides such services as professional links, professional development, an online library, practice support, and discussion groups.

## Clinician Engagement and Informatics Communities

Many Canadian and international health informatics communities exist that offer opportunities for participation, support, educational programs, and networking.

18. The following is a list of several important health informatics communities. Describe the role of each organization in influencing NI.

   a. CNA:

   _____

   _____

   _____

   b. Canadian Nursing Informatics Association:

   _____

   _____

   _____

   c. COACH:

   _____

   _____

   _____

In addition to formal organizations, numerous informal communities are devoted to NI, including blogs, Wikis, listserv and discussion groups, and social networks.

## Review Questions

Select the appropriate answer, and cite the rationale for choosing that particular answer.

1. As a new graduate, you have just started a new position and find in orientation that the EHR is often cited. You know from your reading that this refers to the
   a. Events of health risk
   b. Electronic health record
   c. Entries of the health record
   d. Electronic histogram response

   Answer:_____ Rationale: _____
   _____
   _____

2. You have volunteered to be part of a Standards Collaborative Working Group working on delivery of care. On what type of data would you most likely be developing standards?
   a. Public health investigations
   b. Wait times
   c. Prescribing of medications
   d. Clinical observations

   Answer:_____ Rationale: _____
   _____
   _____

3. Which of the following is *not* one of the benefits of standards to patients?
   a. Enhanced patient outcomes
   b. Improved coordination of care
   c. Reduced duplication of tests and procedures
   d. Accessible personal health history

   Answer:_____ Rationale: _____
   _____
   _____

4. Which of the following is *not* one of the HI:NC categories?
   a. Nursing diagnosis
   b. Patient outcome
   c. Primary nurse identifier
   d. Nursing resource intensity

   Answer:_____ Rationale: _____
   _____
   _____

5. According to ICNP® terminology, nursing outcomes must contain a term from the
   a. Means and Action axes
   b. Action and Location axes
   c. Focus and Judgement axes
   d. Judgement and Patient axes

Answer:_____ Rationale: _____
_____
_____

6. When patients indicate to you that they are afraid that their health information will not be kept confidential, you correctly respond that all nurses are bound by confidentiality in the
   a. CNA *Code of Ethics*
   b. *PIPEDA*
   c. *Privacy Act*
   d. All of the above

Answer:_____ Rationale: _____
_____
_____

# 17

# Communication

## *Preliminary Reading*

Chapter 17, pages 242–261

## *Comprehensive Understanding*

1. Communication is a lifelong process. This process allows

   _____
   _____.

Competency in communication helps the nurse to develop and maintain therapeutic relationships, to promote collaboration and interdisciplinary teamwork, and to meet ethical, legal, and clinical standards of care.

2. Communication is essential to the nurse–patient relationship because

   a. _____
   _____

   b. _____
   _____

## Communication and Interpersonal Relationships

Communication is the means to establishing helping–healing relationships.

3. Nurses with expertise in communication can express caring by

   _____
   _____
   _____.

## Developing Communication Skills

4. Briefly explain the qualities of critical thinking in relation to the communication process.

   _____
   _____
   _____
   _____

Critical thinking can help you overcome perceptual biases.
   Nurses use communication skills to gather, analyze, and transmit information and to accomplish the work of each step of the process.

## Levels of Communication

5. Summarize the following communication interactions.

   a. *Intrapersonal*:

   _____
   _____

   b. *Interpersonal*:

   _____
   _____

   c. *Transpersonal*:

   _____
   _____

d. *Small group*:

_____

_____

e. *Public*:

_____

_____

## Basic Elements of the Communication Process

6. Briefly summarize the following elements of communication.

a. *Referent*:

_____

_____

b. *Sender*:

_____

_____

c. *Receiver*:

_____

_____

d. *Message*:

_____

_____

e. *Channels*:

_____

_____

f. *Feedback*:

_____

_____

g. *Interpersonal variables*:

_____

_____

h. *Environment*:

_____

_____

## Forms of Communication

Messages are conveyed verbally, nonverbally, concretely, and symbolically.

### Verbal Communication

Verbal communication involves spoken or written words. Verbal language is a code that conveys specific meaning as words are combined.

7. Briefly explain the important aspects of verbal communication listed below.

a. Vocabulary:

_____

_____

b. Denotative and connotative meaning:

_____

_____

c. Pacing:

_____

_____

d. Intonation:

_____

_____

e. Clarity and brevity:

_____

_____

f. Timing and relevance:

_____

_____

### Nonverbal Communication

8. Nonverbal communication includes

_____

_____.

Nonverbal communication is much more powerful than verbal communication.

Nonverbal communication is communicated in a cultural context.

9. Becoming an astute observer of nonverbal behaviour takes practice, concentration, and sensitivity to others. Briefly explain the following nonverbal behaviours.

a. Personal appearance:

_____
_____

b. Posture and gait:

_____
_____

c. Facial expression:

_____
_____

d. Eye contact:

_____
_____

e. Gestures:

_____
_____

f. Sounds:

_____
_____

g. Personal space:

_____
_____

10. Identify the zones of personal space.

_____
_____
_____
_____

11. Identify the zones of touch.

_____
_____
_____
_____

**Symbolic Communication**

12. Summarize *symbolic communication*.

_____
_____
_____
_____

**Metacommunication**

13. Define *metacommunication*.

_____
_____
_____

## Professional Nursing Relationships

14. Professional relationships are created through _____, _____, and _____.

**Nurse–Patient Helping Relationships**

The nurse–patient relationship is therapeutic, promoting a psychological climate that facilitates positive change and growth.

15. Acceptance conveys a

_____
_____.

16. The nurse–patient relationship is characterized by four goal-directed phases. Explain the phases.

a. Preinteraction phase:

_____
_____

b. Orientation phase:

_____
_____

c. Working phase:

_____
_____

d. Termination phase:

_____
_____

17. Nurses often encourage patients to share personal stories. This is called _____.

**Nurse–Family Relationships**

18. Summarize the principles related to nurse–family relationships.

_____
_____
_____
_____

**Interprofessional Team Relationships**

19. Communication in nurse–health care team relationships is geared toward _____

_____

_____

_____.

**Nurse–Community Relationships**

20. Communication within the community occurs through channels such as _____

_____

_____

_____.

# Elements of Professional Communication

21. Briefly explain the following elements of professional communication.

a. Courtesy:

_____

_____

b. Use of names:

_____

_____

c. Trustworthiness:

_____

_____

d. Autonomy and responsibility:

_____

_____

e. Assertiveness:

_____

_____

# Communication Within the Nursing Care Process

## Assessment

Assessment of a patient's ability to communicate includes gathering data about the many contextual factors that influence communication.

22. List the contextual factors that influence communication.

a. _____

b. _____

c. _____

d. _____

e. _____

23. Identify the psychophysiological contextual factors that influence communication.

_____

_____

_____

24. List four environmental barriers to communication.

a. _____

b. _____

c. _____

d. _____

## Developmental Factors

25. Explain how developmental factors influence communication.

_____

_____

_____

_____

## Sociocultural Factors

26. Summarize how sociocultural factors influence communication.

_____

_____

_____

_____

## Gender

27. Gender influences communication. Explain how communication differs in regard to gender.

a. Male: _____

b. Female: _____

## Nursing Diagnosis

28. List three nursing diagnoses appropriate for a patient with alterations in communication.

    a. _____

    b. _____

    c. _____

## Planning

29. What factors must be considered as you design a responsive approach and nursing care plan?

    a. _____

    b. _____

    c. _____

    d. _____

    e. _____

### Goals and Outcomes

It is important to identify expected outcomes for all patients, particularly when impaired communication is a concern.

### Setting of Priorities

It is essential for the nurse to be available for communication with some immediacy so that the patient is able to express any pressing needs or problems.

## Implementation

### Therapeutic Communication Techniques

30. Therapeutic communication techniques are specific responses that encourage the expression of feelings and ideas while conveying the nurse's acceptance and respect. Briefly explain the following techniques.

    a. *Active listening*: _____

    b. *Sharing observations*: _____

    c. *Sharing empathy*: _____

    d. *Sharing hope*: _____

    e. *Sharing humour*: _____

    f. *Sharing feelings*: _____

    g. *Using touch*: _____

    h. *Using silence*: _____

    i. *Providing information*: _____

    j. *Clarifying*: _____

    k. *Focusing*: _____

    l. *Paraphrasing*: _____

    m. *Asking relevant questions*: _____

    n. *Summarizing*: _____

    o. *Self-disclosure*: _____

    p. *Confrontation*: _____

31. Certain communication techniques can hinder or damage professional relationships. These techniques are referred to as *nontherapeutic*. Briefly explain the following nontherapeutic techniques.

    a. Asking personal questions:

    _____
    _____

    b. Giving personal opinions:

    _____
    _____

    c. Changing the subject:

    _____
    _____

    d. Automatic responses:

    _____
    _____

    e. False reassurance:

    _____
    _____

    f. Sympathy:

    _____
    _____

    g. Asking for explanations:

    _____
    _____

    h. Approval or disapproval:

    _____
    _____

    i. Defensive responses:

    _____
    _____

    j. Passive or aggressive responses:

    _____
    _____

    k. Arguing:

    _____
    _____

32. Briefly identify the communication techniques to use with the patient who has special needs.

    a. Patients who cannot speak clearly:

    _____
    _____

    b. Patients who are cognitively impaired:

    _____
    _____

    c. Patients who are hearing impaired:

    _____
    _____

    d. Patients who are visually impaired:

    _____
    _____

    e. Patients who are unresponsive:

    _____
    _____

    f. Patients who do not speak English:

    _____
    _____

## Evaluation

33. List four expected outcomes for the patient with impaired communication.

    a. _____
    b. _____
    c. _____
    d. _____

## Review Questions

Select the appropriate answer, and cite the rationale for choosing that particular answer.

1. *Transpersonal communication* is
    a. Interaction that occurs within a person's spiritual domain
    b. One-to-one interaction between the nurse and the patient
    c. Communication within groups
    d. Self-talk

    Answer:_____ Rationale: _____

    _____
    _____

2. In demonstrating the method for deep-breathing exercises, you place your hands on the patient's abdomen to explain diaphragmatic movement. This technique involves the use of which communication element?
   a. Feedback
   b. Tactile channel
   c. Referent
   d. Message

Answer:_____ Rationale: _____

_____

_____

3. Which statement about nonverbal communication is correct?
   a. It is easy for a nurse to judge the meaning of a patient's facial expression.
   b. The nurse's verbal messages should be reinforced by nonverbal cues.
   c. The physical appearance of the nurse rarely influences nurse–patient interaction.
   d. Words convey meanings that are usually more significant than nonverbal communication.

Answer:_____ Rationale: _____

_____

_____

4. The term referring to all of the relational aspects of a message is called
   a. Nonverbal communication
   b. Metacommunication
   c. Connotative meaning
   d. Denotative meaning

Answer:_____ Rationale: _____

_____

_____

5. The referent in the communication process is
   a. That which motivates the communication
   b. The means of conveying messages
   c. Information shared by the sender
   d. The person who initiates the communication

Answer:_____ Rationale: _____

_____

_____

# 18

# Caring in Nursing Practice

## Preliminary Reading

Chapter 18, pages 262–272

## Comprehensive Understanding

1. _____ and _____ that are at the heart of competent nursing practice must be valued and embraced.

## Theoretical Views on Caring

Caring in nursing has been studied from a variety of philosophical and ethical perspectives.

### Caring Is Primary

2. Benner and Wrubel (1989) offer nurses a rich, holistic understanding of nursing practice and caring through the interpretation of

_____.

3. Briefly summarize how Benner and Wrubel described the relationship between health, illness, and disease.

_____

_____

_____

_____

### The Essence of Nursing and Health

4. Explain Leininger's concept of care from a *transcultural* perspective.

_____

_____

_____

_____

5. Define *acts of caring* according to Leininger.

_____

_____

_____

According to Leininger, caring is a universal phenomenon, but the expressions, processes, and patterns of caring vary among cultures.

### Transpersonal Caring

6. Summarize Watson's transpersonal caring theory (transformative model).

_____

_____

_____

_____

### Swanson's Theory of Caring

7. Swanson's theory of caring consists of five categories. Explain each.

a. Knowing:

_____

_____

b. Being with:

_____

_____

c. Doing for:

_____

_____

d. Enabling:

_____

_____

e. Maintaining belief:

_____

_____

**The Human Act of Caring**

8. Roach's theory contains five concepts. Briefly describe each.

a. Compassion:

_____

_____

b. Competence:

_____

_____

c. Confidence:

_____

_____

d. Conscience:

_____

_____

e. Commitment:

_____

_____

**Summary of Theoretical Views**

9. Identify the common themes among the many nursing theories.

_____

_____

_____

_____

## Patient's Perceptions of Caring

10. Establishing a _____, _____, and _____ are recurrent caring behaviours that researchers have identified.

When patients believe that health care providers are sensitive, sympathetic, compassionate, and interested in them as people, they usually become active partners in the plan of care.

You need to consider how patients perceive caring and the best approaches to providing care.

## Ethic of Care

Caring is a moral imperative.

In any patient encounter, you must know what behaviour is ethically appropriate.

11. Define *ethic of care*.

_____

_____

_____

## Caring in Nursing Practice

As you deal with health and illness in your practice, your ability to care grows.

12. Nurse behaviours that have been shown to be related to caring include

_____

_____.

**Providing Presence**

13. Summarize the concept of *presence*.

_____

_____

_____

14. Identify ways you can establish presence with your patients.

_____

_____

_____

**Touch**

The use of touch is one comforting approach whereby the nurse reaches out to patients to communicate concern and support.

15. Give some examples of protective and task-oriented touch.

_____

_____

_____

_____

**Listening**

Listening conveys your full attention and interest. Listening to the meaning of what a patient says helps create a mutual relationship.

You must be able to give patients your full, focused attention as they tell their stories.

When an ill person chooses to tell his or her story, the person is reaching out to another human being.

16. Briefly summarize Frank's view of the clinical relationship the nurse and the patient share.

_____
_____
_____
_____

17. Describe what listening involves.

_____
_____
_____
_____

**Knowing the Patient**

18. Knowing a patient means that the nurse

_____, _____, and _____.

Knowing the patient is at the core of the process by which you make clinical decisions. When you establish a caring relationship, the mutuality that develops helps you better know the patient as an individual and then choose the most appropriate and helpful nursing therapies.

19. Describe the following nurses and how they differ in knowing their patients.

a. Expert nurse:

_____
_____

b. Novice nurse:

_____
_____

**Spiritual Caring**

20. Spiritual health is achieved when

_____
_____.

21. Spirituality offers a sense of connection

_____, _____, and _____.

22. When a caring relationship is established, the patient and the nurse come to know one another so that both move toward a healing relationship by

a. _____
b. _____
c. _____

**Family Care**

23. Success with nursing interventions often depends on the family's willingness to

_____
_____
_____
_____

24. List the ten caring behaviours that are perceived as most hopeful by families of cancer patients.

a. _____
b. _____
c. _____
d. _____
e. _____
f. _____
g. _____
h. _____
i. _____
j. _____

## The Challenge of Caring

Caring motivates people to become nurses, and it becomes a source of satisfaction when they know they have made a difference in their patients' lives.

25. Summarize the challenges facing nursing in today's health care system.

_____
_____
_____
_____

## Review Questions

Select the appropriate answer, and cite the rationale for choosing that particular answer.

1. Leininger's care theory states that the patient's caring values and behaviours are derived largely from
   a. Experience
   b. Gender
   c. Culture
   d. Religious beliefs

   Answer: _____ Rationale: _____
   _____
   _____

2. The central common theme of the caring theories is
   a. Pathophysiology and self-care abilities
   b. Compensation for patient disabilities
   c. The nurse–patient relationship and psychosocial aspects of care
   d. Maintenance of patient homeostasis

   Answer: _____ Rationale: _____
   _____
   _____

3. To effectively listen to the patient, you need to
   a. Sit with the legs crossed
   b. Lean back in the chair
   c. Respond quickly with appropriate answers to the patient
   d. Maintain good eye contact

   Answer: _____ Rationale: _____
   _____
   _____

4. You can demonstrate caring by
   a. Helping family members become active participants in the care of the patient
   b. Doing all the necessary tasks for the patient
   c. Following all of the physician's orders accurately
   d. Maintaining a professional distance at all times

   Answer: _____ Rationale: _____
   _____
   _____

5. Illness is best described as
   a. A disease state that manifests as an abnormality at the cellular, tissue, or organ level
   b. An abnormal condition at the cellular, tissue, or organ level that can be acute or chronic
   c. The patient's personal experience of sickness
   d. The physical experience of disease and disability

   Answer: _____ Rationale: _____
   _____
   _____

6. One of the main concepts for the human act of caring theory is
   a. Cultivating sensitivity of oneself and others
   b. Being with and being emotionally present to the other
   c. Viewing health as a state of being that people define according to their values, personality, and lifestyle
   d. Viewing conscience as a state of moral awareness

   Answer: _____ Rationale: _____
   _____
   _____

# 19

# Family Nursing

## Preliminary Reading

Chapter 19, pages 273–289

## Comprehensive Understanding

1. Define the concept of *family nursing*.

   _____

   _____

   _____

2. Describe the goal of family nursing.

   _____

   _____

   _____

## What Is a Family?

3. The *family* can be defined as a _____, as

   a _____, or as a _____.

To effectively provide care, you must understand that individual attitudes about family are deeply ingrained and deserve respect.

   To provide individualized care, you must understand that families take many forms and have diverse cultural and ethnic orientations.

## Current Trends in the Canadian Family

### Family Forms

4. Summarize the various *family forms*.

   a. Nuclear family:

      _____

      _____

   b. Extended family:

      _____

      _____

   c. Step-family:

      _____

      _____

   d. Blended family:

      _____

      _____

   e. Lone-parent family:

      _____

      _____

   f. Other family forms:

      _____

      _____

### Family Changes and Challenges: Understanding the Influence of Sociocultural Contexts

5. Identify at least three current trends that challenge the family.

   a. _____

   b. _____

   c. _____

6. Explain the following trends and social factors that impact the structure and function of the family.

   a. Domestic roles:

      _____

      _____

b. Economic status:

_____

_____

c. Aboriginal families:

_____

_____

d. Family caregivers:

_____

_____

## The Family and Health

7. The health of the family is influenced by many factors, such as

a. _____

b. _____

c. _____

d. _____

e. _____

f. _____

The family's beliefs, values, and practices influence the health-promoting behaviours of its members. In turn, the health status of each individual influences how the family unit functions and its ability to achieve goals.

Family environment is crucial because health behaviour reinforced in early life has a strong influence on later health practices.

### Attributes of Healthy Families

8. The crisis-proof, or effective, family is able to integrate the need for stability with the need for growth and change. Explain.

_____

_____

_____

_____

9. Define *family hardiness*.

_____

_____

10. Define *family resiliency*.

_____

_____

## Family Nursing Care

11. List the three things that nurses should examine when they consider how a health problem or illness affects a family and how a family affects a health problem or illness.

a. _____

b. _____

c. _____

12. Briefly explain the following two focuses proposed for family nursing practice.

a. Family as *context*:

_____

_____

_____

b. Family as *patient*:

_____

_____

_____

### Understanding Family in Context: Family Nursing as Relational Inquiry

Family nursing as *relational inquiry* invites nurses to consider the ways in which families and nurses are embedded within diverse and complex life contexts. A relational inquiry approach asks nurses to expand their contextual knowledge of families, developing a more in-depth and comprehensive consideration of the historical, economic, political, social, environmental, and geographical influences at play when families encounter illness or other difficulties related to life transitions.

## Assessing the Challenges, Strengths, and Needs of the Family: The Calgary Family Assessment Model

13. Summarize the following three major categories of family life that the Calgary Family Assessment Model offers as a framework for nurses to follow when conducting family assessments.

a. Structural dimension:

_____

_____

b. Developmental dimension:

_____

_____

c. Functional dimension:

_____

_____

**Structural Assessment**

14. Explain these terms.

 a. *Internal structure*:

 _____

 _____

 b. *External structure*:

 _____

 _____

 c. *Context*:

 _____

 _____

15. Explain the purpose of a *genogram*.

 _____

 _____

 _____

 _____

16. Explain the purpose of an *ecomap*.

 _____

 _____

 _____

 _____

**Developmental Assessment**

17. Listed below are McGoldrick and Carter's family life stages. Describe the emotional process of transition associated with each stage.

 a. Leaving Home: Emerging Young Adults:

 _____

 _____

 b. Joining of Families Through Marriage:

 _____

 _____

 c. Family With Young Children:

 _____

 _____

 d. Family With Adolescents:

 _____

 _____

 e. Launching Children and Moving on at Midlife:

 _____

 _____

 f. Family in Late Middle Age:

 _____

 _____

18. What does McGoldrick and Carter's model *not* address?

 _____

 _____

**Functional Assessment**

A functional assessment focuses mainly on how family members interact and behave toward each other.

19. Describe the two subcategories of family functioning.

 a. Instrumental functioning:

 _____

 _____

 b. Expressive functioning:

 _____

 _____

## Family Intervention: The Calgary Family Intervention Model

20. Describe the goal of family intervention.

 _____

 _____

 _____

21. Name the three domains of family functioning that the Calgary Family Intervention Model (CFIM) focuses on promoting and improving.

 a. _____

 b. _____

 c. _____

## Asking Interventive Questions

The practice of asking questions leads family members to reflect on their situation, clarify their opinions and ideas, and understand how they are affected by their family member's illness or condition.

22. Describe the two types of interventive questions.

    a. *Linear questions*:

    _____

    _____

    b. *Circular questions*:

    _____

    _____

## Offering Commendations

23. Describe the meaning of a *commendation* and why it is important for nurses to make commendations to families.

    _____

    _____

    _____

    _____

24. List five common family strengths.

    a. _____

    b. _____

    c. _____

    d. _____

    e. _____

## Providing Information

One of the roles nurses need to adopt is that of educator.

25. Family and patient needs for information may be elicited through direct questioning, but they

    are often _____.

26. When you assume a humble, caring position instead of coming across as an authority on the subject, this attitude often decreases the patient's

    _____ and invites the family to listen

    without feeling _____.

## Validating or Normalizing Emotional Responses

27. What is the purpose of validating emotional responses?

    _____

    _____

    _____

## Encouraging Illness Narratives

28. Describe an *illness narrative*.

    _____

    _____

    _____

## Encouraging Family Support

29. You can enhance family functioning by encouraging and assisting family members

    to listen to each other's _____ and

    _____.

## Supporting Family Caregivers

30. Describe the concept of *reciprocity*.

    _____

    _____

    _____

    _____

31. What are some of the benefits of *reciprocity*?

    _____

    _____

    _____

## Encouraging Respite

32. List nine community resources that may be beneficial to caregivers.

    a. _____

    b. _____

    c. _____

    d. _____

    e. _____

    f. _____

    g. _____

    h. _____

    i. _____

**Interviewing the Family**

33. When interviewing the family, the nurse must display keen perceptual, conceptual, and executive skills. Describe each of these skills in the space provided below.

   a. Perceptual skills:

      _____

      _____

   b. Conceptual skills:

      _____

      _____

   c. Executive skills:

      _____

      _____

34. List five ways to engage in purposeful conversations with families.

   a. _____

   b. _____

   c. _____

   d. _____

   e. _____

## Review Questions

Select the appropriate answer, and cite the rationale for choosing that particular answer.

1. Family functioning can best be described as
   a. The processes that a family uses to meet its goal
   b. The way the family members communicate with each other
   c. Interrelated with family structure
   d. Adaptive behaviours that foster health

Answer:_____ Rationale: _____

_____

_____

2. Family structure can best be described as
   a. A basic pattern of predictable stages
   b. Flexible patterns that contribute to adequate functioning
   c. The pattern of relationships and ongoing membership
   d. A complex set of relationships

Answer:_____ Rationale: _____

_____

_____

3. "Skip-generation" families (grandparents caring for grandchildren), "nonfamilies" (adults living alone), and same-sex couples (with or without children) are considered
   a. Other family forms
   b. Blended families
   c. Extended families
   d. Step-families

Answer:_____ Rationale: _____

_____

_____

4. The majority of families today
   a. Consist of a mother, a father, and one or more children
   b. Include stepchildren
   c. Include a mother who works outside the home
   d. Are very similar to families of the past

Answer:_____ Rationale: _____

_____

_____

5. When planning care for a patient and using the concept of family as patient, you
   a. Consider the developmental stage of the patient and not the family
   b. Realize that cultural background is an important variable when assessing the family
   c. Include only the patient and his or her significant other
   d. Understand that the patient's family will always be a help to the patient's health goals

Answer:_____ Rationale: _____

_____

_____

6. Interventions recommended by the CFIM include
   a. Providing solutions for problems as they arise
   b. Validating emotional responses, encouraging illness narratives, and encouraging the patient to request help from his or her family
   c. Asking interventive questions, offering commendations, providing information, and encouraging respite
   d. Administering nursing care in a manner that provides an opportunity for change

Answer:_____ Rationale: _____

_____

_____

# 20

# Patient Education

## Preliminary Reading

Chapter 20, pages 290–308

## Comprehensive Understanding

Patient education is one of the most important roles for nurses in any health care setting.

### Goals of Patient Education

1. Comprehensive patient education includes which three important goals?

   a. _____

   b. _____

   c. _____

#### Maintaining and Promoting Health and Preventing Illness

The nurse is a visible, competent resource for patients who are intent on improving their physical and psychological well-being. In the school, home, clinic, or workplace, the nurse provides information and skills that will allow people to maintain and improve their health.

2. Greater knowledge can result in _____.

   When patients become more _____,

   they are more likely to _____ of health problems.

#### Restoring Health

3. Many patients seek _____ and _____ that will help them regain or maintain their levels of health.

4. The _____ is a vital part of a patient's return to health, and family members may need as much information as the patient.

You should not assume that the family should be involved and must first assess the patient–family relationship.

#### Coping With Impaired Functioning

5. The family's ability to provide support can result from _____, which begins as soon as the patient's needs are identified and the family displays a willingness to help.

### Teaching and Learning

#### Role of the Nurse in Teaching and Learning

6. Nurses have an _____ responsibility to teach their patients.

The nurse clarifies information provided by physicians and other health care providers, and may become the primary source of information for adjusting to health problems.

#### Teaching as Communication

7. Effective teaching depends on _____.

### Domains of Learning

8. List the three domains in which learning occurs:

   a. _____

   b. _____

   c. _____

The characteristics of learning within each domain affect the teaching and evaluation methods used.

**Cognitive Learning**

9. *Cognitive learning* (Bloom, 1956) classifies cognitive behaviours in an ordered hierarchy. Summarize each one.

   a. Remembering:

   _____

   _____

   b. Understanding:

   _____

   _____

   c. Application:

   _____

   _____

   d. Analysis:

   _____

   _____

   e. Evaluating:

   _____

   _____

   f. Creating:

   _____

   _____

**Affective Learning**

Affective learning deals with the expression of feelings and the acceptance of attitudes, opinions, or values.

10. Summarize the following hierarchy of *affective learning* behaviours.

   a. Receiving:

   _____

   _____

   b. Responding:

   _____

   _____

   c. Valuing:

   _____

   _____

   d. Organizing:

   _____

   _____

   e. Characterizing:

   _____

   _____

**Psychomotor Learning**

Psychomotor learning involves acquiring skills that require the integration of mental and muscular activity.

11. Summarize the following hierarchy of *psychomotor learning* behaviours.

   a. Perception:

   _____

   _____

   b. Set:

   _____

   _____

   c. Guided response:

   _____

   _____

   d. Mechanism:

   _____

   _____

   e. Complex overt response:

   _____

   _____

   f. Adaptation:

   _____

   _____

   g. Origination:

   _____

   _____

## Basic Learning Principles

Before nurses can teach, they must understand how people learn.

### Learning Environment

12. Factors in the physical environment where teaching takes place can make learning pleasant or difficult. List three factors to consider when selecting the learning setting.

    a. _____

    b. _____

    c. _____

### Ability to Learn

13. Summarize how each of the following influences the ability to learn.

    a. Emotional capability:

    b. Intellectual capability:

    c. Physical capability:

    d. Developmental stage:

### Learning Style and Preferences

14. Everyone has different learning preferences and styles. You should ask patients their preferred method for learning. In a group, you should _____.

### Motivation to Learn

15. Motivation is defined as _____.

16. Briefly explain how the following distractions influence the ability to learn.

    a. Physical discomfort:

    b. Anxiety:

    c. Environment:

17. Briefly explain how the following can affect motivation.

    a. Social motives:

    b. Task mastery:

    c. Physical motives:

### Motivation and Social Learning Theory

18. Define *self-efficacy*.

### Motivation and Transtheoretical Model of Change

19. By identifying the patient's stage of change and by focusing learning activities to match the patient's stage, you facilitate the learner's motivation to change and his or her transition from one stage to the next. Identify the five stages used in smoking cessation activities:

    a. _____

    b. _____

    c. _____

    d. _____

    e. _____

## Integrating the Nursing and Teaching Processes

20. Differentiate between the nursing process and the teaching process.

21. The teaching process requires _____.

22. The nurse sets specific learning objectives and implements the teaching plan using teaching and learning principles to ensure

_____.

## Assessment

23. The patient requires the nurse to assess the following factors. Summarize each one.

*Learning needs:*

   a. _____

   b. _____

   c. _____

*Ability to learn:*

   a. _____

   b. _____

   c. _____

   d. _____

   e. _____

*Motivation to learn:*

   a. _____

   b. _____

   c. _____

   d. _____

   e. _____

   f. _____

   g. _____

   h. _____

   i. _____

*Teaching environment:*

   a. _____

   b. _____

   c. _____

*Resources for learning:*

   a. _____

   b. _____

   c. _____

   d. _____

   e. _____

## Nursing Diagnosis

Classifying diagnoses according to the three learning domains helps you focus specifically on subject matter and teaching methods.

## Planning

24. After determining the nursing diagnoses that identify a patient's learning needs, you develop a teaching plan, determine goals and expected outcomes, and involve the patient in a teaching method. Expected outcomes guide the

_____.

### Developing Learning Objectives

25. A learning objective identifies the _____ of a planned learning experience and helps

_____ for learning.

26. A learning objective includes the same criteria as goals or outcomes in a nursing care plan. These are

   a. _____

   b. _____

   c. _____

   d. _____

27. The principles of teaching are techniques that incorporate the principles of learning. Explain the following principles.

   a. Setting priorities:

   _____

   _____

   b. Timing:

   _____

   _____

   c. Organizing teaching material:

   _____

   _____

   d. Maintaining attention and promoting participation:

   _____

   _____

e. Building on existing knowledge:

_____

_____

f. Selecting teaching methods:

_____

_____

g. Selecting resources:

_____

_____

h. Writing teaching plans:

_____

_____

## Implementation

### Teaching Approaches

28. Briefly explain the following teaching approaches.

a. Telling:

_____

_____

b. Selling:

_____

_____

c. Participating:

_____

_____

d. Entrusting:

_____

_____

e. Reinforcing:

_____

_____

### Implementing Teaching Methods

29. Summarize the following instructional methods.

a. One-on-one discussion:

_____

_____

b. Group instruction:

_____

_____

c. Preparatory instruction:

_____

_____

d. Demonstrations:

_____

_____

e. Analogies:

_____

_____

f. Role playing:

_____

_____

g. Simulation

_____

_____

30. Identify some teaching tools to be used with the following.

a. Illiteracy and learning disability:

_____

_____

b. Cultural diversity:

_____

_____

c. Children:

_____

_____

d. Older adults:

_____

_____

## Evaluation

Evaluation reinforces correct behaviour by the learner, helps learners realize how they should change incorrect behaviour, and helps you determine the adequacy of teaching.

31. Identify some evaluation measures.

    _____

    _____

    _____

    _____

32. List three areas to be included when documenting patient teaching.

    a. _____

    b. _____

    c. _____

## Review Questions

Select the appropriate answer, and cite the rationale for choosing that particular answer.

1. An internal impulse that causes a person to take action is
   a. Anxiety
   b. Motivation
   c. Compliance
   d. Adaptation

   Answer:_____ Rationale: _____

   _____

   _____

2. Demonstration of the principles of body mechanics used when transferring patients from bed to chair would be classified under which domain of learning?
   a. Cognitive
   b. Social
   c. Psychomotor
   d. Affective

   Answer:_____ Rationale: _____

   _____

   _____

3. Which of the following patients is most ready to begin a patient-teaching session?
   a. Ms. Benoit, who is unwilling to accept that her back injury may result in permanent paralysis
   b. Mr. Chang, a patient who recently received a diagnosis of diabetes, who is complaining that he was awake all night because of his noisy roommate
   c. Mrs. Ho, a patient with irritable bowel syndrome, who has just returned from a morning of testing in the gastroenterology laboratory
   d. Mr. Cinelli, a patient who had a heart attack 4 days ago and now seems somewhat anxious about how this will affect his future

   Answer:_____ Rationale: _____

   _____

   _____

4. As a nurse, you work with pediatric patients who have diabetes. Which is the youngest age group to which you can effectively teach psychomotor skills such as insulin administration?
   a. Toddler
   b. Adolescent
   c. School age
   d. Preschool

   Answer:_____ Rationale: _____

   _____

   _____

5. Which of the following is an appropriately stated learning objective for Mr. Chang, who has just received a diagnosis of type 2 diabetes?
   a. Mr. Chang will be taught self-administration of insulin by May 2.
   b. Mr. Chang will perform blood glucose monitoring with the EZ-Check Monitor by the time of discharge.
   c. Mr. Chang will know the signs and symptoms of low blood sugar by May 5.
   d. Mr. Chang will understand diabetes.

   Answer:_____ Rationale: _____

   _____

   _____

# 21

# Developmental Theories

## *Preliminary Reading*

Chapter 21, pages 309–325

## *Comprehensive Understanding*

### Growth and Development

1. Define *growth*.

   _____

   _____

   _____

2. Define *development*.

   _____

   _____

   _____

#### Factors Influencing Growth and Development

3. Identify the major factors influencing growth and development.

   a. _____

   b. _____

   c. _____

### Traditions of Developmental Theories

4. List the five traditions of developmental theories.

   a. _____

   b. _____

   c. _____

   d. _____

   e. _____

### Organicism

5. Define *organicism*.

   _____

   _____

   _____

#### Biophysical Developmental Theories

*Biophysical developmental theories* describe and explain how the physical body grows and changes.

6. Briefly summarize Gesell's theory of maturational development.

   _____

   _____

   _____

7. Identify and describe the mechanisms of Gesell's theory.

   a. _____

   _____

   b. _____

   _____

8. Briefly describe Chess and Thomas's theory of temperament development.

   _____

   _____

   _____

9. Identify and describe the three categories of temperament in Chess and Thomas's theory.

   a. _____

   b. _____

   c. _____

10. Identify and describe the mechanisms of Chess and Thomas's theory.

   _____

   _____

   _____

## Cognitive Developmental Theories

*Cognitive developmental theories* focus on reasoning and thinking processes, including the changes in how people perform intellectual operations.

11. Briefly summarize *Piaget's theory of cognitive development.*

   _____

   _____

   _____

12. Identify and describe the mechanisms of Piaget's theory.

   a. _____

   b. _____

13. Explain the four stages of Piaget's theory of cognitive development.

   a. Sensorimotor:

   _____

   _____

   b. Preoperational:

   _____

   _____

   c. Concrete operations:

   _____

   _____

   d. Formal operations:

   _____

   _____

## Moral Developmental Theories

14. Moral developmental theories try to explain

   _____

   _____.

### Piaget's Theory of Moral Development

15. Explain the three stages of Piaget's moral development theory.

   a. *Premoral stage*:

   _____

   _____

   b. *Conventional stage*:

   _____

   _____

   c. *Autonomous stage*:

   _____

   _____

### Kohlberg's Theory of Moral Development

16. Explain the six stages of *Kohlberg's theory of moral development.*

   a. Level I: Preconventional level

   Stage 1: _____

   Stage 2: _____

   b. Level II: Conventional level

   Stage 3: _____

   Stage 4: _____

   c. Level III: Postconventional level

   Stage 5: _____

   Stage 6: _____

### Kohlberg's Critics

17. Identify the limitations to Kohlberg's research.

   _____

   _____

   _____

18. Briefly explain Gilligan's argument against Kohlberg's theory.

_____
_____
_____

## Psychoanalytic and Psychosocial Tradition

19. What do theories in the psychoanalytic and psychosocial tradition describe?

_____
_____
_____

### Sigmund Freud

20. Briefly summarize Freud's theory of personality development.

_____
_____
_____

### Mechanisms of Freud's Theory

21. Identify and describe the mechanisms of Freud's theory.

a. _____
b. _____
c. _____

22. Explain the five stages of Freud's theory.

a. _____
_____
b. _____
_____
c. _____
_____
d. _____
_____
e. _____
_____

### Erikson's Theory of Eight Stages of Life

23. Briefly summarize Erikson's theory of psychosocial development.

_____
_____
_____

### Mechanisms of Erikson's Theory

24. Identify and describe the mechanisms of Erikson's theory.

a. _____
b. _____

25. Explain the following eight stages of Erikson's theory.

a. Trust versus mistrust:

_____
_____

b. Autonomy versus shame and doubt:

_____
_____

c. Initiative versus guilt:

_____
_____

d. Industry versus inferiority:

_____
_____

e. Identity versus role confusion:

_____
_____

f. Intimacy versus isolation:

_____
_____

g. Generativity versus self-absorption and stagnation:

_____
_____

h. Integrity versus despair:

_____

_____

### John Bowlby

Bowlby developed *attachment and separation theory*. The conflict between attachment and separation must be resolved to produce healthy social and emotional developmental outcomes across the lifespan.

### Patricia Crittenden

26. Define *attachment* according to Crittenden's dynamic maturational model.

_____

_____

_____

### Havighurst's Developmental Tasks

27. Briefly summarize Havighurst's theory of development.

_____

_____

_____

28. Identify a limitation to Havighurst's theory.

_____

_____

_____

29. Havighurst defined a series of essential tasks that arise from predictable and external pressures.

These pressures include _____,

_____, and _____.

## Mechanistic Tradition

30. Briefly explain the *mechanistic tradition*.

_____

_____

_____

## Contextualism

31. Developmental theories within the *contextual tradition* focus on

_____

_____.

### Bioecological Theory

32. Briefly summarize Bronfenbrenner's theory of bioecological development.

_____

_____

_____

33. Explain the four "layers" of environment in Bronfenbrenner's theory.

    a. _____

    b. _____

    c. _____

    d. _____

#### Mechanisms of the Bioecological Theory

34. Identify and describe the mechanisms of Bronfenbrenner's theory.

_____

_____

## Dialecticism

35. Briefly explain the *dialectic tradition*.

_____

_____

_____

### Keating and Hertzman's Population Health Theory

36. Briefly summarize Keating and Hertzman's *population health approach*.

_____

_____

_____

**Mechanisms of Population Health Theory**

37. Identify and describe the mechanisms of Keating and Hertzman's theory.

a. _____

b. _____

c. _____

**Resilience Theory**

38. Briefly describe the *resilience* approach to development.

_____

_____

_____

**Mechanisms of Resilience**

39. Identify and describe the mechanisms of resilience theory.

a. _____

b. _____

## Review Questions

Select the appropriate answer, and cite the rationale for choosing that particular answer.

1. According to Piaget, the school-aged child is in the third stage of cognitive development, which is characterized by
   a. Conventional thought
   b. Concrete operations
   c. Identity versus role diffusion
   d. Postconventional thought

   Answer:_____ Rationale: _____
   _____
   _____

2. According to Bronfenbrenner's developmental theory, the individual and his or her environment are seen as mutually influential. Development of a national child care policy is an example of an intervention at which level?
   a. Microsystem
   b. Mesosystem
   c. Exosystem
   d. Macrosystem

   Answer:_____ Rationale: _____
   _____
   _____

3. According to Erikson's developmental theory, the primary developmental task of the middle adult years is to
   a. Achieve generativity
   b. Achieve intimacy
   c. Establish a set of personal values
   d. Establish a sense of personal identity

   Answer:_____ Rationale: _____
   _____
   _____

4. Which of the following behaviours is most characteristic of the concrete operations stage of cognitive development?
   a. There is progression from reflex activity to imitative behaviour.
   b. There is inability to put oneself in another's place.
   c. Thought processes become increasingly logical and coherent.
   d. The ability to think in abstract terms and draw logical conclusions develops.

   Answer:_____ Rationale: _____
   _____
   _____

5. According to Kohlberg, children develop moral reasoning as they mature. Which of the following is most characteristic of a preschooler's stage of moral development?
   a. It is important to obey the rules of correct behaviour.
   b. Showing respect for authority is important behaviour.
   c. Behaviour that pleases others is considered good.
   d. Actions are determined as good or bad in terms of their consequences.

   Answer:_____ Rationale: _____
   _____
   _____

# 22

# Conception Through Adolescence

## *Preliminary Reading*

Chapter 22, pages 326–360

## *Comprehensive Understanding*

Human growth and development are continuous, intricate, and complex processes that are often divided into stages organized by age groups.

### Selecting a Developmental Framework for Nursing

Providing nursing care that is developmentally appropriate is easier when planning on a theoretical framework.

A developmental approach encourages organized care directed at the child's current level of functioning to motivate self-direction and health promotion.

### Conception

#### Intrauterine Life

1. Define the following terms or events.

   a. *Nagele's rule:*

   _____

   _____

   b. *Fertilization:*

   _____

   _____

   c. *Zygote:*

   _____

   _____

   d. *Morula:*

   _____

   _____

   e. *Blastocyst:*

   _____

   _____

   f. *Embryo:*

   _____

   _____

   g. *Placenta:*

   _____

   _____

   h. *Implantation:*

   _____

   _____

2. Explain the development process and health concerns for the following trimesters.

   a. First trimester

   Physical changes:

   _____

   _____

   Health promotion:

   _____

   _____

   Teratogens:

   _____

   _____

b. Second trimester

Physical changes:

_____

_____

Health promotion:

_____

_____

c. Third trimester

Physical changes:

_____

_____

Health promotion:

_____

_____

## Transition From Intrauterine to Extrauterine Life

3. _____, _____, and _____ changes all contribute to the infant's adaptation to neonatal life.

### Physical Changes

4. An immediate assessment of the neonate's condition is performed because the first concern is

_____.

5. List the five physiological parameters evaluated through the Apgar assessment.

   a. _____

   b. _____

   c. _____

   d. _____

   e. _____

### Psychosocial Changes

6. Which two factors are most important in promoting closeness of the parents and the neonate?

   a. _____

   b. _____

7. Define *bonding*.

_____

_____

### Health Risks

8. Briefly explain the three most important physical needs of the newborn in each category.

   a. Airway:

   _____

   _____

   b. Temperature:

   _____

   _____

   c. Prevention of infection:

   _____

   _____

## Newborn

9. The neonatal period is defined as

_____.

### Physical Changes

10. Identify the normal characteristics of the newborn.

    a. Height: _____

    b. Weight: _____

    c. Head circumference: _____

    d. Vital signs: _____

    _____

    e. Physical characteristics: _____

    _____

    f. Neurological function: _____

    _____

    g. Behavioural characteristics: _____

    _____

**Cognitive Changes**

Early cognitive development begins with innate behaviour, reflexes, and sensory functions.

11. Identify the sensory functions that contribute to cognitive development in the newborn.

_____

_____

**Psychosocial Changes**

12. Explain the interactions that foster deep attachment between the infant and the parents.

_____

_____

**Health Risks**

13. Define *hyperbilirubinemia*.

_____

_____

**Health Concerns**

14. Screening for inborn errors of metabolism applies to

_____

_____.

15. Circumcision is a common and controversial procedure. Identify the risks of this procedure.

_____

_____

## Infant

16. Infancy is the period from _____ to

_____.

**Physical Changes**

17. Summarize the normal characteristics of the infant.

 a. Physical growth:

   _____

   _____

 b. Vital signs:

   _____

   _____

 c. Gross motor skills:

   _____

   _____

 d. Fine motor skills:

   _____

   _____

**Cognitive Changes**

18. Summarize the cognitive development of an infant.

_____

_____

_____

**Psychosocial Changes**

During the first year, infants begin to differentiate themselves from others as separate beings capable of acting on their own.

Erikson describes the psychosocial developmental crisis for the infant as trust versus mistrust.

19. Define *play*.

_____

_____

20. Identify activities appropriate at this stage of development.

_____

_____

_____

**Health Risks**

21. Identify the common types of injury and possible prevention strategies.

_____

_____

_____

22. Child maltreatment includes

_____.

**Health Concerns**

The quality of nutrition influences the infant's growth and development.

23. Identify the feeding alternatives for an infant.

_____

_____

_____

_____

24. Identify some supplementation needs of an infant.

_____

_____

25. Briefly explain health concerns related to the following.

    a. Dentition:

    _____

    _____

    b. Immunizations:

    _____

    _____

    c. Sleep:

    _____

    _____

## Toddler

26. Toddlerhood ranges from _____ to _____.

**Physical Changes**

27. Summarize the normal characteristics of a toddler.

    a. Self-care activities:

    _____

    _____

    b. Motor skills:

    _____

    _____

    c. Vital signs:

    _____

    _____

    d. Weight:

    _____

    _____

    e. Height:

    _____

    _____

**Cognitive Changes**

28. Summarize Piaget's *preoperational* thought stage.

    _____

    _____

    _____

    _____

**Language**

29. Describe language ability at this stage.

    _____

    _____

    _____

**Psychosocial Changes**

30. Identify Erikson's psychosocial development stage.

    _____

    _____

    _____

    _____

31. Explain the parental implications of the following developmental states.

    a. Independence:

    _____

    _____

    b. Social interactions:

    _____

    _____

    c. Play:

    _____

    _____

**Health Risks**

32. Describe some developmental abilities for this age period.

    _____

    _____

    _____

    _____

33. Identify injury prevention strategies.

_____
_____
_____
_____

**Health Concerns**

34. Briefly explain the nutrition requirements for this age group.

_____
_____
_____

# Preschooler

35. The preschool period refers to

_____.

**Physical Changes**

36. Summarize the normal characteristics of the preschooler.

a. Vital signs:

_____
_____

b. Weight:

_____
_____

c. Height:

_____
_____

d. Coordination:

_____
_____

**Cognitive Changes**

Preschoolers continue to master the preoperational stage of cognition.

37. The first phase of this period (2 to 4 years) is characterized by _____.

38. Define *artificialism*.

_____
_____
_____

39. Define *animism*.

_____
_____

40. Define immanent justice.

41. Summarize the intuitive phase of preoperational thought (4 years).

_____
_____
_____
_____

42. The greatest fear of this age group is

_____.

43. Summarize this group's moral development.

_____
_____
_____
_____

**Language**

44. Describe the language ability for this age group.

_____
_____
_____

**Psychosocial Changes**

The preschooler's world expands beyond the family into the neighbourhood, where preschoolers meet other children and adults.

45. Identify some dependent behaviours that preschoolers may revert to during stress or illness.

_____
_____

**Play**

46. Summarize the pattern of play for the preschooler.

_____
_____
_____
_____

**Health Risks**

Guidelines for injury prevention in the toddler also apply to the preschooler.

47. _____ and _____ remain the leading causes of injury for this age group.

**Health Concerns**

48. Explain health concerns related to the following for this group.

    a. Nutrition:

    _____

    _____

    b. Sleep:

    _____

    _____

    c. Vision:

    _____

    _____

# School-Age Children and Adolescents

## School-Age Child

49. The school-age years range from _____ to _____.

50. _____ signals the end of middle childhood.

The school and home influence growth and development, and adjustments by the parents and child are required.

    Parents must learn to allow their child to make decisions, accept responsibility, and learn from life's experiences.

**Physical Changes**

51. Summarize the normal characteristics of the school-age child.

    a. Weight:

    _____

    _____

    b. Height:

    _____

    _____

    c. Cardiovascular functioning:

    _____

    _____

    d. Neuromuscular functioning:

    _____

    _____

    e. Skeletal growth:

    _____

    _____

**Cognitive Changes**

Cognitive changes provide the school-age child with the ability to think in a logical manner about the here and now. They are not yet capable of abstract thinking.

52. Define the cognitive skills that are developing in this group.

    _____

    _____

    _____

    _____

**Language Development**

53. Describe language development during middle childhood.

    _____

    _____

    _____

    _____

**Psychosocial Changes**

54. The developmental task for school-age children is _____ versus _____.

55. Summarize psychosocial development in relation to the following.

    a. Moral development:

    _____

    _____

    b. Peer relationships:

    _____

    _____

c. Sexual identity:

_____

_____

**Health Risks**

56. _____ and _____ are the leading causes of death or injury.

Infections account for the majority of all childhood illnesses; respiratory infections are the most prevalent.

57. Identify the specific health concerns of children living in poverty.

_____

_____

_____

**Health Concerns**

School-age children are aware of their bodies and are sensitive about being exposed. Provide for privacy and offer explanations of common procedures.

**Health Education**

58. Identify five critical functions of a school-based health promotion program.

a. _____

b. _____

c. _____

d. _____

e. _____

59. Identify at least five health promotion activities that are appropriate for the school-age child.

a. _____

b. _____

c. _____

d. _____

e. _____

**Safety**

Accidents are the leading cause of death and injury in the school-age period. Children should be encouraged to take responsibility for their own safety.

**Nutrition**

60. Identify the nutritional requirements for the school-age child.

_____

_____

_____

_____

## Adolescent

61. Adolescence is the period of development

_____.

62. Define *puberty* and explain the changes that occur at this time.

_____

_____

_____

**Physical Changes**

63. List the four major physical changes associated with sexual maturation.

a. _____

b. _____

c. _____

d. _____

64. The hormones responsible for the development of secondary sex characteristics are _____ and _____.

65. Summarize the weight and skeletal changes that occur during adolescence.

_____

_____

_____

_____

_____

66. Explain the effects of physical changes on peer interactions.

_____

_____

_____

## Cognitive Changes

67. Changes that occur within the mind and the widening social environment of the adolescent result in _____, the highest level of intellectual development.

During this period of cognitive development, the adolescent develops the ability to solve problems through logical operations.

For the first time, the young person can move beyond the physical or concrete properties of a situation and use reasoning powers to understand the abstract.

68. Briefly explain the cognitive abilities of this group.

_____
_____
_____
_____
_____

## Language Skills

69. Describe the language skills of the adolescent.

_____
_____
_____

## Psychosocial Changes

70. The search for _____ is the major task of adolescent psychosocial development.

Teenagers must establish close peer relationships or risk remaining socially isolated.

71. Explain identity versus role confusion (Erikson).

_____
_____
_____

72. Behaviours indicating a lack of resolution are _____ and _____.

73. Explain the following components of total identity.

a. Gender identity: _____

b. Group identity: _____

c. Family identity: _____

d. Vocational identity: _____

e. Moral identity: _____

f. Health identity: _____

## Health Risks

### Injuries

74. Identify the leading cause of death and its sources among adolescents.

_____
_____
_____

### Suicide

75. Suicide is the second leading cause of death among adolescents. List the six warning signs of suicide for this group.

a. _____

b. _____

c. _____

d. _____

e. _____

f. _____

### Substance Abuse

76. Substance abuse is a major concern. Adolescents most at risk are those coming from _____.

### Eating Disorders

77. Define the two eating disorders that follow.

a. Anorexia nervosa:

_____
_____

b. Bulimia nervosa:

_____
_____

### Obesity and Physical Inactivity

Overweight and obesity, together with a decrease in physical activity, are becoming serious public health problems in Canada.

### Sexual Experimentation

78. _____, _____, and _____ expectations contribute to early heterosexual and homosexual relations.

79. Briefly explain the two prominent consequences of adolescent sexual activity.

    a. Sexually transmitted infections (STIs):

    _____

    _____

    b. Pregnancy:

    _____

    _____

**Health Concerns**

To help adolescents form healthy habits of daily living, you need to emphasize the importance of exercise, sleep, nutrition, and stress reduction.

**Health Education**

80. Identify health promotion interventions for the adolescent in regard to the following.

    a. Unintentional injuries:

    _____

    _____

    b. Firearm use and violence:

    _____

    _____

    c. Substance abuse:

    _____

    _____

    d. Suicide:

    _____

    _____

    e. Sexual activity:

    _____

    _____

81. Identify the health concerns of the following.

    a. Adolescents in rural communities:

    _____

    _____

    b. Minority adolescents:

    _____

    _____

    c. Aboriginal adolescents:

    _____

    _____

    d. Lesbian, gay, and bisexual adolescents:

    _____

    _____

## *Review Questions*

Select the appropriate answer, and cite the rationale for choosing that particular answer.

1. Which statement about human growth and development is accurate?
   a. Growth and development processes are unpredictable.
   b. Growth and development begin with birth and end after adolescence.
   c. All individuals progress through the same phases of growth and development.
   d. All individuals accomplish developmental tasks at the same pace.

Answer: _____ Rationale: _____

_____

_____

2. The mother of a 2-year-old expresses concern that her son's appetite has diminished and that he seems to prefer milk to solid foods. Which response reflects your knowledge of the principles of communication and nutrition?
   a. "Oh, I wouldn't be too worried; children tend to eat when they're hungry. I just wouldn't give him dessert unless he eats his meal."
   b. "That is not uncommon in toddlers. You might consider increasing his milk to 2 L per day to be sure he gets enough nutrients."
   c. "Have you considered feeding him when he doesn't seem interested in feeding himself?"
   d. "A toddler's rate of growth normally slows down. It's common to see a toddler's appetite diminish in response to decreased calorie needs."

Answer: _____ Rationale: _____

_____

_____

3. Which neonatal assessment finding would be considered abnormal?
   a. Cyanosis of the hands and feet during activity
   b. Palpable anterior and posterior fontanels
   c. Soft, protuberant abdomen
   d. Absence of the rooting, grasping, and sucking reflexes

Answer: _____ Rationale: _____
_____
_____

4. To stimulate cognitive and psychosocial development of the toddler, it is important for parents to
   a. Set firm and consistent limits
   b. Foster sharing of toys with playmates and siblings
   c. Provide clarification about what is right and wrong
   d. Allow complete freedom for exploration of the environment

Answer: _____ Rationale: _____
_____
_____

5. Which of the following statements is true of the developmental behaviours of school-age children?
   a. Formal and informal peer group membership is the key to forming self-esteem.
   b. Fears centre on the loss of self-control.
   c. Positive feedback from parents and teachers is crucial to development.
   d. A full range of defence mechanisms is used, including rationalization and intellectualization.

Answer: _____ Rationale: _____
_____
_____

6. Adolescents have mastered age-appropriate sexuality when they feel comfortable with their sexual
   a. Behaviours
   b. Choices
   c. Relationships
   d. All of the above

Answer: _____ Rationale: _____
_____
_____

# 23

# Young to Middle Adulthood

## Preliminary Reading

Chapter 23, pages 361–373

## Comprehensive Understanding

1. Young adulthood is the period from _____ to _____.

2. Individuals in young adulthood _____, _____, and _____.

3. Middle age occurs from _____ to _____.

4. Middle-aged adults become aware of changes in _____ and _____ abilities. This is a time when individuals may reassess _____.

## Young Adulthood

### Physical Changes

5. The young adult has completed physical growth by the age of 20. List the characteristics of young adults.

   a. _____
   b. _____
   c. _____
   d. _____

6. Identify the main components of a personal life-style assessment of a young adult.

   _____
   _____
   _____

### Cognitive Changes

7. Formal and informal education, life experiences, and work opportunities increase the young adult's _____ and _____.

8. Choosing an occupation is a _____ of young adults and involves knowing their _____, _____, and _____.

### Psychosocial Changes

9. The emotional health of the young adult is related to the individual's ability to address and resolve personal and social tasks. Explain the patterns of change that are common in the following age groups.

   a. 23 to 28 years:

   _____
   _____

   b. 29 to 34 years:

   _____
   _____

10. _____ and _____ issues influence an adult's life and can pose challenges for nursing care.

11. Identify the six major developmental tasks of adulthood.

   a. _____

   b. _____

   c. _____

   d. _____

   e. _____

   f. _____

12. For young men and women, successful employment ensures _____ and promotes _____, _____, _____, and _____.

13. Two-career marriages are _____.

14. The average age for first marriage for women is _____ years and for men is _____ years.

15. Close friends and associates of the single young adult may also be viewed as the individual's _____.

16. Identify five tasks to be completed by a couple before marriage.

   a. _____

   b. _____

   c. _____

   d. _____

   e. _____

17. Identify three changing norms and values in Canada related to alternative family structures.

   a. _____

   b. _____

   c. _____

**Hallmarks of Emotional Health**

18. During a psychological assessment of young adults, the nurse can assess for _____ of emotional health that indicate successful maturation in this developmental stage.

**Social Support in Health and Illness**

A current trend in health care is the use of *peer navigators* to facilitate well-being.

**Health Risks**

19. Briefly explain the risk factors for young adults in regard to the following.

   a. Lifestyle:

   _____

   _____

   b. Family history:

   _____

   _____

   c. Accidental death and injury:

   _____

   _____

   d. Substance abuse:

   _____

   _____

   e. Unplanned pregnancies:

   _____

   _____

   f. Sexually transmitted infections:

   _____

   _____

   g. Environmental and occupational factors:

   _____

   _____

**Health Concerns**

20. Give examples of nursing assessment and interventions for young adults related to the following areas of health.

   a. Infertility:

   _____

   _____

   b. Exercise:

   _____

   _____

   c. Routine health screening:

   _____

   _____

21. The psychosocial concerns of the young adult are often related to stress. Briefly explain each of the following sources of stress.

 a. Job stress:

 _____
 _____

 b. Family stress:

 _____
 _____

**Pregnancy**

22. Explain the health practices that you would discuss with a woman anticipating pregnancy.

 _____
 _____
 _____
 _____
 _____
 _____

**Prenatal Care**

23. Prenatal care is

 _____.

**Physiological Changes**

24. Explain the physiological changes that occur during pregnancy and the puerperium.

 a. First trimester:

 _____
 _____

 b. Second trimester:

 _____
 _____

 c. Third trimester:

 _____
 _____

 d. Puerperium:

 _____
 _____

**Psychosocial Changes**

25. Explain the implications for nursing associated with the following psychosocial changes that occur during pregnancy.

 a. Body image:

 _____
 _____

 b. Role changes:

 _____
 _____

 c. Sexuality:

 _____
 _____

 d. Coping mechanisms:

 _____
 _____

 e. Stresses during puerperium:

 _____
 _____

 f. Postpartum blues and depression:

 _____
 _____

**Acute Care**

26. Provide examples of when acute care might be required for young adults.

 _____
 _____
 _____

**Restorative and Continuing Care**

27. Describe the effect of chronic illness and disability on the young adult.

 _____
 _____
 _____
 _____

## Middle Adulthood

28. Briefly explain the characteristics of the middle adult years.

_____
_____
_____
_____

### Physical Changes

29. Briefly explain the major physiological changes that occur between 40 and 65 years of age.

_____
_____
_____
_____

### Perimenopause and Menopause

30. Define *menopause.*

_____
_____

### Psychosocial Changes

31. Define *sandwich generation.*

_____
_____

32. Summarize the psychosocial development of the middle-aged adult in the following areas.

a. Career transition:

_____
_____

b. Sexuality:

_____
_____

c. Family types:

_____
_____

d. Singlehood:

_____
_____

e. Marital changes:

_____
_____

f. Family transitions:

_____
_____

g. Care of aging parents

_____
_____

### Health Concerns

33. Briefly explain each of the following physiological concerns for the middle-aged adult and suggest appropriate nursing assessment and interventions.

a. Stress and stress reduction:

_____
_____

b. Obesity:

_____
_____

### Forming Positive Health Habits

34. List some positive health habits that support health for the middle-aged adult.

_____
_____
_____
_____

35. _____ and _____ are often directed at improving health habits.

36. Identify three external barriers to change.

a. _____
b. _____
c. _____

37. Identify four internal barriers to change.

a. _____
b. _____
c. _____
d. _____

38. Summarize two psychosocial concerns of the middle-aged adult, and provide the appropriate nursing assessment and interventions.

a. Anxiety:

_____
_____
_____

b. Depression:

_____

_____

_____

**Primary Health Care Programs**

39. Primary health care programs for young and middle adults are designed to _____, _____, and _____.

**Acute Care**

40. Identify examples of acute illnesses and injuries (similar to the young adult) that occur in middle adulthood.

_____

_____

_____

**Restorative and Continuing Care**

41. Identify some chronic illnesses or issues that occur in middle adulthood.

_____

_____

_____

## Review Questions

Select the appropriate answer, and cite the rationale for choosing that particular answer.

1. The leading cause of injury and death in the young adult population is
   a. Sexually transmitted infection
   b. Accidents
   c. Cardiovascular disease
   d. Substance abuse

   Answer: _____ Rationale: _____

   _____

   _____

2. Psychosocial changes of pregnancy commonly involve all of the following areas, except
   a. Altered body image
   b. Reduced stress
   c. Role changes
   d. Sexuality

   Answer: _____ Rationale: _____

   _____

   _____

3. Which physiological change would be a normal assessment finding in a middle-aged adult?
   a. Increased breast size
   b. Abdominal tenderness
   c. Increased thoracic diameter
   d. Reduced auditory acuity

   Answer: _____ Rationale: _____

   _____

   _____

4. Which of the following is most likely to affect the overall level of health of a patient in middle adulthood?
   a. Stress due to life changes
   b. Decreased visual acuity
   c. Declining sexual interest
   d. Onset of menopause

   Answer: _____ Rationale: _____

   _____

   _____

5. In planning patient education for Fran Higuchi, a 45-year-old woman who had an ovarian cyst removed, which of the following facts is true about the sexuality of the middle-aged adult?
   a. Menstruation ceases after menopause.
   b. Estrogen is produced after menopause.
   c. Middle-aged men are unable to produce fertile sperm.
   d. With removal of an ovarian cyst, pregnancy cannot occur.

   Answer: _____ Rationale: _____

   _____

   _____

# 24

# Older Adulthood

Preliminary Reading

## Preliminary Reading

Chapter 24, pages 374–395

## Comprehensive Understanding

1. Briefly summarize demographic trends of older Canadians.

   _____

   _____

   _____

   _____

## Variability Among Older Adults

2. Briefly explain the changes of the older adult.

   a. Physiological:

   _____

   _____

   b. Cognitive and psychosocial:

   _____

   _____

   _____

   _____

## Terminology

3. Explain the following terminology.

   a. Geriatrics:

   _____

   _____

   b. Gerontology:

   _____

   _____

   c. Gerontological nursing:

   _____

   _____

   d. Gerontic nursing:

   _____

   _____

## Myths and Stereotypes

4. Identify at least five myths or stereotypes regarding the older adult.

   a. _____

   b. _____

   c. _____

   d. _____

   e. _____

5. Define *ageism*.

   _____

   _____

## Nurses' Attitudes Toward Older Adults

6. The attitude of the nurse toward older adults comes

   in part from _____, _____,

   _____, and _____.

## Theories of Aging

7. Give a brief description of the following biological theories.

   a. *Stochastic theories*:

   _____
   _____

   b. *Nonstochastic theories*:

   _____
   _____

8. Describe the three classic psychosocial theories of aging.

   a. _____
   b. _____
   c. _____

### Developmental Tasks for Older Adults

9. List the seven developmental tasks of the older adult.

   a. _____
   b. _____
   c. _____
   d. _____
   e. _____
   f. _____
   g. _____

## Aging Well and Quality of Life

10. Older adults are considered to be _____ when they are _____.

## Community-Based and Institutional Health Care Services

11. Briefly describe the following health services that are used by the older population.

   a. Long-term care facilities:

   _____
   _____

   b. Assisted-living facilities:

   _____
   _____

   c. Personal care homes:

   _____
   _____

## Assessing the Needs of Older Adults

12. Nurses need to take into account five key points to ensure an age-specific approach.

   a. _____
   b. _____
   c. _____
   d. _____
   e. _____

13. List some techniques to use for the older adult with visual impairments.

   a. _____
   b. _____
   c. _____

14. List some techniques to use with the older adult with hearing impairment.

   a. _____
   b. _____
   c. _____
   d. _____
   e. _____

### Physiological Changes

15. Identify the physiological changes that occur in the older adult with regard to the following.

   a. General survey:

   _____
   _____

   b. Integumentary system:

   _____
   _____

   c. Head and neck:

   _____
   _____

   d. Thorax and lungs:

   _____
   _____

e. Heart and vascular system:

_____

_____

f. Breasts:

_____

_____

g. Gastrointestinal system and abdomen:

_____

_____

h. Reproductive system:

_____

_____

i. Urinary system:

_____

_____

j. Musculoskeletal system:

_____

_____

k. Neurological system:

_____

_____

**Functional Changes**

16. Functional status in older adults ordinarily refers to the capacity and safe performance of activities of daily living, and it is a sensitive indicator of health or illness in older adults. Factors that promote the highest level of functioning in all areas include:

a. _____

b. _____

c. _____

d. _____

e. _____

f. _____

**Cognitive Changes**

The structural and physiological changes that occur in the brain during aging do not necessarily affect adaptive and functional abilities.

17. Define the following terms.

   *a. Delirium:*

   _____

   _____

   _____

   b. *Dementia*:

   _____

   _____

   _____

   c. *Depression*:

   _____

   _____

   _____

18. Identify the characteristic progressive symptoms of *Alzheimer's disease.*

   a. _____

   b. _____

   c. _____

   d. _____

**Psychosocial Changes**

**Retirement**

19. Identify at least five areas that should be addressed when counselling an older adult about retirement.

   a. _____

   b. _____

   c. _____

   d. _____

   e. _____

**Social Isolation**

20. Briefly explain some of the reasons older adults experience social isolation.

_____

_____

_____

_____

**Abuse**

21. *Elder abuse* is the mistreatment of an older adult by other people who are in a position of trust or power or who are responsible for the adult's care. List the six types of abuse, and discuss the role of the nurse.

a. _____

b. _____

c. _____

d. _____

e. _____

f. _____

**Sexuality**

22. Briefly describe the sexual changes that occur in the older adult.

_____

_____

_____

_____

**Housing and Environment**

23. List four factors to assess when assisting older adults with housing needs.

a. _____

b. _____

c. _____

d. _____

# Addressing the Health Concerns of Older Adults

24. The two most common causes of death in the older adult are _____ and

_____.

**Health Promotion and Maintenance: Physiological Health Concerns**

25. Summarize the physiological health concerns related to each of the following.

a. Cancer:

_____

_____

b. Heart disease:

_____

_____

c. Stroke:

_____

_____

d. Smoking:

_____

_____

e. Alcohol abuse:

_____

_____

f. Nutrition:

_____

_____

g. Dental problems:

_____

_____

h. Exercise:

_____

_____

i. Arthritis:

_____

_____

j. Falls:

_____

_____

k. Sensory impairments:

_____

_____

l. Pain:

_____

_____

m. Medication use:

_____

_____

**Health Promotion and Maintenance: Psychosocial Health Concerns**

26. Briefly describe the interventions used to maintain the psychosocial health of the older adult.

   a. Therapeutic communication:

   _____

   _____

   _____

   b. Touch:

   _____

   _____

   _____

   c. Cognitive stimulation:

   _____

   _____

   _____

   d. Reminiscence:

   _____

   _____

   _____

   e. Body-image interventions:

   _____

   _____

   _____

## Older Adults and the Acute Care Setting

27. Explain why the older adult is at risk for each of the following.

   a. Delirium:

   _____

   _____

   b. Dehydration:

   _____

   _____

   c. Malnutrition:

   _____

   _____

   d. Health care–associated (or nosocomial) infections:

   _____

   _____

   e. Urinary incontinence:

   _____

   _____

   f. Falls:

   _____

   _____

## Older Adults and Restorative Care

28. Summarize the two types of ongoing care for the older adult, and identify the focus of each.

   _____

   _____

   _____

   _____

## *Review Questions*

Select the appropriate answer, and cite the rationale for choosing that particular answer.

1. Which statement about older adults is accurate?
   a. Older adults are institutionalized.
   b. Most older adults live on a fixed income.
   c. Most older adults cannot learn to care for themselves.
   d. Most older adults have no sexual desire.

Answer:_____ Rationale: _____

_____

_____

2. Which statement describing *delirium* is correct?
   a. Persons with delirium may experience hallucinations.
   b. The onset of delirium is slow and insidious.
   c. Symptoms of delirium are stable and unchanging.
   d. Symptoms of delirium are irreversible.

Answer:_____ Rationale: _____

_____

_____

3. Katherine Dale states that she does not need the television turned on because she cannot see very well. Normal visual changes in older adults include all of the following, *except*
   a. Decreased visual acuity
   b. Decreased accommodation to darkness
   c. Double vision
   d. Sensitivity to glare

Answer:_____ Rationale: _____
_____
_____

4. Stephen DeLonghi states that he is worried about his parents' plans to retire. All of the following would be an appropriate response regarding retirement of the older adult, *except*
   a. Positive adjustment is often related to how much a person planned for the retirement

b. Retirement for most persons represents a sudden shock that is irreversibly damaging to self-image and self-esteem
c. Reactions to retirement are influenced by the importance that has been attached to the work role
d. Retirement may affect an individual's physical and psychological functioning

Answer:_____ Rationale: _____
_____
_____

# 25

# Self-Concept

## *Preliminary Reading*

Chapter 25, pages 396–414

## *Comprehensive Understanding*

### Nursing Knowledge Base

**Development of Self-Concept**

1. Each stage of development has specific activities that assist the patient in developing a positive self-concept. Identify some activities for each stage.

   a. 0 to 1 year:

   _____

   _____

   b. 1 to 3 years:

   _____

   _____

   c. 3 to 6 years:

   _____

   _____

   d. 6 to 12 years:

   _____

   _____

   e. 12 to 20 years:

   _____

   _____

   f. Mid-20s to mid-40s:

   _____

   _____

   g. Mid-40s to mid-60s:

   _____

   _____

   h. Late 60s on:

   _____

   _____

2. Self-concept is a dynamic perception that is based on the following:

   a. _____

   b. _____

   c. _____

   d. _____

   e. _____

   f. _____

   g. _____

   h. _____

   i. _____

   j. _____

   k. _____

   l. _____

   m. _____

**Components and Interrelated Terms of Self-Concept**

A healthy self-concept has a high degree of stability, generates positive or negative feelings toward the self, and helps individuals adapt positively to stressors.

3. Briefly explain the four significant components of self-concept.

   a. Identity:

   _____
   _____
   _____

   b. Body image:

   _____
   _____
   _____

   c. Self-esteem:

   _____
   _____
   _____

   d. Role performance:

   _____
   _____
   _____

4. List the processes through which a child learns appropriate behaviours.

   a. _____
   b. _____
   c. _____
   d. _____
   e. _____

**Stressors Affecting Self-Concept**

Stressors challenge a person's adaptive capacities.

5. A self-concept stressor is any

   _____.

Being able to adapt to stressors is likely to lead to a positive sense of self, whereas failure to adapt may lead to a negative sense of self.
   Any change in health can be a stressor that affects self-concept.

A physical change in the body leads to an altered body image. Identity and self-esteem can also be affected.
   A crisis occurs when a person cannot overcome obstacles with the usual methods of problem solving and adapting.

6. Define *identity*.

   _____
   _____
   _____
   _____

7. Define *identity confusion*.

   _____
   _____
   _____
   _____

8. Changes in the appearance, structure, or function of a body part will require a change in body image. Identify at least five stressors that affect body image.

   a. _____
   b. _____
   c. _____
   d. _____
   e. _____

9. Transitions within one's roles may lead to the following. Explain.

   a. Role conflict:

   _____
   _____

   b. Role ambiguity:

   _____
   _____

   c. Role strain:

   _____
   _____

   d. Role overload:

   _____
   _____

## The Family's Effect on Development of Self-Concept

The family plays a key role in creating and maintaining its members' self-concepts.

Children learn from their parents and siblings a basic sense of who they are and how they are expected to live.

## The Nurse's Effect on the Patient's Self-Concept

A nurse's acceptance of a patient with an altered self-concept helps stimulate positive rehabilitation.

10. List five areas you must clarify and assess about yourself in order to promote a positive self-concept in patients.

   a. _____
   b. _____
   c. _____
   d. _____
   e. _____

## Self-Concept and the Nursing Process

### Assessment

11. In assessing self-concept, you should focus on each component of self-concept: behaviours suggestive of _____, actual and potential self-concept _____, and _____ patterns.

Many of the data regarding self-concept are most effectively gathered through observation of a patient's nonverbal behaviour and by paying attention to the content of the patient's conversation rather than through direct questioning.

12. The nursing assessment should include consideration of previous coping behaviours: the _____, _____, and _____ of the stressors; and the patient's _____ and _____ resources.

As the nurse identifies previous coping patterns, it is useful to consider if these patterns have contributed to healthy functioning or created more problems.

Exploring resources and strengths, such as helpful significant others or prior use of community resources, can be important in formulating a realistic and effective plan.

13. Asking the patient how he or she believes interventions will make a difference in the problem can provide useful information regarding the patient's expectations and can provide an opportunity to discuss the patient's goals. Give an example.

   _____
   _____

## Nursing Diagnosis

Accurate development of a nursing diagnosis requires discussing the problem with the patient and the family.

## Planning

The nurse, patient, and family need to plan care directed at helping the patient regain or maintain a healthy self-concept.

Interventions focus on helping the patient and on coping methods.

The nurse looks for strengths in both the individual and the family, and provides resources and education to turn limitations into strengths.

14. Before involving the family, you need to consider the _____ and _____.

## Implementation

### Health Promotion

15. List some healthy lifestyle measures that contribute to a healthy self-concept.

   _____
   _____
   _____
   _____

**Acute Care**

16. In acute care, the nurse is likely to encounter patients who are experiencing _____ to their self-concept due to the nature of the treatment and diagnostic procedure.

17. Identify ways a nurse can assist a patient in the adjustment to a change in physical appearance.

_____

_____

_____

_____

**Restorative Care**

18. Identify goals to help a patient attain a more positive self-concept.

a. _____

b. _____

c. _____

d. _____

e. _____

19. Identify seven nursing interventions for the patient to engage in self-exploration.

a. _____

b. _____

c. _____

d. _____

e. _____

f. _____

g. _____

## Evaluation

20. Patient care evaluates the actual care delivered by the health team based on expected outcomes. Briefly explain the expected outcomes for a self-concept disturbance.

_____

_____

_____

_____

21. Patient expectations evaluate care from the patient's perspective. Give an example.

_____

_____

## Review Questions

Select the appropriate answer, and cite the rationale for choosing that particular answer.

1. Which developmental stage is particularly crucial for identity development?
   a. Infancy
   b. Preschool age
   c. Adolescence
   d. Young adulthood

Answer:_____ Rationale: _____

_____

_____

2. Which of the following statements about body image is correct?
   a. Physical changes are quickly incorporated into a person's body image.
   b. Body image refers only to the external appearance of a person's body.
   c. Body image involves attitudes related to the body, including physical appearance, structure, or function.
   d. Perceptions by other persons have no influence on a person's body image.

Answer:_____ Rationale: _____

_____

_____

3. Sandeep, who is 2 years old, is praised for using his potty instead of wetting his pants. This is an example of learning a behaviour by:
   a. Identification
   b. Imitation
   c. Substitution
   d. Reinforcement–extinction

Answer:_____ Rationale: _____

_____

_____

4. Mrs. Watson has just undergone a radical mastectomy. You are aware that Mrs. Watson will probably have considerable anxiety over
   a. Role performance
   b. Self-identity
   c. Body image
   d. Self-esteem

Answer:_____ Rationale: _____
_____
_____

5. Which of the following statements demonstrates that your self-concept is positively affecting the Patient?
   a. "You've got to take a more active part in caring for your ostomy."
   b. "I know your ostomy is difficult to look at, but you will get used to it in time."
   c. (While grimacing) "Ostomy care isn't so bad."
   d. "Let me show you how to place the bag on your stoma."

Answer:_____ Rationale: _____
_____
_____

## Critical Thinking Model for Nursing Care Plan for Disturbed Body Image

Imagine that you are the student nurse in the Nursing Care Plan on page 405 of your text. Complete the *assessment phase* of the critical thinking model by writing in the appropriate boxes on the model shown. Think about the following:

- In developing Ms. Johnson's plan of care, what knowledge did you apply?

- In what way might your previous experience apply in this case?

- What intellectual or professional standards were applied to Ms. Johnson?

- What critical thinking attitudes were used in assessing Ms. Johnson?

- As you review your assessment, what key areas did you cover?

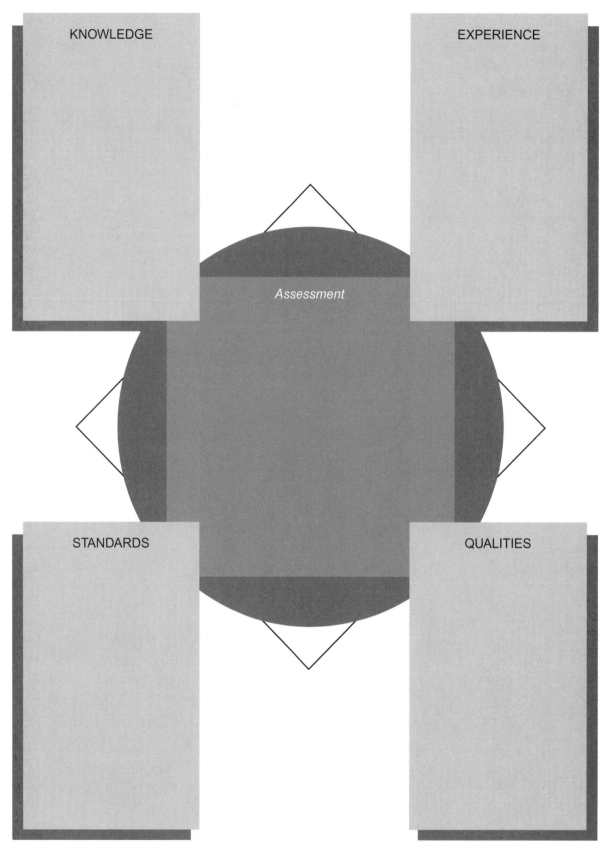

KNOWLEDGE

EXPERIENCE

*Assessment*

STANDARDS

QUALITIES

CHAPTER 25   Critical Thinking Model for Nursing Care Plan for *Disturbed Body Image*
See answers on Evolve site.

# 26

# Sexuality

## *Preliminary Reading*

Chapter 26, pages 415–432

## *Comprehensive Understanding*

1. Sexual health requires a _____ and _____ approach to sexuality and sexual relationships, as well as to the possibility of having pleasurable and _____ sexual experiences, free of _____, _____ and _____.

_____

_____.

## Scientific Knowledge Base

### Sexual and Gender Identity

2. Define the following.

   a. *Sexual identity*:

   _____

   _____

   b. *Gender identity*:

   _____

   _____

   c. *Transsexuality*:

   _____

   _____

### Sexual Orientation

3. Define *sexual orientation*.

   _____

   _____

4. Define *heterosexuality*.

   _____

   _____

5. Define *homosexuality*.

   _____

   _____

6. Define *bisexuality*.

   _____

   _____

You must not assume that you know your patients' gender identity or sexual orientation.

   If you learn of a patient's sexual orientation, you should not assume that you may tell anyone else or include it in the medical record without the patient's knowledge.

7. Define *homophobia*.

   _____

   _____

The nurse who is nonjudgemental and equipped with an appropriate knowledge base can help address the problems of homophobia and provide nursing care that does not discriminate against the patient's sexual orientation.

## Sexual Development

8. Each stage of development brings changes in sexual functioning and the role of sexuality in relationships. Explain each stage.

    a. Infancy and childhood:

    _____
    _____
    _____
    _____

    b. Puberty and adolescence:

    _____
    _____
    _____
    _____

    c. Adulthood:

    _____
    _____
    _____
    _____

    d. Older adulthood:

    _____
    _____
    _____
    _____

## Sexual Response Cycle

9. The four phases of the sexual response cycle are

    _____, _____,

    _____, and _____.

10. These phases are the result of vasocongestion and muscle contraction. Explain the physiological responses for each of the four phases.

    a. Female:

    _____
    _____

    b. Male:

    _____
    _____

## Sexual Behaviour

Sexual behaviour comprises the broad array of sexual activities in which people participate. It is difficult to say what is "normal" or "abnormal" because wide variation exists between cultures and at different times in society.

### High-Risk Sexual Behaviour

11. Define *safer sex*.

    _____
    _____

12. List three examples of unsafe sex practices.

    a. _____

    b. _____

    c. _____

## Sexually Transmitted Infections

13. A major problem in dealing with sexually transmitted infections (STIs) is _____

    _____.

14. List the prevalent STIs.

    a. _____

    b. _____

    c. _____

    d. _____

    e. _____

    f. _____

15. People most likely to contract an STI are those who

    a. _____

    b. _____

    c. _____

    d. _____

16. Condoms reduce the risk of most STIs (including HIV infection). A condom acts as a barrier to

    keep _____, _____, and

    _____ from passing from one person

    to another.

## Contraception

17. Numerous contraceptive options are available. Briefly list the options available under the following categories.

    a. Nonprescriptive methods:

    _____
    _____

b. Methods requiring a health care provider:

_____

_____

18. Emergency contraception pills are most effective up to _____ hours following intercourse and are recommended to _____.

### Abortion

Since 1988, Canada has been one of the few countries without any criminal law restricting abortion.

Two-thirds of abortions are performed in hospitals; the remaining one-third are performed in abortion clinics and health centres.

Health care providers must reflect on personal values related to abortion. The health care provider is entitled to personal views and should not be forced to participate in counselling or procedures contrary to his or her beliefs or values.

## Nursing Knowledge Base

### Sociocultural Dimensions of Sexuality

Global cultural diversity creates considerable variability in sexual norms and represents a wide spectrum of beliefs and values.

19. Common areas of diversity include the following:

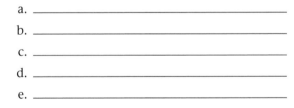

a. _____

b. _____

c. _____

d. _____

e. _____

### Discussing Sexual Issues

20. Identify the issues regarding the difficulty the nurse has in discussing sexuality with patients.

a. _____

b. _____

c. _____

d. _____

e. _____

### Alterations in Sexual Health

21. Explain the following issues.

a. Infertility:

_____

_____

b. Sexual abuse:

_____

_____

c. Sexual dysfunction:

_____

_____

### Patients With Particular Sexual Health Concerns

22. Describe the possible sexual concerns that should be considered for each of the following patients.

a. Pregnant and postpartum women:

_____

_____

b. Patients recovering from surgery:

_____

_____

c. Patients with illness or disabilities:

_____

_____

## Critical Thinking

Patients may have customs and values different from yours. Professional standards call for you to respect each patient as an individual.

## Sexuality and the Nursing Process

A person's sexuality has physical, psychological, social, and cultural elements.

## Assessment

### Factors Affecting Sexuality

23. Briefly explain the following factors that affect sexuality.

a. Physical:

_____

_____

b. Self-concept:

_____

_____

c. Relationship:

_____

_____

d. Self-esteem:

_____

_____

### Sexual Health History

24. List the questions you may use to elicit a brief sexual history from an adult.

a. _____

b. _____

c. _____

d. _____

When taking a health history, you should include a few questions related to sexual functioning to determine whether the patient has any sexual concerns. It is important to ask these questions once you have established rapport with the patient, and the sexual history is usually taken at the end of the general history.

### Physical Assessment

25. Briefly explain the physical assessment in evaluating the cause of sexual concerns or problems.

_____

_____

_____

## Nursing Diagnosis

26. Identify clues that may signal risk for or an actual nursing diagnosis related to sexuality.

a. _____

b. _____

c. _____

d. _____

e. _____

## Planning

### Goals and Outcomes

It is especially important to maintain a patient's dignity and identity when you develop the care plan. Together, you and the patient set realistic goals for care.

### Setting Priorities

27. The "PLISSIT" model developed by Annon (1974) guides the planning phases. Explain each of the following parts of the abbreviation.

a. *P*:

_____

_____

b. *LI*:

_____

_____

c. *SS*:

_____

_____

d. *IT*:

_____

_____

## Implementation

### Health Promotion

28. Topics of education vary depending on the defining characteristics and related factors. Describe some situations.

_____

_____

### Acute Care

29. Nursing interventions that address alterations in sexuality are aimed at _____, _____, _____, or _____.

The patient should be encouraged to investigate and acknowledge social and ethical values and analyze the role of sexuality in his or her self-concept.

30. Identify situational and developmental crises that prompt education.

_____
_____
_____
_____

**Restorative Care**

In the home, it is important to assist individuals in creating an environment comfortable for sexual activity.

In the long-term care setting, facilities should make proper arrangements for privacy during residents' sexual experiences.

## Evaluation

**Patient Care**

Patient care evaluates the actual care delivered by the health care team based on the expected outcomes.

Patient or spouse verbalizations determine if goals and outcomes have been achieved.

Sexuality is felt more than observed, and sexual expression requires an intimacy not amenable to observation.

All people involved may need to be reminded of the individual nature of sexual expression and the multiple factors that affect perceptions and responses.

**Patient Expectations**

31. Patient expectations evaluate care from the patient's perspective. Briefly explain the patient's perspective with respect to resolution of his or her sexual concerns.

_____
_____
_____
_____

## *Review Questions*

Select the appropriate answer, and cite the rationale for choosing that particular answer.

1. At what developmental stage is it particularly important for children reared in lone-parent families to be exposed to same-sex adults?
   a. Neonatal
   b. Toddlerhood and preschool years
   c. School age
   d. Adolescence

Answer:_____ Rationale: _____
_____
_____

2. In the school-age child, learning and reinforcement of gender-appropriate behaviours are not commonly derived from:
   a. Parents
   b. Teachers
   c. Siblings
   d. Peers

Answer:_____ Rationale: _____
_____
_____

3. Why is it often more difficult to discuss sexuality issues with older patients?
   a. Older people are less likely to be sexually active.
   b. They are more likely to have complex causes for sexual problems.
   c. They may have more difficulty discussing intimate issues.
   d. They are frequently deaf, and it is difficult to talk about this in a loud voice.

Answer:_____ Rationale: _____
_____
_____

4. The least effective means of preventing pregnancy is
   a. Coitus interruptus
   b. Birth control patch
   c. Body temperature method
   d. Mucous method

Answer:_____ Rationale: _____
_____
_____

5. The only 100% effective method to avoid contracting a disease through sex is
   a. Using condoms
   b. Avoiding sex with partners at risk
   c. Knowing the sexual partner's health history
   d. Abstinence

Answer:_____ Rationale: _____
_____
_____

## Critical Thinking Model for Nursing Care Plan for Sexual Dysfunction

Imagine that you are Jack, the nursing student in the Nursing Care Plan on page 428 of your text. Complete the *assessment* phase of the critical thinking model by writing your answers in the appropriate boxes of the model shown. Think about the following:

- In developing Mr. Clements's plan of care, what knowledge did you apply?

- In what way might your previous experience assist in this case?

- What intellectual or professional standards were applied in caring for Mr. Clements?

- What critical thinking attitudes did you utilize in assessing Mr. Clements?

- As you review your assessment, what key areas did you cover?

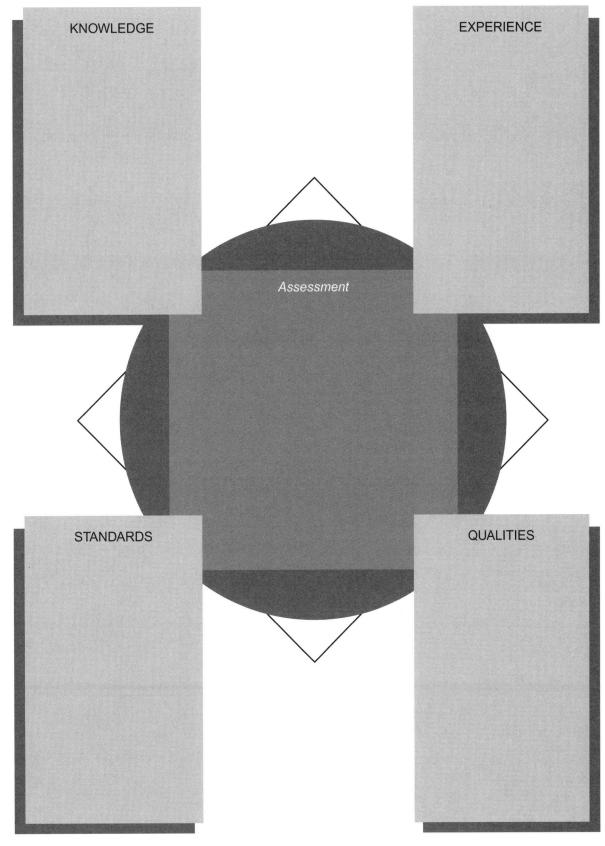

KNOWLEDGE

EXPERIENCE

*Assessment*

STANDARDS

QUALITIES

CHAPTER 26    Critical Thinking Model for Nursing Care Plan for *Sexual Dysfunction*
See answers on Evolve site.

# 27

# Spiritual Health

*Preliminary Reading*

Chapter 27, pages 433–446

## Comprehensive Understanding

1. Define *spirituality*.

   _____

   _____

   _____

2. Describe the association between spirituality and health.

   _____

   _____

   _____

### Historical Perspectives

3. Identify four historical milestones related to spirituality and nursing.

   _____

   _____

   _____

   _____

### Spirituality and Health: Empirical Evidence

4. Define *spiritual health*.

   _____

   _____

5. There is increasing evidence that spirituality has the_____.

**Mind–Body Connection and Psycho-neuro-immunology**

6. Briefly discuss *holism*.

   _____

   _____

7. Rituals and other practices that support spiritual and religious expression provide the following benefits:

   a. _____

   b. _____

### Spirituality and Nursing Theory

8. Some scholars are challenging the idea that spirituality should be _____.

9. Absence of an idealized spiritual state does not dictate some _____.

10. We need to be cautious about creating _____, particularly those based on _____.

### Conceptualizing Spirituality and Religion

11. Identify the common themes of spirituality in health care.

    _____

    _____

12. Discuss the challenge of defining spirituality for nursing.

_____

_____

13. A person's spirituality may be expressed in religious and philosophical beliefs and practices, and these may differ widely, depending _____.

14. Explain the differences between the terms *spirituality* and *religion*.

_____

_____

_____

_____

15. Explain the concept of *faith*.

_____

_____

_____

16. The belief that comes with faith involves _____, or an awareness of that which one cannot see or know in ordinary ways.

17. Explain how the following view spirituality.

a. *Atheists*:

_____

_____

b. *Agnostics*:

_____

_____

## Spirituality and the Life Journey

18. It is not unusual for youth who have been reared in a religious tradition to _____ as they search for _____.

19. Evidence of healthy spirituality is _____ for others and self.

20. A _____ may help to protect older adults from _____ and _____ that occur with aging.

21. Briefly explain how each of the following may impact a patient's spiritual journey.

a. Unexpected or chronic illness:

_____

_____

_____

b. Terminal illness:

_____

_____

_____

22. Briefly discuss what patients expect from nurses regarding their spiritual care.

_____

_____

_____

_____

## Critical Thinking

23. The nurse's approach to spirituality begins with _____.

### Understanding Patients' Spirituality

24. Spiritual care is _____ from the _____ aspects of care. Spirituality contains an element of _____ that cannot be _____ and _____ in the same way that you might treat a physical problem. _____ and _____ in a patient's spirituality may be considered _____ and _____.

25. Describe the nurse's role in understanding a patient's spirituality.

_____

_____

_____

_____

26. Briefly explain shared community and *compassion*.

_____

_____

27. Discuss the purpose of spiritual screening.

_____

_____

28. Identify six ways to try to understand a patient's spirituality:

a. _____

b. _____

c. _____

d. _____

e. _____

f. _____

**Ethical Spiritual Care**

Discrimination is not a conscious process but rather an unchallenged set of biases that cause us to react to others in less than caring ways.

An important part of ethical spiritual care is constantly working with your own potential biases as a nurse.

29. Describe the importance of reflective practice.

_____

_____

30. Identify two ethical issues that emerge when nurses engage in spiritual care.

_____

_____

31. Discuss how the *Code of Ethics for Registered Nurses* can be applied to boundaries and the provision of spiritual care.

_____

_____

32. Competencies for spiritual care include

_____.

Although nurses can provide a caring context for patients' spirituality, this should not in any way be misconstrued to suggest that nurses have expertise in spiritual care.

33. Describe how nurses are prepared to provide a good context for spiritual care.

_____

_____

_____

_____

There is great variability even among common religions, and individuals will pick and choose the practices they adhere to within that religion. You need not be afraid to ask. Many religious individuals will gladly talk about their faith and practices if you are open.

## Providing Spiritual Care

34. Spiritual care is often overlooked in the provision of nursing care. Identify some perceived barriers to nurses offering spiritual care.

a. _____

b. _____

c. _____

d. _____

e. _____

f. _____

35. Spiritual nursing care, at its foundation, is

_____.

36. Briefly describe spiritual care.

_____

_____

_____

37. _____ that undergird all of nursing practice are the same skills that create the

_____.

Nurses grow in their ability to provide spiritual care.

38. The beginning point of spiritual care is _____ and _____ and _____ to enter into conversations about what is meaningful and important to each patient.

**Facilitating Spiritual Practices**

Rituals that bring meaning to life are spiritual practices. They are integrated throughout a person's daily activities.

39. Give three examples of how a nurse can facilitate spiritual care.

_____

_____

_____

_____

## Reflecting on Nurses' Spiritual Care

Scholars have proposed that it is not normally within the nursing role to "evaluate" whether patients achieve connectedness, meaning, peace, hope, or other indicators of spirituality.

40. Identify six spiritual "interventions."

a. _____

b. _____

c. _____

d. _____

e. _____

f. _____

Nurses need to be cautious about entering into the areas of mystery, particularly if we are sensing our own need to explain or control patients' suffering.

## *Review Questions*

Select the appropriate answer, and cite the rationale for choosing that particular answer.

1. When planning care to include spiritual needs for a patient of the Hindu faith, the religious practices you should understand include all of the following, *except*
   a. Public prayer is important
   b. Modesty is important
   c. Religious symbols should not be removed
   d. Same-sex caregivers are preferred

   Answer:_____ Rationale: _____
   _____
   _____

2. The role of the nurse in spiritual care is to
   a. Assess, diagnose, and treat
   b. Delve into the intimate layers of spirituality
   c. Seek to understand and become a co-learner
   d. Not discuss but refer to religious leaders

   Answer:_____ Rationale: _____
   _____
   _____

3. A patient who is an Orthodox Jew may
   a. Keep a cross and prayer beads at the bedside
   b. Refuse treatment on the Sabbath
   c. Prefer to have pork with meals
   d. Choose death over breaking kosher

   Answer:_____ Rationale: _____
   _____
   _____

4. *Spiritual* is
   a. Defined by the individual
   b. The same as religion
   c. An organized system of beliefs
   d. Important to agnostics

   Answer:_____ Rationale: _____
   _____
   _____

5. Mr. Lanois is 90 years old and recently received a diagnosis of a malignant tumour. Staff members have observed him crying on several occasions, and now he cries as he reads from his Bible. Interventions to help Mr. Lanois cope with his illness would include
   a. Asking the parish nurse from his congregation to visit him
   b. Engaging Mr. Lanois in diversional activities to reduce feelings of hopelessness
   c. Discouraging family from being involved in activities and planning
   d. Praying with Mr. Lanois as often as possible

   Answer:_____ Rationale: _____
   _____
   _____

# 28

# The Experience of Loss, Death, and Grief

## Preliminary Reading

Chapter 28, pages 447–471

## Comprehensive Understanding

Loss and grief are experiences that affect not only patients and their families but the nurses who care for them as well.

### Scientific Knowledge Base

**Loss**

1. Give an example of the five categories of loss.

   a. *Necessary loss:*

   _____

   _____

   _____

   b. *Actual loss:*

   _____

   _____

   _____

   c. *Perceived loss:*

   _____

   _____

   _____

   d. *Maturational loss:*

   _____

   _____

   _____

   e. *Situational loss:*

   _____

   _____

   _____

**Grief**

2. Describe the following terms.

   a. *Grief:*

   _____

   _____

   _____

   b. *Bereavement:*

   _____

   _____

   _____

**Selected Theories of Grief**

3. List the phases of the grieving process proposed by each of the theorists listed below.

   a. Kübler-Ross's Stages of Grief:

   i. _____

   ii. _____

   iii. _____

   iv. _____

   v. _____

   b. Bowlby's Phases of Mourning:

   i. _____

   ii. _____

   iii. _____

   iv. _____

c. Worden's Four Tasks of Mourning

i. _____

ii. _____

iii. _____

iv. _____

**Types of Grief**

4. Briefly describe the following types of grief.

a. Normal grief:

_____

_____

b. Anticipatory grief:

_____

_____

c. Complicated grief:

_____

_____

d. Disenfranchised grief:

_____

_____

**Application of Grief Theory to Other Types of Loss**

Although grief theories apply mainly to the way that individuals cope with the death of a loved one, they also apply to other losses.

## Nursing Knowledge Base

**Factors Influencing Loss and Grief**

5. Briefly explain the factors that influence loss and grief.

a. Human development:

_____

_____

_____

b. Psychosocial perspectives:

_____

_____

_____

c. Socioeconomic status:

_____

_____

_____

d. Personal relationships:

_____

_____

e. Nature of the loss:

_____

_____

_____

f. Culture and ethnicity:

_____

_____

_____

g. Spiritual beliefs:

_____

_____

_____

**Coping With Grief and Loss**

6. Explain how the mechanism of *hope* is used to cope with grief and loss.

_____

_____

_____

_____

## The Nursing Process and Grief

## Assessment

**Type and Stage of Grief**

It is important for you to assess how a patient *is reacting* rather than how the patient *should be* reacting. A single behaviour can represent various types of grief. Therefore, the identification of the type and stage of grief should be used only to guide your assessment and not to judge the outcomes of the grieving process.

**Grief Reactions**

7. Identify some symptoms of normal grief feelings.

_____

_____

_____

_____

### Factors That Affect Grief

8. List four of the factors that affect grief.

_____

_____

_____

_____

### End-of-Life Decisions

9. Briefly explain end-of-life decisions.

_____

_____

_____

_____

### Nurses' Experience With Grief

Nurses may not always identify maladaptive coping behaviours themselves, and the entire team has a responsibility to recognize and support ineffective coping in their colleagues.

10. Assess your own experience with grief.

_____

_____

_____

## Nursing Diagnosis

11. List four possible nursing diagnoses for patients or families experiencing grief.

a. _____

b. _____

c. _____

d. _____

## Planning

Grieving is the natural response to loss and thus has a therapeutic value.

### Goals and Outcomes

12. List three goals appropriate for a patient dealing with loss.

a. _____

b. _____

c. _____

### Setting Priorities

13. Briefly explain how to prioritize the needs of the grieving patient.

_____

_____

_____

## Implementation

### Health Promotion

Nurses help patients and families deal with loss, make decisions about the patient's health care, and adjust to any disappointment, frustration, and anxiety created by their loss.

### Therapeutic Communication

14. Describe five therapeutic communication strategies you can use to help patients discuss and work through their loss.

a. _____

b. _____

c. _____

d. _____

e. _____

### Promoting Hope

15. Give an example of a nursing strategy to promote hope for each dimension.

a. Affective dimension:

_____

_____

b. Cognitive dimension:

_____

_____

c. Behavioural dimension:

_____

_____

d. Affiliative dimension:

_____

_____

e. Temporal dimension:

_____

_____

f. Contextual dimension:

_____

_____

**Facilitating Mourning**

16. Identify the nursing strategies to facilitate mourning for the patient and family.

    a. _____

    b. _____

    c. _____

    d. _____

    e. _____

    f. _____

    g. _____

**Acute Care**

**Palliative Care**

17. According to the World Health Organization, when health care providers deliver palliative care, they do the following:

    a. _____

    b. _____

    c. _____

    d. _____

    e. _____

    f. _____

    g. _____

18. Give examples of how the following contribute to comfort for the dying patient.

    a. Symptom control:

    _____

    _____

    b. Maintaining dignity and self-esteem:

    _____

    _____

    c. Preventing abandonment and isolation:

    _____

    _____

    d. Providing a comfortable and peaceful environment:

    _____

    _____

**Support for the Grieving Family**

The family may be the primary caregivers when the patient chooses to die at home. Family members need your support, and they benefit from being taught ways to care for their loved one.

**Hospice Care**

19. Identify the components of hospice care.

    a. _____

    b. _____

    c. _____

    d. _____

    e. _____

    f. _____

    g. _____

    h. _____

**Care After Death**

Care after death includes caring for the body with dignity and sensitivity, and in a manner consistent with the patient's religious or cultural beliefs.

20. Explain how you can support the family through the organ and tissue request or donation process.

    _____

    _____

    _____

    _____

21. The family becomes _____ when the

    _____, and the shift _____
    to the living family.

**The Grieving Nurse**

When you have cared for a patient for a period of time, it is possible to have deep personal feelings of loss and sadness when the patient dies. Your self-care is crucial for your survival and recovery from loss, not only for your sake but also for the sake of future patients.

# Evaluation

**Patient Care**

You care for patients and families at every phase of the grief process. This requires you to remain aware of signs and symptoms of grief, even when patients are not specifically seeking care directly related to a loss.

It is important for the patient and family to share experiences and be active participants in the evaluation process.

### Patient Expectations

The patient expects individualized care, including relief of symptoms, preservation of dignity, and support of the family to maximize quality of life.

## Review Questions

Select the appropriate answer, and cite the rationale for choosing that particular answer.

1. Which statement about loss is accurate?
   a. Loss is experienced only when something valued is actually absent.
   b. The more an individual has invested in what is lost, the less the feeling of loss.
   c. Loss may be maturational, situational, or both.
   d. The degree of stress experienced is unrelated to the type of loss.

Answer: _____ Rationale:_____

_____

_____

2. A hospice program emphasizes
   a. Curative treatment and alleviation of symptoms
   b. Palliative treatment and control of symptoms
   c. Hospital-based care
   d. Prolongation of life

Answer: _____ Rationale:_____

_____

_____

3. Trying uncertain forms of complementary therapy is a behaviour that is characteristic of which stage of dying?
   a. Anger
   b. Depression
   c. Bargaining
   d. Acceptance

Answer: _____ Rationale:_____

_____

_____

4. All of the following are crucial needs of the dying patient *except*
   a. Control of pain
   b. Preservation of dignity and self-worth
   c. Love and belonging
   d. Freedom from decision making

Answer:_____ Rationale: _____

_____

_____

## Critical Thinking Model for Nursing Care Plan for Ineffective Coping

Imagine that you are the student nurse in the Nursing Care Plan on pages 459–460 of your text. Complete the *evaluation* phase of the critical thinking model by writing your answers in the appropriate boxes of the model shown. Think about the following:

- In evaluating Mrs. Miller's plan of care, what knowledge did you apply?

- In what way might your previous experience influence your evaluation of Mrs. Miller's care?

- During evaluation, what intellectual and professional standards were applied to Mrs. Miller's care?

- In what way do critical thinking attitudes play a role in how you approach evaluation of Mrs. Miller's care?

- How might you adjust Mrs. Miller's care?

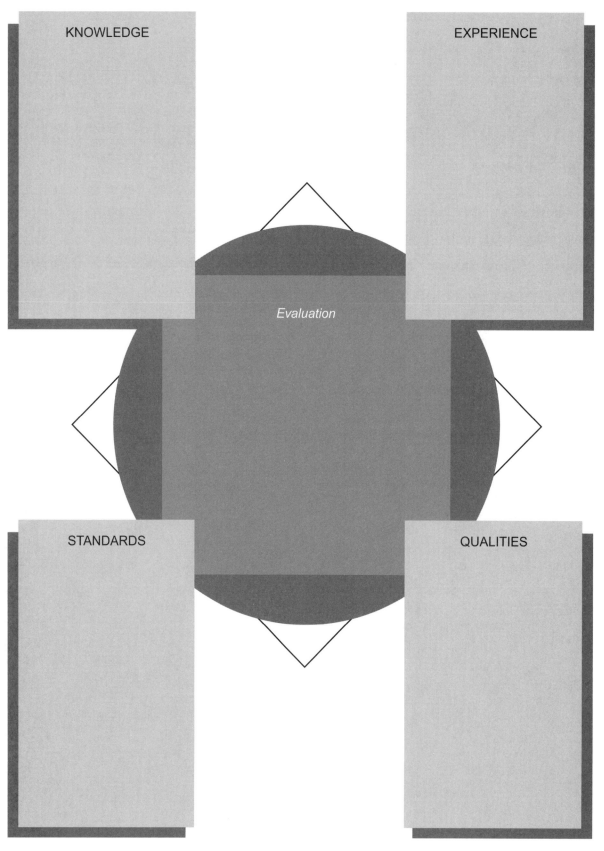

KNOWLEDGE

EXPERIENCE

*Evaluation*

STANDARDS

QUALITIES

CHAPTER 28   Critical Thinking Model for Nursing Care Plan for *Ineffective Coping*
See answers on Evolve site.

# 29

# Stress and Adaptation

## Preliminary Reading

Chapter 29, pages 472–488

## Comprehensive Understanding

1. Define the term *stress*.

2. *Stressors* are _____.

Physical and psychological health can be severely affected by serious or chronic stressors, and these effects can be long-standing and pervasive.

## Conceptualizations of Stress

### Physiological Conceptualizations

3. Explain the *fight-or-flight* response to stress.

_____
_____
_____

4. List (in sequence) and briefly describe the three stages of the *general adaptation syndrome*.

   a. _____
   b. _____
   c. _____

5. Define *homeostasis*.

_____
_____

### Psychological Conceptualizations

The roles of perception and appraisal in stress response are integral in the framework of stress. A person is under stress only if the person evaluates the event or circumstances as personally significant.

6. Explain the following terms.

   a. *Primary appraisal:*

   _____
   _____

   b. *Secondary appraisal:*

   _____
   _____

   c. *Coping:*

   _____
   _____

7. If previous ways of coping are not effective, a crisis may occur, in which the person faces a turning point in life and the person must change. Explain the two types of crisis.

   a. *Developmental crisis:*

   _____
   _____

   b. *Situational crisis:*

   _____
   _____

## Stress Response Systems

### Sympathetic-Adrenal-Medullary (SAM) System

8. Explain how the following areas of the brain are involved in the stress response.

   a. Reticular formation:

   _____

   _____

   b. Limbic system:

   _____

   _____

   c. Midbrain and pons:

   _____

   _____

   d. Medulla oblongata:

   _____

   _____

### Hypothalamic-Pituitary-Adrenal Axis

9. Describe the activation process of the HPA axis.

   _____

   _____

   _____

   _____

10. Briefly describe the areas of the brain involved in the stress response system.

   a. _____

   b. _____

   c. _____

## Stress and the Immune System

Dysregulation or chronic activation of the SAM system and the HPA axis may increase the risk of stress-related mental illnesses, as well as cardio-vascular disease, insulin resistance (which in turn can increase risk for type 2 diabetes), metabolic syndromes, and autoimmune illnesses.

## The Relationship Between Type of Stressor and Health

11. Distinguish between the different types of stress:

   a. *Eustress:*

   _____

   _____

   b. *Distress:*

   _____

   _____

   c. *Trauma:*

   _____

   _____

   d. *Post-traumatic growth:*

   _____

   _____

### Stress-Related Disorders

12. Explain the following stress-related disorders:

   a. *Acute stress disorder:*

   _____

   _____

   b. *Post-traumatic stress disorder (PTSD):*

   _____

   _____

## Nursing Knowledge Base

Nurses have proposed theories related to stress and coping. Because stress plays a role in vulnerability to disease, symptoms of stress often necessitate nursing intervention.

### Nursing Theory and the Role of Stress

13. Summarize the following models related to stress and coping.

   a. Neuman's systems model:

   _____

   _____

   _____

   _____

b. Pender et al.'s health promotion model:

_____

_____

_____

_____

**Situational, Maturational, and Sociocultural Factors**

14. The following factors can potentially be stressors. Explain.

a. Situational factors:

_____

_____

_____

b. Maturational factors:

_____

_____

_____

c. Sociocultural factors:

_____

_____

_____

## Nursing Process

## Assessment

When assessing a patient's stress level and coping resources, you must ask the patient to share personal and sensitive information. Therefore, you must first establish a trusting nurse–patient relationship.

**Subjective Findings**

15. Give an example of each of the following factors to assess.

a. Perception of stressor:

_____

b. Available coping resources:

_____

c. Maladaptive coping used:

_____

d. Adherence to healthy practices:

_____

**Objective Findings**

16. Identify six objective indicators of stress.

a. _____

b. _____

c. _____

d. _____

e. _____

f. _____

**Patient Expectations**

It is crucial that you understand the meaning the patient attaches to the precipitating event and how stress responses are affecting the patient's life.

## Nursing Diagnosis

Stress can result in multiple diagnostic statements.

17. Give two examples of nursing diagnostic statements related to stress.

_____

_____

_____

_____

## Planning

**Goals and Outcomes**

18. Desirable outcomes for persons experiencing stress are

a. _____

b. _____

c. _____

d. _____

## Implementation

**Health Promotion**

19. Identify the primary modes of intervention for stress.

a. _____

b. _____

c. _____

20. Explain how the following methods reduce stressors.

   a. Regular exercise:

      _____

      _____

   b. Support systems:

      _____

      _____

   c. Time management:

      _____

      _____

   d. Guided imagery and visualization:

      _____

      _____

   e. Progressive muscle relaxation:

      _____

      _____

   f. Assertiveness training:

      _____

      _____

   g. Journal writing:

      _____

      _____

   h. Stress management in your workplace:

      _____

      _____

**Acute Care**

**Crisis Intervention**

21. Crises occur _____.

22. Crisis intervention is _____.

**Restorative and Continuing Care**

23. Briefly explain when recovery from stress occurs.

   _____

   _____

   _____

## Evaluation

24. Briefly explain the patient's care in relation to

   a. Patient's perceptions of stress:

      _____

      _____

      _____

   b. Patient's expectations:

      _____

      _____

      _____

## *Review Questions*

Select the appropriate answer, and cite the rationale for choosing that particular answer.

1. Which definition *does not* characterize stress?
   a. Any situation in which a nonspecific demand requires an individual to respond or take action
   b. A phenomenon affecting social, psychological, developmental, spiritual, and physiological dimensions
   c. A condition eliciting an intellectual, behavioural, or metabolic response
   d. Efforts to maintain relative constancy within the internal environment

Answer: _____ Rationale: _____

_____

_____

2. Which statement about homeostasis is *not* accurate?
   a. Homeostatic mechanisms provide long-term and short-term control over the body's equilibrium.
   b. Homeostatic mechanisms are self-regulatory.
   c. Homeostatic mechanisms function through negative feedback.
   d. Illness may inhibit normal homeostatic mechanisms.

Answer: _____ Rationale: _____

_____

_____

3. Major homeostatic mechanisms are controlled by all of the following *except*
   a. Thymus gland
   b. Medulla oblongata
   c. Reticular formation
   d. Pituitary gland

Answer: _____ Rationale: _____

_____

_____

4. Which of the following is a stage of the general adaptation syndrome?
   a. Alarm reaction
   b. Fight-or-flight response
   c. Coping mechanisms
   d. Inflammatory response

Answer: _____ Rationale: _____

_____

_____

5. Crisis intervention is a specific measure used for helping a patient resolve a particular, immediate stress problem. This approach is based on
   a. The ability of the nurse to solve the patient's problems
   b. An in-depth analysis of a patient's situation
   c. Teaching the patient how to help make the mental connection between the stressful event and his or her reaction to it
   d. Effective communication between the nurse and the patient

Answer: _____ Rationale: _____

_____

_____

## Critical Thinking Model for Nursing Care Plan for Caregiver Role Strain

Imagine that you are the student nurse in the Nursing Care Plan on pages 482-483 of your text. Complete the *evaluation* phase of the critical thinking model by writing your answers in the appropriate boxes of the model shown. Think about the following:

• In evaluating the care of Carl and Evelyn, what knowledge did you apply?

• In what way might your previous experience influence the evaluation of Carl's care?

• During evaluation, what intellectual and professional standards were applied to Carl's care?

• In what way do critical thinking attitudes play a role in how you approach the evaluation of Carl's care?

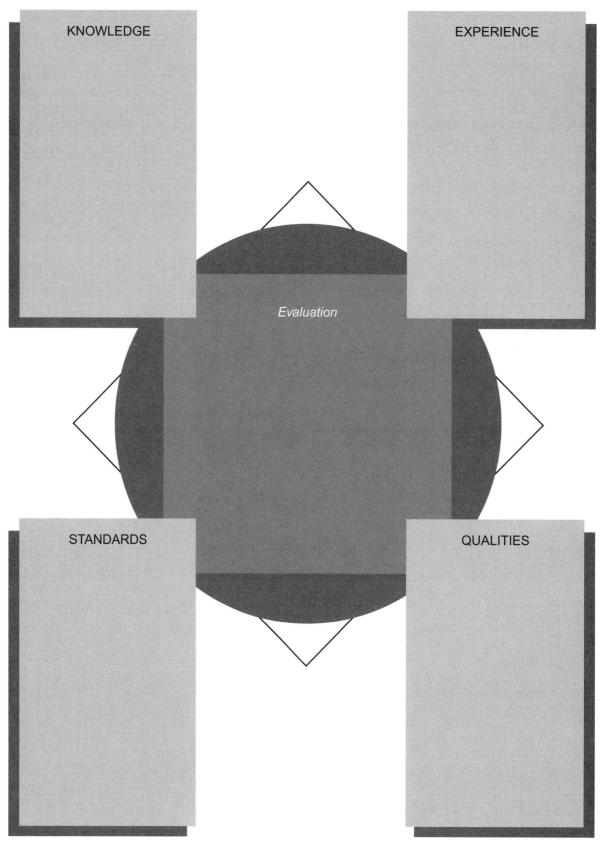

KNOWLEDGE

EXPERIENCE

Evaluation

STANDARDS

QUALITIES

CHAPTER 29    Critical Thinking Model for Nursing Care Plan for *Caregiver Role Strain*
See answers on Evolve site.

# 30

# Vital Signs

## *Preliminary Reading*

Chapter 30, pages 489–536

## *Comprehensive Understanding*

Vital signs provide important data to determine the usual state of health (baseline data). A change in vital signs indicates a change in physiological function, which may signal the need for medical or nursing intervention.

### Guidelines for Measuring Vital Signs

1. Identify the guidelines that assist you to incorporate vital sign measurement into practice.

   a. _____

   b. _____

   c. _____

   d. _____

   e. _____

   f. _____

   g. _____

   h. _____

   i. _____

   j. _____

   k. _____

### Body Temperature

#### Physiology

2. The body temperature is the difference between the _____ and the _____.

3. Define *core temperature*.

   _____

   _____

   _____

#### Regulation

4. Define *thermoregulation*.

   _____

   _____

   _____

#### Neural and Vascular Control

5. Briefly summarize how neural and vascular mechanisms control body temperature.

   _____

   _____

   _____

   _____

#### Heat Production

6. List four sources, or mechanisms, for heat production.

   a. _____

   b. _____

   c. _____

   d. _____

**Heat Loss**

7. Explain the following mechanisms of body heat loss, and give an example of each.

   a. *Radiation*:

   _____

   _____

   _____

   b. *Conduction*:

   _____

   _____

   _____

   c. *Convection*:

   _____

   _____

   _____

   d. *Evaporation*:

   _____

   _____

   _____

   e. *Diaphoresis*:

   _____

   _____

   _____

**Skin in Temperature Regulation**

8. Briefly explain the skin's role in temperature regulation.

   a. Insulation of the body:

   _____

   _____

   _____

   b. Vasoconstriction:

   _____

   _____

   _____

   c. Temperature sensation:

   _____

   _____

   _____

**Behavioural Control**

9. Identify four factors that must be present for a person to control body temperature.

   a. _____

   b. _____

   c. _____

   d. _____

**Factors Affecting Body Temperature**

10. Changes in body temperature within the normal range occur when the relationship between heat production and heat loss is altered by physiological or behavioural variables. Summarize the following variables.

   a. Age:

   _____

   _____

   b. Exercise:

   _____

   _____

   c. Hormone level:

   _____

   _____

   d. Circadian rhythm:

   _____

   _____

   e. Stress:

   _____

   _____

   f. Environment:

   _____

   _____

**Temperature Alterations**

11. Temperature alterations can be related to

   _____, _____, _____,

   _____, or any combination of these alterations.

**Fever**

12. *Pyrexia*, or *fever*, occurs because _____
_____ .

13. Explain how a fever works as an important defence mechanism.
_____
_____
_____
_____

14. Explain how a fever serves a diagnostic purpose.
_____
_____
_____
_____

15. Explain how a fever affects metabolism.
_____
_____
_____
_____

**Hyperthermia**

16. Define the following terms.

    a. *Hyperthermia*:
    _____
    _____

    b. *Malignant hyperthermia*:
    _____
    _____

*Heatstroke*

17. Define and explain the causes of *heatstroke*.
_____
_____
_____
_____

*Heat Exhaustion*

18. Define and explain the causes of *heat exhaustion*.
_____
_____
_____
_____

**Hypothermia**

19. Define and explain the causes of *hypothermia*.
_____
_____
_____
_____

20. *Frostbite* occurs when _____
_____ .

## Assessment

**Sites**

21. List the routine assessment sites for intermittent temperature measurement.

    a. _____
    b. _____
    c. _____
    d. _____

**Thermometers**

22. Identify three types of thermometers, and list advantages and disadvantages of each.

    a. _____
    _____
    _____

    b. _____
    _____
    _____

    c. _____
    _____
    _____

## Nursing Diagnosis

23. Identify three nursing diagnoses related to thermoregulation.

    a. _____
    b. _____
    c. _____

## Planning

Match patients' needs with interventions that are supported and recommended in the clinical research literature.

## Implementation

### Health Promotion

24. Health promotion for patients at risk of altered temperature is directed toward _____.

25. Identify the risk factors for hypothermia.

_____

_____

_____

_____

### Acute Care

### Fever

The procedures used to intervene and treat an elevated temperature depend on the fever's cause; its adverse effects; and its strength, intensity, and duration of the elevation.

26. Explain the differences related to febrile states in each of the following.

   a. Children:

   _____

   _____

   _____

   b. Hypersensitivity to medications:

   _____

   _____

   _____

27. Give three examples of each type of fever therapy.

   Pharmacological:

   a. _____

   b. _____

   c. _____

   Nonpharmacological:

   a. _____

   b. _____

   c. _____

28. Identify an independent and a dependent nursing intervention to control shivering.

   _____

   _____

   _____

   _____

### Heatstroke

29. First aid treatment for heatstroke includes _____, _____, _____, and _____.

### Hypothermia

30. Summarize the treatment for hypothermia.

   _____

   _____

   _____

### Restorative and Continuing Care

31. Summarize the patient teaching in regard to the treatment of a fever.

   _____

   _____

   _____

   _____

## Evaluation

### Pulse

32. Define *pulse*.

   _____

   _____

   _____

### Physiology and Regulation

33. Define the following terms.

   a. *Stroke volume*:

   _____

   _____

   _____

   b. *Cardiac output*:

   _____

   _____

   _____

### Assessment of Pulse

34. Identify the two most common peripheral pulse sites to assess.

   a. _____

   b. _____

**Use of a Stethoscope**

35. Identify the five major parts of the stethoscope.

   a. _____

   b. _____

   c. _____

   d. _____

   e. _____

**Character of the Pulse**

36. List four characteristics to identify during peripheral pulse assessment. Using an asterisk, specify the two characteristics to identify when assessing an apical pulse.

   a. _____

   b. _____

   c. _____

   d. _____

37. Define the following.

   a. *Tachycardia*:

   _____

   _____

   _____

   b. *Bradycardia*:

   _____

   _____

   _____

   c. *Pulse deficit*:

   _____

   _____

   _____

   d. *Dysrhythmia*:

   _____

   _____

   _____

## Respiration

38. Define the following.

   a. *Ventilation*:

   _____

   _____

   b. *Diffusion*:

   _____

   _____

   c. *Perfusion*:

   _____

   _____

**Physiological Control**

Breathing is a passive process. The respiratory centre in the brain stem regulates the involuntary control of respirations.

39. Ventilation is regulated by levels of _____, _____, and _____ in the arterial blood.

40. The most important factor in the control of ventilation is the level of _____.

41. *Hypoxemia* occurs when _____.

**Mechanics of Breathing**

42. Briefly summarize the process of inspiration.

   _____

   _____

   _____

   _____

43. Define the following terms.

   a. *Tidal volume*:

   _____

   _____

   b. *Eupnea*:

   _____

   _____

**Assessment of Ventilation**

44. Accurate measurement of ventilation requires _____ and _____ movements.

45. List three objective measurements used in respiratory status assessment.

   a. _____

   b. _____

   c. _____

46. Define the following alterations in breathing patterns.

a. Bradypnea:

b. Tachypnea:

c. Hyperpnea:

d. Apnea:

e. Hyperventilation:

f. Hypoventilation:

g. Cheyne-Stokes respiration:

h. Kussmaul's respiration:

i. Biot's respiration:

**Assessment of Diffusion and Perfusion**

The respiratory processes of diffusion and perfusion can be evaluated by measuring the oxygen saturation of the blood.

47. The percentage of oxygen saturation of arterial blood is _____ and of venous blood is _____.

**Measurement of Arterial Oxygen Saturation**

48. Explain the purpose of a pulse oximeter.

49. List three things that can affect the accuracy of an oxygen saturation reading.

a. 

b. 

c. 

## Blood Pressure

50. Define the following terms.

a. *Blood pressure*:

b. *Systolic*:

c. *Diastolic*:

51. The difference between the systolic and diastolic pressure is the _____.

**Physiology of Arterial Blood Pressure**

52. Blood pressure reflects the interrelationships of the following. Briefly explain each.

a. Cardiac output:

b. Peripheral vascular resistance:

c. Blood volume:

d. Blood viscosity:

_____

_____

_____

e. Artery elasticity:

_____

_____

_____

**Factors Influencing Blood Pressure**

53. List six factors that influence blood pressure.

a. _____

b. _____

c. _____

d. _____

e. _____

f. _____

**Hypertension**

54. Identify the criteria for the diagnosis of hypertension in an adult.

_____

_____

_____

_____

55. Briefly summarize the physiology of hypertension.

_____

_____

_____

_____

56. List five risk factors that are linked to hypertension.

a. _____

b. _____

c. _____

d. _____

e. _____

**Hypotension**

57. Identify the criteria for the diagnosis of hypotension in an adult.

_____

_____

_____

_____

58. Explain the physiology of hypotension and its causes.

_____

_____

_____

_____

59. Orthostatic hypotension occurs when

_____.

60. Explain how you would assess a patient for orthostatic hypotension.

_____

_____

_____

_____

**Measurement of Blood Pressure**

61. Identify two methods for measuring blood pressure.

a. _____

_____

b. _____

_____

**Blood Pressure Equipment**

62. Identify the two types of *sphygmomanometers*, and list their advantages and disadvantages.

a. _____

b. _____

**Auscultation**

63. The sounds heard over an artery distal to the blood pressure cuff are Korotkoff sounds. Describe each.

a. First:

_____

_____

b. Second:

_____

_____

c. Third:

_____

_____

d. Fourth:

_____

_____

e. Fifth:

_____

_____

64. During the initial assessment, you should obtain and record the blood pressure in both arms. Pressure differences between the arms greater than _____ mm Hg indicate vascular problems.

65. Identify five common mistakes in blood pressure assessment.

a. _____

b. _____

c. _____

d. _____

e. _____

**Assessment in Children**

66. Identify four reasons why the measurement of blood pressure in infants and children is difficult.

a. _____

b. _____

c. _____

d. _____

**Ultrasonic Stethoscope**

67. Explain the rationale for the use of an ultrasonic stethoscope.

_____

_____

_____

_____

**Palpation**

68. Identify the method you may use to assess blood pressure when Korotkoff sounds are not audible with the standard stethoscope.

_____

_____

_____

_____

69. Define *auscultatory gap.*

_____

_____

_____

_____

**Lower Extremity Blood Pressure**

70. Give an example of when you would assess a patient's blood pressure using the patient's lower extremities.

_____

_____

**Automatic Blood Pressure Devices**

71. Identify the advantages and disadvantages of using automatic blood pressure devices.

_____

_____

_____

_____

**Self-Measurement of Blood Pressure**

72. List the benefits of blood pressure self-measurement.

a. _____

b. _____

c. _____

d. _____

## Recording Vital Signs

73. Identify at least two variations that are unique to the older adult.

a. Temperature:

_____

_____

b. Pulse rate:

_____

_____

c. Blood pressure:

_____

_____

d. Respirations:

_____

_____

## Review Questions

Select the appropriate answer, and cite the rationale for choosing that particular answer.

1. The skin plays a role in temperature regulation by
   a. Insulating the body
   b. Constricting blood vessels
   c. Sensing external temperature variations
   d. All of the above

Answer: _____ Rationale: _____

_____

_____

2. You minimize coverings on the body of a patient with a fever. This promotes heat loss through
   a. Radiation, convection, and evaporation
   b. Evaporation
   c. Condensation
   d. Radiation

Answer: _____ Rationale: _____

_____

_____

3. You are assessing a patient suspected of having the nursing diagnosis *hyperthermia related to vigorous exercise in hot weather*. In reviewing the data, you know that the most important sign of heatstroke is
   a. Confusion
   b. Hot, dry skin
   c. Excess thirst
   d. Muscle cramps

Answer: _____ Rationale: _____

_____

_____

4. When taking a patient's radial pulse, you note a dysrhythmia. The most appropriate action is to
   a. Inform the physician immediately
   b. Wait 5 minutes and retake the radial pulse
   c. Take the pulse apically for 1 full minute
   d. Check the patient's record for the presence of a previous dysrhythmia

Answer: _____ Rationale: _____

_____

_____

5. You are auscultating Mrs. McKinnon's blood pressure. You inflate the cuff to 180 mm Hg. At 156 mm Hg, you hear the onset of a tapping sound. At 130 mm Hg, the sound changes to a murmur or swishing. At 100 mm Hg, the sound momentarily becomes sharper, and at 92 mm Hg, it becomes muffled. At 88 mm Hg, the sound disappears. Mrs. McKinnon's blood pressure is:
   a. 180/92
   b. 180/130
   c. 156/88
   d. 130/88

Answer: _____ Rationale: _____

_____

_____

# 31

# Health Assessment and Physical Examination

## Preliminary Reading

Chapter 31, pages 537–617

## Comprehensive Understanding

### Social and Cultural Considerations

Cultural assessment data inform culturally safe physical assessments, by providing information that helps the nurse think critically about the political, social, and economic contexts of patients' lives, and how inequities in power and access to resources for health influence the health of individuals.

### Purposes of Physical Examination

1. Physical assessment enables the nurse to _____ and _____.

2. List the five nursing purposes for performing a physical assessment.

    a. _____
    _____

    b. _____
    _____

    c. _____
    _____

    d. _____
    _____

    e. _____
    _____

### Gathering a Health History

The main objective of interacting with patients is to find out what their concerns are and to help them find solutions.

### Developing Nursing Diagnoses and a Care Plan

After gathering information about the patient's health from the health history, a subsequent physical assessment can reveal information that refutes, confirms, or supplements the history.

### Skills of Physical Assessment

#### Inspection

3. Define *inspection*.

    _____
    _____
    _____

4. List six principles to facilitate accurate inspection of body parts.

    a. _____
    _____

    b. _____
    _____

    c. _____
    _____

    d. _____
    _____

    e. _____
    _____

    f. _____
    _____

## Palpation

5. Define *palpation*.

_____

_____

_____

6. Identify the parts of the hand to use to assess each of the following:

    a. Temperature: _____

    b. Moisture: _____

    c. Turgor: _____

    d. Tenderness and thickness: _____

## Percussion

7. Identify the information obtained through percussion.

_____

_____

_____

## Auscultation

8. Define *auscultation*.

_____

_____

_____

_____

9. Briefly explain the following characteristics of sound.

    a. Frequency: _____

    b. Loudness: _____

    c. Quality: _____

    d. Duration: _____

## Olfaction

While assessing a patient, become familiar with the nature and source of body odours. Olfaction helps to detect abnormalities that you cannot recognize by any other means.

## Preparation for the Physical Examination

### Infection Control

Examination techniques cause the nurse to contact body fluids and discharge. Standard precautions should be used throughout the examination.

### Environment

10. List at least three environmental factors that the nurse should attempt to control before performing a physical examination.

    a. _____

    b. _____

    c. _____

### Equipment

Handwashing is done before equipment preparation and before the examination.

All equipment should be checked to see that it functions properly.

11. Briefly explain the following pre-examination preparations:

    a. Physical: _____

    b. Positioning: _____

    c. Psychological: _____

### Assessment of Age Groups

12. List seven ways to facilitate data collection when examining children:

    a. _____

    b. _____

    c. _____

    d. _____

    e. _____

    f. _____

    g. _____

## Organization of the Examination

13. List eight principles to follow for a well-organized examination.

a. _____

b. _____

c. _____

d. _____

e. _____

f. _____

g. _____

h. _____

## General Survey

### General Appearance and Behaviour

14. List at least eight specific observations of the patient's general appearance and behaviour that should be reviewed.

a. _____

b. _____

c. _____

d. _____

e. _____

f. _____

g. _____

h. _____

15. Identify the questions related to the following acronym.

C _____

A _____

G _____

E _____

### Height and Weight

16. List three actions that should be taken to ensure accurate weight measurement of a hospitalized patient.

a. _____

b. _____

c. _____

## The Integumentary System—Skin, Hair, and Nails

### Skin

17. List the risks for skin lesions in the hospitalized patient.

_____

_____

18. Define the following terms:

a. *Melanoma*:

_____

_____

b. *Pigmentation*:

_____

_____

19. For each skin colour variation, identify the mechanism that produces colour change, common causes of the variation, and the optimal sites for assessment (see the following table).

| Skin Colour | Condition | Causes | Assessment Locations |
|---|---|---|---|
| Cyanosis | | | |
| Pallor | | | |
| Jaundice | | | |
| Erythema | | | |

20. Identify two conditions that are due to excessive skin dryness.

    a. _____

    b. _____

The temperature of the skin depends on the amount of blood circulating through the dermis. Increased or decreased skin temperature indicates an increase or decrease in blood flow. Always assess skin temperature for patients at risk of having impaired circulation.

21. Define the following terms.

    a. *Indurated*:

        _____

        _____

    b. *Turgor*:

        _____

        _____

    c. *Petechiae:*

        _____

        _____

    d. *Edema*:

        _____

        _____

    e. *Senile keratosis*:

        _____

        _____

    f. *Cherry angiomas*:

        _____

        _____

22. Briefly describe the following primary skin lesions, and give an example of each.

    a. Macule:

        _____

        _____

    b. Papule:

        _____

        _____

    c. Nodule:

        _____

        _____

    d. Tumour:

        _____

        _____

    e. Wheal:

        _____

        _____

    f. Vesicle:

        _____

        _____

    g. Pustule:

        _____

        _____

    h. Ulcer:

        _____

        _____

    i. Atrophy:

        _____

        _____

Cancerous lesions frequently undergo changes in colour and size. *Report abnormal lesions to the health care provider for further examination.*

**Hair and Scalp**

**Inspection**

23. Name the three types of lice.

    a. _____

    b. _____

    c. _____

**Nails**

24. Briefly describe the following abnormalities of the nail bed.

    a. Clubbing:

        _____

        _____

    b. Beau's lines:

        _____

        _____

    c. Koilonychia:

        _____

        _____

d. Splinter hemorrhages:

_____

_____

e. Paronychia:

_____

_____

*Capillary refill* is a test that applies gentle, firm, quick pressure with the thumb to the nail bed; release and observe the results. As you apply pressure, the nail bed will appear white or blanched; however, the pink colour should return immediately on release of pressure. Failure of the pinkness to return promptly indicates circulatory insufficiency.

## Head and Neck

### Head

25. Define the following head abnormalities.

a. *Hydrocephalus*:

_____

_____

b. *Acromegaly*:

_____

_____

### Eyes

26. Define the following common eye and visual abnormalities.

a. Hyperopia:

_____

_____

b. Myopia:

_____

_____

c. Presbyopia:

_____

_____

d. Retinopathy:

_____

_____

e. Strabismus:

_____

_____

f. Amblyopia:

_____

_____

g. Cataracts:

_____

_____

h. Glaucoma:

_____

_____

i. Macular degeneration:

_____

_____

## External Eye Structures

27. Examination of the eye includes assessment of five areas. Name them.

a. _____

b. _____

c. _____

d. _____

e. _____

28. Identify the structures of the external eye that you would inspect.

a. _____

b. _____

c. _____

d. _____

e. _____

f. _____

g. _____

29. Define the following terms related to the external eye.

a. *Exophthalmos*:

_____

_____

b. *Ptosis*:

_____

_____

c. *Ectropion*:

_____

_____

d. *Entropion*:

_____

_____

e. *Conjunctivitis*:

_____

_____

f. *Arcus senilis*:

_____

_____

g. *PERRLA*:

_____

_____

**Internal Eye Structures**

30. Identify the internal eye structures that you would examine with an ophthalmoscope.

_____

_____

_____

_____

**Extraocular Movements**

As the patient gazes in each direction, observe for parallel eye movement, the position of the upper eyelid in relation to the iris, and the presence of abnormal movements. Disturbances in eye movement reflect local injury to eye muscles and supporting structures or a disorder of the cranial nerves innervating the muscles.

**Visual Acuity**

31. The assessment of visual acuity, the ability to see small details, tests central vision. Near vision is assessed by _____. Distance vision is assessed using a _____.

**Ears**

32. Identify the parts of the ear canal.

a. _____

b. _____

c. _____

33. List the steps of hearing (sound travelling through the ear by air and bone conduction).

a. _____

b. _____

c. _____

d. _____

e. _____

**Hearing Acuity**

34. Identify three types of hearing loss.

a. _____

b. _____

c. _____

35. Explain the following tuning fork tests.

a. Weber's test:

_____

_____

b. Rinne test:

_____

_____

**Nose and Sinuses**

36. Define the following terms that relate to the nose.

a. *Excoriation*:

_____

_____

_____

b. *Polyps*:

_____

_____

_____

**Mouth and Pharynx**

37. Define the following terms that relate to the oral cavity.

a. *Leukoplakia*:

_____

_____

_____

b. *Varicosities*:

_____

_____

_____

c. *Exostosis*:

_____

_____

_____

**Pharynx**

Perform an examination of pharyngeal structures to rule out infection, inflammation, or lesions.

**Neck**

38. Assessment of the neck includes _____.

## Thorax and Lungs

**Posterior Thorax**

39. Define *vocal* or *tactile fremitus*.

_____
_____
_____

40. Define the following normal breath sounds heard over the posterior thorax.

a. Vesicular:

_____
_____
_____

b. Bronchovesicular:

_____
_____
_____

c. Bronchial:

_____
_____
_____

41. Complete the following table of adventitious breath sounds.

| Sounds | Site Auscultated | Cause | Character |
|---|---|---|---|
| Crackles | | | |
| Rhonchi (sonorous wheeze) | | | |
| Wheezes (sibilant wheeze) | | | |
| Pleural friction rub | | | |

**Anterior Thorax**

Inspect the anterior thorax for the same features as the posterior thorax.

## Heart

42. Explain the following terms related to assessment of the heart.

a. Point of maximal impulse:

_____
_____

b. $S_1$:

_____
_____

c. $S_2$:

_____
_____

d. $S_3$:

_____
_____

e. $S_4$:

_____
_____

**Inspection and Palpation**

43. Identify the appropriate sites for inspection and palpation of the following.

a. Angle of Louis:

_____

_____

b. Aortic area:

_____

_____

c. Pulmonic area:

_____

_____

d. Second pulmonic area:

_____

_____

e. Tricuspid area:

_____

_____

f. Mitral area:

_____

_____

g. Epigastric area

_____

_____

**Auscultation**

44. Auscultation of the heart detects normal

_____, _____, and _____.

45. Define *murmur*.

_____

_____

_____

46. List the six factors to assess when a murmur is detected.

a. _____

b. _____

c. _____

d. _____

e. _____

f. _____

## Vascular System

47. Explain the following conditions that are related to the vascular system.

a. *Syncope*:

_____

_____

b. *Occlusion*:

_____

_____

c. *Atherosclerosis*:

_____

_____

d. *Bruit*:

_____

_____

**Jugular Veins**

48. Explain the steps the nurse would use to assess venous pressure.

a. _____

b. _____

c. _____

d. _____

e. _____

Peripheral Arteries and Veins

49. Complete the following table by listing the signs of venous and arterial insufficiency.

| Assessment Criterion | Venous | Arterial |
|---|---|---|
| Colour | | |
| Temperature | | |
| Pulse | | |
| Edema | | |
| Skin changes | | |

50. Describe how you would assess for phlebitis.

_____

_____

_____

_____

## Breasts

51. The Canadian Cancer Society Steering Committee (2010) recommends the following guidelines for the early detection of breast cancer:

    a. _____

    b. _____

    c. _____

    d. _____

**Palpation**

52. Define the following terms.

    a. *Metastasize*:

    _____

    _____

    b. *Benign (fibrocystic) breast disease*:

    _____

    _____

## Abdomen

53. Define the following terms related to the abdomen.

    a. *Striae*:

    _____

    _____

    b. *Hernias*:

    _____

    _____

    c. *Distension*:

    _____

    _____

    d. *Peristalsis*:

    _____

    _____

    e. *Paralytic ileus*:

    _____

    _____

    f. *Borborygmi*:

    _____

    _____

    g. *Rebound tenderness*:

    _____

    _____

h. *Aneurysm*:

_____

_____

## Female Genitalia and Reproductive Tract

54. Describe the following terms related to the female genitourinary tract.

a. *Chancres*:

_____

_____

b. *Papanicolaou specimen*:

_____

_____

## Male Genitalia

55. Identify the common symptoms of testicular cancer.

_____

_____

_____

_____

## Rectum and Anus

56. The purpose of the digital examination is.

_____

_____

_____

_____.

## Musculoskeletal System

### General Inspection

57. Define the following terms.

a. *Kyphosis*:

_____

_____

_____

b. *Lordosis*:

_____

_____

_____

c. *Scoliosis*:

_____

_____

_____

d. *Osteoporosis*:

_____

_____

_____

e. *Goniometer*:

_____

_____

_____

### Muscle Tone and Strength

58. Identify the correct range of motion for the following terms.

a. Flexion: _____

b. Extension: _____

c. Hyperextension: _____

d. Pronation: _____

e. Supination: _____

f. Abduction: _____

g. Adduction: _____

h. Internal rotation: _____

i. External rotation: _____

j. Eversion: _____

k. Inversion: _____

l. Dorsiflexion: _____

m. Plantar flexion: _____

59. Define the following terms related to muscle tone and strength.

a. *Hypertonicity*:

_____

_____

_____

b. *Hypotonicity*:

_____

_____

_____

c. *Atrophy*:

_____

_____

_____

## Neurological System

### Mental and Emotional Status

60. The purpose of the Mini-Mental State Examination is to measure _____ and _____.

61. Delirium is characterized by _____, _____, and _____.

62. The purpose of the Glasgow Coma Scale is to _____.

63. Briefly explain the two types of aphasia.

    a. Receptive:

    _____

    _____

    b. Expressive:

    _____

    _____

### Intellectual Function

Intellectual function includes memory, knowledge, abstract thinking, association, and judgement.

### Cranial Nerve Function

64. Identify the 12 cranial nerves.

    a. _____

    b. _____

    c. _____

    d. _____

    e. _____

    f. _____

    g. _____

    h. _____

    i. _____

    j. _____

    k. _____

    l. _____

### Sensory Function

65. The sensory pathways of the central nervous system conduct what type of sensations?

    _____

    _____

66. Identify how to assess sensory nerve function.

    _____

    _____

### Motor Function

67. Identify the functions of the cerebellum.

    _____

    _____

### Reflexes

68. Identify the two types of normal reflexes.

    a. _____

    b. _____

## Review Questions

Select the appropriate answer, and cite the rationale for choosing that particular answer.

1. The component that should receive the highest priority before a physical examination is
   a. Preparation of the equipment
   b. Preparation of the environment
   c. Physical preparation of the patient
   d. Psychological preparation of the patient

   Answer: _____ Rationale: _____

   _____

   _____

2. The nurse assesses the skin turgor of the patient by
   a. Inspecting the buccal mucosa with a penlight
   b. Palpating the skin with the dorsum of the hand
   c. Grasping a fold of skin on the back of the forearm and releasing
   d. Pressing the skin for 5 seconds, releasing, and noting each centimetre of depth

   Answer: _____ Rationale: _____

   _____

   _____

3. While examining Mr. Polanzky, the nurse notes a circumscribed elevation of skin filled with serous fluid on his upper lip. The lesion is 0.4 cm in diameter. This type of lesion is called a
   a. Macule
   b. Nodule
   c. Vesicle
   d. Pustule

   Answer: _____ Rationale: _____

   _____

   _____

4. When assessing a patient's thorax, the nurse should
   a. Complete the left side and then the right side
   b. Compare symmetrical areas from side to side
   c. Begin with the posterior lobes on the right side
   d. Change the position of the stethoscope between inspiration and expiration

Answer: _____ Rationale: _____
_____
_____

5. In a patient with pneumonia, the nurse hears high-pitched, continuous musical sounds over the bronchi and bronchioles that become louder on expiration. These sounds are called
   a. Rhonchi
   b. Crackles
   c. Wheezes
   d. Friction rubs

Answer: _____ Rationale: _____
_____
_____

6. The second heart sound (S$_2$) occurs when
   a. Systole begins
   b. There is rapid ventricular filling
   c. The mitral and tricuspid valves close
   d. The aortic and pulmonic valves close

Answer: _____ Rationale: _____
_____
_____

# 32

# Infection Control

*Preliminary Reading*

Chapter 32, pages 618–661

## *Comprehensive Understanding*

Practices or techniques that control or prevent transmission of infection help to create an environment that protects patients and health care workers from disease.

### Scientific Knowledge Base

1. An infection is _____.

2. Define *communicable*.

   _____

   _____

   _____

### Chain of Infection

3. Development of an infection occurs in a cycle that depends on the following elements:

   a. _____

   b. _____

   c. _____

   d. _____

   e. _____

   f. _____

### Infectious Agents

4. Microorganisms include _____,

   _____, _____, and

   _____.

5. Define the following.

   a. *Virulence*:

   _____

   _____

   b. *Immunocompromised*:

   _____

   _____

6. The potential for microorganisms to cause disease depends on four factors. Name them.

   a. _____

   b. _____

   c. _____

   d. _____

### Reservoir

7. Define *reservoir*.

   _____

   _____

   _____

8. Define *carriers*.

   _____

   _____

   _____

9. To thrive, organisms require the following. Briefly explain each one.

  a. Food:

  _____

  _____

  b. Oxygen (or lack of oxygen):

  _____

  _____

  c. Water:

  _____

  _____

  d. Temperature:

  _____

  _____

  e. pH:

  _____

  _____

  f. Minimal light:

  _____

  _____

**Portal of Exit**

10. What is a portal of exit? Give examples.

  _____

  _____

  _____

  _____

**Modes of Transmission**

11. List the major modes of transmission of micro-organisms from the reservoir to the host.

  _____

  _____

  _____

  _____

**Portal of Entry**

Organisms can enter the body through the same routes they use to exit.

**Susceptible Host**

12. Explain *susceptibility*.

  _____

  _____

**The Infectious Process**

13. The severity of the patient's illness depends on the _____, the _____, and the _____.

14. Describe the two types of infections.

  a. Localized:

  _____

  _____

  b. Systemic:

  _____

  _____

**Defences Against Infection**

15. The immune response is _____ _____.

16. Explain the normal body's defences against infection.

  a. Normal flora:

  _____

  _____

  b. Body system defences:

  _____

  _____

  _____

  c. Inflammation:

  _____

  _____

  _____

17. For each body system or organ in the grid that follows, identify at least one defence mechanism and the primary action to prevent infection.

| System/Organ | Defence Mechanism | Action |
|---|---|---|
| Skin | | |
| Mouth | | |
| Eye | | |
| Respiratory tract | | |
| Urinary tract | | |
| Gastrointestinal tract | | |
| Vagina | | |

18. The *inflammatory response* includes the following. Explain each briefly.

   a. Vascular and cellular responses:

   _____
   _____
   _____

   b. Inflammatory exudates:

   _____
   _____
   _____

   c. Tissue repair:

   _____
   _____
   _____

19. Briefly explain the following vascular and cellular responses.

   a. *Edema*:

   _____
   _____

   b. *Phagocytosis*:

   _____
   _____

**Health Care–Associated Infections**

20. Define *health care–associated infection (HAI) or nosocomial infection.*

   _____
   _____
   _____
   _____

21. Define the following types of HAIs.

   a. *Exogenous*:

   _____
   _____

   b. *Endogenous*:

   _____
   _____

22. Identify at least three factors that increase a hospitalized patient's risk of acquiring an HAI.

   a. _____
   b. _____
   c. _____

23. Identify the major sites for nosocomial infection (HAI).

_____

_____

_____

_____

## Nursing Process in Infection Control

### Assessment

Nurses assess the patient's defence mechanisms, susceptibility, and knowledge of infections.

Knowing the factors that increase the patient's susceptibility or risk for infection, you are better able to plan preventive therapy that includes aseptic technique.

#### Status of Defence Mechanisms

You can determine the status of the patient's normal defence mechanisms against infection through a review of the physical assessment findings and the patient's medical condition.

24. Any reduction in the body's primary or secondary defences against infection places a patient at risk. List at least four risk factors of each.

a. Inadequate primary defences:

_____

_____

b. Inadequate secondary defences:

_____

_____

#### Patient Susceptibility

25. The following factors influence patient susceptibility to infection. Explain each one.

a. Age:

_____

_____

_____

b. Nutritional status:

_____

_____

_____

c. Stress:

_____

_____

_____

d. Disease process:

_____

_____

_____

e. Medical therapy:

_____

_____

_____

#### Clinical Appearance

26. Describe the signs and symptoms of each type of infection.

a. Localized infection:

_____

_____

_____

b. Systemic infection:

_____

_____

_____

27. Describe how an infection is manifested in an older adult.

_____

_____

_____

_____

#### Laboratory Data

28. List at least five laboratory values that may indicate infection.

a. _____

b. _____

c. _____

d. _____

e. _____

**Patient With Infection**

29. The ways in which infection can affect the patient's and family's needs may be _____, _____, _____, or _____.

# Nursing Diagnosis

You may diagnose a risk for infection or make diagnoses that result from the effects of infection on health status.

# Planning

**Goals and Outcomes**

30. Four common goals of care relating to infection include

    a. _____

    b. _____

    c. _____

    d. _____

# Implementation

**Health Promotion**

31. List five ways you may prevent an infection from developing or spreading.

    a. _____

    b. _____

    c. _____

    d. _____

    e. _____

32. List preventive interventions to protect a patient from invasion by pathogens.

    _____

    _____

    _____

    _____

**Acute Care Measures**

Treatment of an infectious process includes eliminating the infectious organisms and supporting the patient's defences.

**Asepsis**

33. Define the following terms.

    a. *Asepsis:*

    _____

    _____

    b. *Medical asepsis:*

    _____

    _____

You are responsible for providing the patient with a safe environment. Your failure to be meticulous places the patient at risk for an infection that can seriously impair recovery or lead to death.

**Control or Elimination of Infectious Agents**

34. Explain the following methods of controlling or eliminating infectious agents.

    a. Cleaning:

    _____

    _____

    _____

    b. Disinfection:

    _____

    _____

    _____

    c. Sterilization:

    _____

    _____

    _____

    d. Control or elimination of reservoirs:

    _____

    _____

    _____

    e. Control of portals of exit:

    _____

    _____

    _____

    f. Control of transmission:

    _____

    _____

    _____

g. Hand hygiene:

_____

_____

_____

35. Describe the Centers for Disease Control and Prevention (CDC) guidelines on handwashing and the use of alcohol-based waterless antiseptics.

a. _____

b. _____

c. _____

d. _____

e. _____

f. _____

g. _____

h. _____

i. _____

**Control of Portals of Entry**

36. Many measures that control the exit of microorganisms also control the entrance of pathogens. Give at least five examples.

a. _____

b. _____

c. _____

d. _____

e. _____

**Protection of the Susceptible Host**

37. A patient's resistance to infection improves as the nurse protects the body's normal defences against infection. Explain.

_____

_____

_____

_____

**Isolation Guidelines**

38. Standard precautions or routine practices call for the appropriate use of protective devices and clothing, including _____,

_____, _____, and

_____.

39. Barrier protection is indicated for use with all patients because every patient has the potential

to _____.

40. The CDC's (1996) and Health Canada's (1999) isolation guidelines contain a two-tiered approach. Explain.

a. Standard precautions (first tier):

_____

_____

_____

b. Transmission-based (isolation) precautions (second tier):

_____

_____

_____

41. List four basic principles common to all categories of isolation precautions.

a. _____

b. _____

c. _____

d. _____

Psychological Implications of Isolation Precautions

42. Briefly summarize the psychological implications of isolation.

_____

_____

_____

_____

_____

_____

Specimen Collection

43. Explain the techniques for collecting specimens from the patient with a suspected infection.

a. Wound:

_____

_____

b. Blood:

_____

_____

c. Stool:

_____

_____

d. Urine:

_____

_____

44. Explain Health Canada's recommendations for bagging waste or linen.

_____

_____

_____

_____

Transporting Patients

45. Describe how you would transport a patient with an infection.

_____

_____

_____

_____

**Role of the Infection-Control Professional**

46. List eight responsibilities of the infection control professional.

a. _____

b. _____

c. _____

d. _____

e. _____

f. _____

g. _____

h. _____

**Patient Education**

47. List six topics you need to discuss with the patient in relation to infection control practices.

a. _____

b. _____

c. _____

d. _____

e. _____

f. _____

Surgical Asepsis

48. Briefly explain what is meant by the concepts of *surgical asepsis* and *medical asepsis*.

_____

_____

_____

_____

49. Explain when surgical asepsis must be used.

_____

_____

_____

_____

Patient Preparation

50. List three teaching points that reduce the risk of patient-associated contamination during sterile procedures or treatments.

a. _____

b. _____

c. _____

Principles of Surgical Asepsis

51. List the seven principles of surgical asepsis.

a. _____

_____

b. _____

_____

c. _____

_____

d. _____

_____

e. _____

_____

f. _____

_____

g. _____

_____

Performing Sterile Procedures

52. List and briefly explain the nine steps in the preparation of a sterile field.

a. _____

b. _____

c. _____

d. _____

e. _____

f. _____

g. _____

h. _____

i. _____

# Evaluation

The success of infection control techniques is measured by determining whether the goals for reducing or preventing infection are achieved.

Two important skills in evaluation are the ability to correctly assess wounds for healing and the ability to conduct a physical assessment of body systems.

A clear description of any signs and symptoms of systemic or local infection is necessary to give all nurses a baseline for comparative evaluation.

The patient at risk for infection must understand the measures needed to reduce or prevent microorganism growth and spread.

## Review Questions

Select the appropriate answer, and cite the rationale for choosing that particular answer.

1. Of the following, which is *not* an element in the chain of infection?
   a. Infectious agent or pathogen
   b. Reservoir for pathogen growth
   c. Mode of transmission
   d. Formation of immunoglobulin

   Answer:_____ Rationale: _____
   _____
   _____

2. Pathogenic organisms include all of the following, *except*:
   a. Bacteria
   b. Leukocytes
   c. Viruses
   d. Fungi

   Answer:_____ Rationale: _____
   _____
   _____

3. The severity of a patient's illness will depend on all of the following *except*
   a. Extent of infection
   b. Pathogenicity of the microorganism
   c. Susceptibility of the host
   d. Incubation period

   Answer:_____ Rationale: _____
   _____
   _____

4. Which of the following best describes an iatrogenic infection or HAI?
   a. It results from a diagnostic or therapeutic procedure.
   b. It occurs when patients are infected with their own organisms as a result of immunodeficiency.
   c. It involves an incubation period of 3 to 4 weeks before it can be detected.
   d. It results from an extended infection of the urinary tract.

   Answer:_____ Rationale: _____
   _____
   _____

5. The nurse sets up a sterile field on the patient's over-bed table. In which of the following instances is the field contaminated?
   a. The nurse keeps the top of the table above his or her waist.
   b. Sterile saline solution is spilled on the field.
   c. Sterile objects are kept within a 2.5-cm border of the field.
   d. The nurse, who has a cold, wears a double mask.

   Answer:_____ Rationale: _____
   _____
   _____

6. When airborne or droplet isolation precautions are being observed for a patient who must be transported to another part of the hospital, which of the following is *not* required of you as the nurse?
   a. Place a mask on the patient before leaving the room.
   b. Obtain a physician's order to prohibit the patient from being transported.
   c. Advise personnel in diagnostic or procedural areas that the patient is under isolation precautions.
   d. Provide the patient with tissues and a bag for proper disposal of secretions.

   Answer:_____ Rationale: _____
   _____
   _____

# 33

# Medication Administration

## *Preliminary Reading*

Chapter 33, pages 662–750

## *Comprehensive Understanding*

A medication is a substance used in the prevention, diagnosis, relief, treatment, or cure of health alterations.

## Scientific Knowledge Base

Medication administration and evaluation are essential to nursing practice; you need to understand the actions and effects of the medications your patients take.

### Pharmacological Concepts

#### Drug Names

1. A single medication may have three different names. Define each one.

   a. Chemical name:

   _____

   _____

   b. Generic name:

   _____

   _____

   c. Trade name:

   _____

   _____

#### Classification

2. A medication classification indicates

   _____.

#### Medication Forms

3. The form of the medication determines its

   _____.

### Medication Legislation and Standards

#### Canadian Drug Legislation

4. Briefly summarize the role of the federal government in medication regulation.

   _____

   _____

   _____

   _____

#### Drug Standards

5. Official publications set standards for medications in the following areas:

   a. _____

   b. _____

   c. _____

   d. _____

   e. _____

   f. _____

#### Control

6. The Health Protection Branch is responsible for

   _____.

**Provincial, Territorial, and Local Regulation of Medications**

7. Summarize the role of the provincial government in medication regulation.

   _____

   _____

   _____

   _____

8. Summarize the role of health care institutions with regard to government medication regulation.

   _____

   _____

   _____

   _____

**Medication Regulation and Nursing Practice**

9. Describe why it is important for registered nurses to be aware of both federal and provincial regulations affecting medication administration in their practice.

   _____

   _____

   _____

   _____

**Pharmacokinetics as the Basis of Medication Actions**

10. _Pharmacokinetics_ is the study of

    _____.

**Absorption**

11. Define _absorption._

    _____

    _____

    _____

12. Briefly explain the following factors that influence drug absorption.

    a. Route of administration:

       _____

       _____

    b. Ability of a medication to dissolve:

       _____

       _____

    c. Blood flow to the site of administration:

       _____

       _____

    d. Body surface area:

       _____

       _____

    e. Lipid solubility of a medication:

       _____

       _____

Before administering any medication, check pharmacology books, drug references, or package inserts, or consult with pharmacists to identify medication–medication interactions or medication–nutrient interactions.

**Distribution**

The rate and extent of distribution depend on the physical and chemical properties of the medication and on the physiology of the person taking the medication.

13. Explain how each of the following affect the rate and extent of medication distribution.

    a. Circulation:

       _____

       _____

    b. Membrane permeability:

       _____

       _____

    c. Protein binding:

       _____

       _____

**Metabolism**

14. Define _biotransformation_, and identify where it occurs.

    _____

    _____

    _____

    _____

15. Explain why biotransformation is an important concept for registered nurses to understand.

    _____

    _____

    _____

    _____

**Excretion**

16. After drugs are metabolized, they exit the body through the following routes:

    _____

    _____

17. Identify the primary organ for medication excretion, and explain what happens if this organ's function declines.

    _____

    _____

## Types of Medication Action

Medications vary considerably in the way they act and in their types of action. Factors other than characteristics of the medication also influence medication actions. A patient does not always respond in the same way to each successive dose of a medication, and the same medication causes very different responses in different patients.

18. Define the following predicted or unintended effects of medications, and provide a nursing practice example.

    a. Therapeutic effects:

    _____

    _____

    b. Side effects:

    _____

    _____

    c. Adverse effects:

    _____

    _____

    d. Toxic effects:

    _____

    _____

    e. Idiosyncratic reactions:

    _____

    _____

    f. Allergic reactions:

    _____

    _____

    g. Anaphylactic reactions:

    _____

    _____

## Medication Interactions

19. Describe the process of a medication–medication interaction, and provide an example from nursing practice.

    _____

    _____

    _____

    _____

20. Describe the concept of a *synergistic effect*, and provide an example from nursing practice.

    _____

    _____

    _____

    _____

## Medication Dose Responses

When a medication is prescribed, the goal is to achieve a constant blood level within a safe therapeutic range.

Repeated doses are required to achieve a constant therapeutic concentration of a medication because a portion of a drug is always being excreted.

21. Define the following.

    a. *Serum concentration*:

    _____

    _____

    b. *Serum half-life*:

    _____

    _____

22. Using the concepts of serum concentration and serum half-life, explain why it is important for both patients and nurses to follow regular dosage schedules and adhere to prescribed doses and dose intervals.

    _____

    _____

    _____

    _____

23. Explain the following time intervals of medication actions.

    a. Onset of drug action:

    _____

    _____

b. Trough:

_____

_____

c. Duration of action:

_____

_____

d. Plateau:

_____

_____

## Routes of Administration

The route prescribed for a medication's administration depends on its properties, the desired effect, and the patient's physical and mental condition.

### Oral Routes

The oral route is the easiest and the most commonly used route.

24. Identify the types of oral routes, explain how the oral routes are used, and identify the effects of using these routes.

_____

_____

_____

_____

_____

_____

### Parenteral Routes

The parenteral route involves administering a drug through injection into body tissues.

25. List the four major sites of parenteral injections.

a. _____

b. _____

c. _____

d. _____

26. Define the following advanced techniques of medication administration.

a. Epidural:

_____

_____

b. Intrathecal:

_____

_____

c. Intraosseous:

_____

_____

d. Intraperitoneal:

_____

_____

e. Intrapleural:

_____

_____

f. Intra-arterial:

_____

_____

g. Intracardiac:

_____

_____

h. Intra-articular:

_____

_____

### Topical Administration

Medications that are applied to the skin and mucous membranes generally have local effects.

27. Identify five methods for applying medications to mucous membranes.

a. _____

b. _____

c. _____

d. _____

e. _____

### Inhalation Route

Medications that are administered by the inhalation route are readily absorbed and work rapidly. Inhaled medications may have either local or systemic effects.

28. Describe the three passages through which *inhalations* can be administered.

a. Nasal:

_____

_____

b. Oral:

_____

_____

c. Endotracheal or tracheal:

_____

_____

**Intraocular Route**

29. Describe the process of intraocular medication delivery.

_____

_____

_____

_____

**Systems of Medication Measurement**

The proper administration of a medication depends on your ability to compute medication doses accurately and to measure medications correctly. Mistakes can lead to a fatal error.

30. The following are measuring systems used in medication therapy. Briefly explain their basic units.

a. *Metric system*:

_____

_____

b. *Household measurements:*

_____

_____

**Household Measurements**

34. Complete the following measurement equivalents.

31. A solution is _____.

**Nursing Knowledge Base**

More people die from medical errors than from motor vehicle accidents, breast cancer, and workplace injuries.

32. To safely administer medications, ensure that

you know _____, _____

and _____.

**Clinical Calculations**

To administer medications safely, you need an understanding of basic arithmetic to calculate medication doses, mix solutions, and perform a variety of other activities. This skill is important because medications are not always dispensed in the unit of measure in which they are ordered.

**Conversions Within One System**

33. Indicate which direction the decimal point is moved for the following mathematical calculations in the metric system, and provide a rationale.

a. Division:

_____

_____

b. Multiplication:

_____

_____

| Metric | Household |
|---|---|
| 1 mL | ___ drops |
| ___ mL | 1 tablespoon |
| 30 mL | ___ tablespoon(s) |
| ___ mL | 1 cup |
| ___ mL | 1 pint |
| ___ mL | 1 quart |

35. Complete the following conversions.

    a. 100 mg = _____ g

    b. 2.5 L   = _____ mL

    c. 500 mL = _____ L

    d. 15 mg   = _____ g

    e. 30 gtt   = _____ mL

    f. 1/6 g   = _____ mg

**Dose Calculations**

36. Write out the formula used to determine the correct dose when preparing solid or liquid forms of medications.

    _____

37. Define the following.

    a. Dose ordered:

    _____

    _____

    b. Dose on hand:

    _____

    _____

    c. Amount on hand:

    _____

    _____

38. Do not _____ tablets because the

    potential _____ .

Liquid medications are often manufactured in volumes greater than 1 mL. In applying the formula, be careful to use the correct concentration to avoid a medication error.

**Pediatric Doses**

39. Write out the formula applied to accurately calculate safe pediatric doses.

    _____

    _____

40. Explain why calculating children's medication doses requires caution.

    _____

    _____

    _____

    _____

41. The nurse who is administering the medications is accountable for

    _____ .

**Prescriber's Role**

42. Identify the primary responsibilities of the prescriber in giving medications to patients.

    _____

    _____

    _____

    _____

43. Identify recommendations to reduce medication errors associated with both verbal medication orders and prescriptions.

    _____

    _____

    _____

    _____

44. Use caution when you use abbreviations because some _____ can lead to

    _____ and the potential for

    _____ .

**Types of Orders**

45. Briefly explain the five common types of medication orders.

    a. Routine:

    _____

    _____

    b. As needed ("prn"):

    _____

    _____

    c. Single (one-time):

    _____

    _____

    d. STAT:

    _____

    _____

    e. Now:

    _____

    _____

**Prescriptions**

46. List the six parts of a prescription.

 a. _____

 b. _____

 c. _____

 d. _____

 e. _____

 f. _____

**Pharmacist's Role**

47. Identify the primary responsibility of the pharmacist in the administration of medications.

 _____
 _____
 _____
 _____

**Distribution Systems**

48. List the three medication distribution systems, and identify the advantages and disadvantages of each.

 a. _____

 b. _____

 c. _____

**Nurse's Role**

49. Summarize the nurse's primary responsibilities when administering medications, and explain why these responsibilities are important in nursing practice.

 _____
 _____
 _____
 _____

50. A medication error is

 _____.

51. Identify steps that registered nurses can take to prevent medication errors.

 _____
 _____
 _____
 _____
 _____
 _____
 _____
 _____

52. Explain what steps you should take if a medication error occurs.

 a. _____

 b. _____

 c. _____

 d. _____

53. Identify sources of medication errors:

 a. _____

 b. _____

 c. _____

 d. _____

 e. _____

 f. _____

 g. _____

 h. _____

 i. _____

54. Briefly describe *medication reconciliation*.

 _____
 _____
 _____

# Critical Thinking

### Knowledge

55. Summarize the knowledge needed from other disciplines to safely administer medications.

 _____
 _____
 _____
 _____

### Experience

Psychomotor skills, the patient's attitudes, knowledge, physical and mental status, and responses can make medication administration a complex experience.

### Cognitive and Behavioural Attributes

56. Demonstrating accountability and responsibility when administering medications means that

 the nurse _____.

**Standards**

57. List the "ten rights" of medication administration, and briefly explain each one.

    a. _____

    b. _____

    c. _____

    d. _____

    e. _____

    f. _____

    g. _____

    h. _____

    i. _____

    j. _____

58. Explain the importance of adhering to agency policies and procedures when administering medications.

    _____

    _____

    _____

    _____

**Maintaining Patients' Rights**

59. Because of the potential risks related to medication administration, patients have the right to the following:

    a. _____

    b. _____

    c. _____

    d. _____

    e. _____

    f. _____

    g. _____

    h. _____

## Nursing Process and Medication Administration

## Assessment

60. Describe the following elements of nursing assessment, and explain each element's significance as related to safe medication administration.

    a. History:

    _____

    _____

    b. History of allergies:

    _____

    _____

    c. Medication data:

    _____

    _____

    d. Diet history:

    _____

    _____

    e. Patient's perceptual or coordination problems:

    _____

    _____

    f. Patient's current condition:

    _____

    _____

    g. Patient's attitude toward medication use:

    _____

    _____

    h. Patient's knowledge and understanding of medication therapy:

    _____

    _____

    i. Patient's learning needs:

    _____

    _____

## Nursing Diagnosis

Assessment provides data on the patient's condition, ability to self-administer medications, and medication use patterns. This information can be used to determine actual or potential problems with medication therapy.

61. Identify potential nursing diagnoses that apply to the process of medication administration.

    _____

    _____

    _____

    _____

    _____

    _____

## Planning

Organize nursing care activities to ensure the safe administration of medications.

### Goals and Outcomes

62. Identify a goal and related outcomes that the nurse or patient needs to meet before the administration of medications, and provide the rationale for each goal and outcome.

_____
_____
_____
_____

### Setting Priorities

Prioritize care when administering medications. Use information gathered from your assessment of the patient to determine whether the administration of medications is appropriate and, if it is, which medication should be given first.

## Implementation

### Health Promotion

63. Identify factors that can influence the patient's compliance with the medication regimen, and provide the rationale for your answers.

_____
_____
_____
_____

64. Identify important information that you should provide to the patient and family in relation to medications, and provide the rationale for your answers.

_____
_____
_____
_____

### Acute Care

65. Identify the necessary components of medication orders.

_____
_____
_____
_____
_____
_____

66. Explain why the following interventions are essential for safe and effective medication administration.

a. Receiving medication orders:

_____
_____

b. Correct transcription and communication of orders:

_____
_____

c. Accurate dose calculation and measurement:

_____
_____

d. Correct administration, adhering to the ten rights of medication administration:

_____
_____

e. Recording medication administration:

_____
_____

### Restorative Care

67. Regardless of the type of medication activity, you are responsible for _____.

### Special Considerations for Administering Medications to Specific Age Groups

#### Infants and Children

68. Identify strategies to address children's psychosocial preparation before administering medications.

_____
_____
_____
_____

#### Older Adults

69. Identify special considerations for older adults when administering medication, and provide rationales.

_____
_____
_____
_____

Polypharmacy

70. *Polypharmacy* occurs when _____,

_____, _____, or

_____.

71. Describe the difference between rational and irrational polypharmacy.

_____

_____

_____

_____

Noncompliance

72. Noncompliance is defined as a _____,

of medication, such as _____ a pre-

scribed medication or _____ the dose of
a medication.

# Evaluation

You must know the therapeutic action and common side effects of each medication in order to monitor a patient's response to that medication.

73. Many different evaluation measures can be used in the context of medication administration. Identify various measures used in practice to evaluate medication administration processes.

_____

_____

_____

_____

74. The most common type of measurement is

_____

# Medication Administration

## Oral Administration

The easiest and most desirable way to administer medications is by mouth.

75. The primary contraindications to giving oral

medications include _____.

76. To protect the patient against possible aspiration, what nursing assessments should be conducted? What nursing interventions should be implemented? Provide rationales for your answers.

_____

_____

_____

_____

## Topical Medication Applications

Topical medications are applied locally, most often to intact skin. They can also be applied to mucous membranes.

### Skin Applications

Many locally applied medications, such as lotions, pastes, and ointments, cause both systemic and local effects; apply these medications using gloves and applicators.

77. Explain the procedure for administering the following skin applications.

a. Ointment:

_____

_____

b. Lotion:

_____

_____

c. Transdermal patch:

_____

_____

### Nasal Instillation

78. Summarize the rationale for nasal instillations.

_____

_____

_____

_____

### Eye Instillation

79. List four principles for administering eye instillations.

a. _____

b. _____

c. _____

d. _____

**Intraocular Administration**

80. Summarize the procedure for administering ophthalmic medications, and provide rationales for steps specific to ophthalmic medication delivery.

_____
_____
_____
_____

**Ear Instillation**

81. Explain the procedure for administering ear instillations.

a. Adults:

_____
_____

b. Children:

_____
_____

82. Identify the significant differences between adults and children when administering ear medications.

_____
_____
_____
_____

**Vaginal Instillation**

83. Vaginal medications are available as

_____, _____, _____,

and _____.

**Rectal Instillation**

84. Explain the differences between vaginal and rectal suppositories, and the reason for these differences.

_____
_____
_____
_____

85. Summarize the procedure for administering rectal suppositories, and provide rationales for steps specific to rectal suppository administration.

_____
_____
_____
_____

**Administering Medications by Inhalation**

86. Identify the most common conditions of patients who are prescribed medications via the inhalation route.

_____
_____
_____
_____

87. Summarize the procedure for teaching patients to self-administer medications via a metered-dose inhaler, and provide the rationale.

_____
_____
_____
_____

**Administering Medications by Irrigations**

88. Identify the principles you must adhere to when performing irrigations, and provide rationales for your answers.

_____
_____
_____
_____

**Administering Parenteral Medications**

When medications are administered parenterally, it is an invasive procedure that must be performed using aseptic techniques.

Each type of injection requires certain skills to ensure that the medication reaches the proper location.

**Equipment**

89. Identify the two major types of syringes.

a. _____
b. _____

90. Identify three factors that must be considered when selecting a needle for an injection.

a. _____
b. _____
c. _____

91. Identify the advantages of using the Tubex® or Carpuject® injection systems.

_____

_____

_____

_____

**Preparing an Injection From an Ampule**

92. An ampule is

_____.

93. Summarize the procedure for withdrawing medication from an ampule, and provide the rationale for each step.

_____

_____

_____

**Preparing an Injection From a Vial**

94. A vial is a

_____.

The vial is a closed system, and air must be injected into it to permit easy withdrawal of the solution.

95. Summarize the procedure for withdrawing medication from a vial and provide a rationale for each step.

_____

_____

_____

_____

**Mixing Medications**

96. If two medications are compatible, it is possible to mix two drugs together into one injection if

_____.

**Mixing Medications From Two Vials**

97. List the three principles to follow when mixing medications from two vials.

a. _____

b. _____

c. _____

**Mixing Medications From One Vial and One Ampule**

98. When mixing medications from an ampule and a vial, which medication should be prepared first? Provide the rationale for your answer.

_____

_____

_____

_____

**Insulin Preparation**

99. Insulin is _____.

100. Explain why insulin must be administered by injection.

_____

_____

_____

_____

101. Insulin is classified by

_____.

Insulin is ordered either by a specific dose at select times or by a sliding scale. A sliding scale dictates a certain dose on the basis of the patient's blood glucose level.

102. Summarize the procedure for mixing two kinds of insulin in the same syringe.

_____

_____

_____

_____

**Administering Injections**

103. The characteristics of the tissues injected influence the

_____.

104. List the techniques used to minimize patient discomfort associated with injections, and provide rationales for your answers.

a. _____

b. _____

c. _____

d. _____

e. _____

f. _____

g. _____

## Subcutaneous Injections

Subcutaneous injections involve placing the medications into the loose connective tissue under the dermis.

105. Explain the differences in absorption between a subcutaneous and an intramuscular (IM) injection.

_____

_____

_____

_____

106. The best sites for subcutaneous injections include _____, _____, and _____.

107. The site chosen for a subcutaneous injection should be free of _____, _____, and _____.

108. Identify the maximum amount of water-soluble medication given by the subcutaneous route.

_____

_____

_____

_____

109. Identify the factors to consider when determining if a subcutaneous injection should be given at a 90- or 45-degree angle.

_____

_____

_____

_____

## Intramuscular Injections

110. Identify some important things to consider when using the IM route.

_____

_____

_____

_____

111. The angle of insertion for an IM injection is _____ degrees.

112. Indicate the maximum volume of medication for IM injection in each of the following groups (provide rationales for your answers).

a. Well-developed adult:

_____

_____

b. Children, older adults, or thin adults:

_____

_____

c. Older infants and small children:

_____

_____

d. Smaller infants:

_____

_____

### Sites

113. List the assessment criteria for selecting an IM site.

a. _____

b. _____

c. _____

d. _____

114. Describe the characteristics, advantages, and disadvantages of the following injection sites.

a. Ventrogluteal:

_____

_____

b. Vastus lateralis:

_____

_____

c. Dorsogluteal:

_____

_____

d. Deltoid:

_____

_____

### Technique for IM Injections

115. Describe the Z-track technique for administering IM injections. Explain the rationale for using the _Z-track method_ of injection.

_____

_____

_____

_____

**Intradermal Injections**

116. Explain the rationale for using the intradermal route to administer medication.

_____

_____

_____

_____

**Safety in Administering Medications by Injection**

**Needleless Devices**

117. Explain the rationale for the use of a needle-less device.

_____

_____

_____

_____

**Intravenous Administration**

118. The nurse administers medications intravenously by the following methods.

a. _____

b. _____

c. _____

119. Discuss the advantages of administering medications by the IV route.

_____

_____

_____

_____

**Large-Volume Infusions**

120. Identify the advantage and disadvantage of the large-volume infusion method (provide rationales for your answers).

_____

_____

_____

_____

**Intravenous Bolus**

121. Explain the advantage and disadvantage of the IV bolus route of administration (provide rationales for your answers).

_____

_____

_____

_____

**Volume-Controlled Infusions**

122. List the advantages of using volume-controlled infusions.

a. _____

b. _____

c. _____

_Volume-Control Administration_

123. Describe the setup and purpose of a volume-control administration set.

_____

_____

_____

_____

_Piggyback_

124. Describe the setup and purpose of a piggyback set.

_____

_____

_____

_____

_Tandem_

125. Describe the setup and purpose of a tandem set.

_____

_____

_____

_____

_Mini-Infusion Pump_

126. Describe the setup and purpose of a mini-infusion pump.

_____

_____

_____

_____

**Intermittent Venous Access**

127. List two advantages of using intermittent venous access devices.

a. _____

b. _____

**Administration of IV Therapy in the Home**

128. When receiving home IV therapy, patient education should include

_____ .

**Subcutaneous Butterfly Catheters**

129. Briefly define *hypodermoclysis*, and list its advantages.

_____

_____

_____

_____

## Review Questions

Select the appropriate answer, and cite the rationale for choosing that particular answer.

1. The study of how medications enter the body, reach their sites of action, are metabolized, and exit from the body is called:
   a. Pharmacology
   b. Pharmacokinetics
   c. Pharmacopoeia
   d. Biopharmaceutica

Answer: _____ Rationale: _____

_____

_____

2. Which statement correctly characterizes medication absorption?
   a. Many medications must enter the systemic circulation to have a therapeutic effect.
   b. Mucous membranes are relatively impermeable to chemicals, making absorption slow.
   c. Oral medications are absorbed more quickly when administered with meals.
   d. Drugs administered subcutaneously are absorbed more quickly than those injected intramuscularly.

Answer: _____ Rationale: _____

_____

_____

3. The onset of medication action is the time it takes for a drug to
   a. Produce a response
   b. Accelerate the cellular process
   c. Reach its highest effective concentration
   d. Produce blood serum concentration and maintenance

Answer: _____ Rationale: _____

_____

_____

4. Which of the following is *not* a parenteral route of administration?
   a. Buccal
   b. Subcutaneous
   c. Intramuscular
   d. Intradermal

Answer: _____ Rationale: _____

_____

_____

5. Using the body surface area formula, what dose of drug X should a child who weighs 12 kg (body surface area = 0.54 m$^2$) receive if the normal adult dose of drug X is 300 mg?
   a. 50 mg
   b. 95 mg
   c. 100 mg
   d. 200 mg

Answer: _____ Rationale: _____

_____

_____

6. The nurse is preparing an insulin injection in which both short-acting (clear) and long-acting (cloudy) insulin will be mixed. Into which vial should the nurse inject air first?
   a. The vial of long-acting insulin
   b. The vial of short-acting insulin
   c. Either vial, as long as long-acting insulin is drawn up first
   d. Neither vial; it is not necessary to put air into vials before withdrawing medication

Answer: _____ Rationale: _____

_____

_____

# 34

# Complementary and Alternative Therapies

## Preliminary Reading

Chapter 34, pages 751–768

## Comprehensive Understanding

People desired a different kind of health care—one that embraced healing, acknowledgement of the spiritual dimensions of health and illness, and openness toward alternative medical systems.

### Complementary and Alternative Medicine Therapies in Health Care

1. Describe the difference between the following terms.

    a. *Complementary therapies*:

    _____
    _____
    _____

    b. *Alternative therapies*:

    _____
    _____
    _____

2. Describe *integrative medicine*.

    _____
    _____

3. Complementary and alternative therapies are often organized into five categories that researchers find useful. List the five categories.

    a. _____
    b. _____
    c. _____
    d. _____
    e. _____

4. Explain the following alternative therapies in the whole medical systems category and give an example of each.

    a. Ayurveda:

    _____
    _____
    _____

    b. Latin American practices:

    _____
    _____
    _____

    c. Traditional Aboriginal medicine:

    _____
    _____
    _____

d. Naturopathic medicine:

_____

_____

_____

e. Traditional Chinese medicine (TCM):

_____

_____

_____

**Public Interest in Complementary and Alternative Medicine Therapies**

5. Describe *integrative medical programs.*

_____

_____

_____

_____

In Canada and worldwide, demand is growing for alternative medicines and the services of alternative health care providers. The persons who use complementary and alternative medicine (CAM) therapies typically are women with a post–high school or college-equivalent education.

**Complementary and Alternative Medicine Therapies and Holistic Nursing**

The practice of holistic nursing regards and treats the patient's mind, body, and spirit. Holistic interventions can augment standard treatments, replace ineffective or debilitating interventions, and promote and maintain health.

6. Discuss the two types of CAM therapies.

_____

_____

## Nursing-Accessible Therapies

Some CAM therapies and techniques use natural processes, such as breathing, concentration, and simple touch, to help patients feel better and cope with their chronic conditions.

7. CAM therapies should be chosen _____

_____.

**Relaxation Therapy**

8. Define the *stress response.*

_____

_____

9. *Relaxation* is _____.

10. *Progressive relaxation* training helps to _____.

11. *Passive relaxation* involves teaching _____.

**Clinical Applications of Relaxation Therapy**

12. Relaxation techniques can lower _____, decrease _____, improve _____, and reduce _____.

13. The type of relaxation intervention should be matched to _____.

**Limitations of Relaxation Therapy**

14. Identify the limitations of relaxation therapy.

_____

_____

_____

_____

**Meditation and Breathing**

15. *Meditation* is _____.

**Clinical Applications of Meditation**

16. Identify the clinical applications of meditation.

_____

_____

_____

_____

**Limitations of Meditation**

17. Identify the limitations of meditation.

_____

_____

_____

_____

**Imagery**

18. *Imagery* is _____.

19. *Creative visualization* is _____.

**Clinical Applications of Imagery**

20. Identify the clinical applications of imagery.

_____

_____

_____

_____

**Limitation of Imagery**

21. Identify the limitations of imagery.

_____

_____

_____

_____

## Training-Specific Therapies

**Biofeedback**

22. *Biofeedback* is _____.

**Clinical Applications of Biofeedback**

23. Identify the clinical applications of biofeedback.

_____

_____

_____

_____

**Limitations of Biofeedback**

24. Identify the limitations of biofeedback.

_____

_____

_____

_____

**Therapeutic Touch**

25. *Therapeutic touch (TT)* is _____.

26. TT consists of five phases. Explain each.

a. Centring:

_____

_____

b. Assessment:

_____

_____

c. Unruffling:

_____

_____

d. Treatment:

_____

_____

e. Evaluation:

_____

_____

27. Identify the physiological indicators of energy imbalance.

_____

_____

_____

_____

**Clinical Applications of Therapeutic Touch**

28. Identify the clinical applications of TT.

_____

_____

_____

_____

**Limitations of Therapeutic Touch**

29. Identify the limitations of TT.

_____

_____

_____

**Chiropractic Therapy**

30. *Chiropractic therapy* is _____.

**Clinical Applications of Chiropractic Therapy**

31. Describe the clinical applications of chiropractic therapy.

_____

_____

_____

_____

**Limitations of Chiropractic Therapy**

32. Identify the limitations of chiropractic therapy.

_____

_____

_____

_____

**Traditional Chinese Medicine**

33. TCM comprises several healing modalities, including

_____

_____.

34. Explain the concept of *yin and yang*.

_____

_____

_____

_____

35. *Qi* is _____.

36. TCM classifies disease into three categories. State the influences of each.

   a. External causes:

   _____

   _____

   b. Internal causes:

   _____

   _____

   c. Nonexternal, noninternal causes:

   _____

   _____

37. Define *meridians*.

_____

_____

**Acupuncture**

38. *Acupuncture* is _____.

**Clinical Applications of Acupuncture**

39. Describe the clinical applications of acupuncture.

_____

_____

_____

_____

**Limitations of Acupuncture**

40. Identify the limitations of acupuncture.

_____

_____

_____

_____

## Role of Nutrition in Disease Prevention and Health Promotion

**Herbal Therapies**

41. The goal of *herbal therapy* is _____.

42. Medication therapy is aimed at _____.

**Clinical Applications of Natural Health Products (NHPs)**

43. Describe the clinical applications of herbal therapy.

_____

_____

_____

_____

44. Explain what a natural product number (NPN) is.

_____

_____

_____

_____

**Limitations of NHPs**

45. Identify the limitations of herbal therapy.

_____

_____

_____

_____

Data does not support the use of these herbs in infants or children, or during pregnancy or lactation.

## Nursing Role in Complementary and Alternative Therapies

46. Summarize the role of the nurse regarding CAM therapies.

_____

_____

_____

_____

## Review Questions

Select the appropriate answer, and cite the rationale for choosing that particular answer.

1. Patients choose to use unconventional therapies because
   a. They are willing to pay to feel better
   b. Such therapies are now widely accepted by Health Canada's Office of Natural Health Products
   c. They are dissatisfied with conventional medicine
   d. They want religious approval for the remedies they use

   Answer: _____ Rationale: _____
   _____
   _____

2. A herb considered safe for the treatment of mild depression is
   a. Milk thistle
   b. St. John's wort
   c. Pokeroot
   d. Hawthorn

   Answer: _____ Rationale: _____
   _____
   _____

3. You can best assess your patient's use of alternative therapies by
   a. Asking the patient true-or-false questions about his or her health
   b. Asking for a thorough medical history
   c. Reviewing laboratory studies that assess levels of certain herbs
   d. Asking open-ended questions on alternative therapies

   Answer: _____ Rationale: _____
   _____
   _____

4. Which of the following steps should you take to be better informed about alternative therapies?
   a. Keep abreast of the current research on alternative therapies.
   b. Familiarize yourself with recent case studies on alternative therapies.
   c. Familiarize yourself with general principles of homeopathics.
   d. Review herb manufacturers' literature on specific herbs.

   Answer: _____ Rationale: _____
   _____
   _____

# 35

# Activity and Exercise

## *Preliminary Reading*

Chapter 35, pages 769–789

## *Comprehensive Understanding*

1. Understanding *body mechanics* and *ergonomics* includes _____.

### Scientific Knowledge Base

#### Physiology of Movement

2. List three systems responsible for coordinating body movements.

   a. _____

   b. _____

   c. _____

#### Skeletal System

3. List five functions of the skeletal system.

   a. _____

   b. _____

   c. _____

   d. _____

   e. _____

4. Describe the four types of bones:

   a. _____

   b. _____

   c. _____

   d. _____

5. Describe the following.

   a. *Joints:*

   _____

   _____

   b. *Synarthrotic joint:*

   _____

   _____

   c. *Cartilaginous joint:*

   _____

   _____

   d. *Fibrous joint:*

   _____

   _____

   e. *Synovial joint:*

   _____

   _____

   f. *Ligaments:*

   _____

   _____

   g. *Tendons:*

   _____

   _____

   h. *Cartilage:*

   _____

   _____

**Skeletal Muscle**

6. Briefly describe how skeletal muscles affect movement.

_____

_____

_____

_____

**Muscles Concerned With Movement**

7. Briefly explain the work of muscles concerned with movement.

_____

_____

_____

**Muscles Concerned With Posture**

8. Briefly explain the work of muscles concerned with *posture*.

_____

_____

_____

**Muscle Groups**

9. The nervous system regulates and coordinates the following different muscle groups. Briefly explain each.

   a. *Antagonistic muscles*:

   _____

   _____

   _____

   b. *Synergistic muscles*:

   _____

   _____

   _____

   c. *Antigravity muscles*:

   _____

   _____

   _____

Skeletal muscles support posture and carry out voluntary movement. These muscles are attached to the skeleton by tendons, which provide strength and permit motion.

**Nervous System**

10. Briefly describe how movement and posture are regulated by the nervous system.

_____

_____

_____

_____

**Proprioception**

11. Define *proprioception*.

_____

_____

_____

_____

**Balance**

12. The structures in the ear that assist in maintaining balance are the _____.

**Principles of Body Mechanics**

13. List five principles of body mechanics.

   a. _____

   b. _____

   c. _____

   d. _____

   e. _____

**Body Alignment**

14. Define body alignment.

_____

_____

_____

_____

**Body Balance**

15. Body balance is achieved when

_____.

16. Define *centre of gravity*.

_____

_____

_____

_____

17. Proper body alignment and posture are maintained by using the following two simple techniques:

    a. _____

    b. _____

**Friction**

18. Define *friction*.

    _____

    _____

    _____

19. List two techniques that minimize friction.

    a. _____

    b. _____

**Pathological Influences on Body Mechanics and Movement**

20. Briefly explain how the following pathological conditions may affect body alignment and mobility.

    a. Congenital abnormalities:

       _____

       _____

       _____

    b. Degenerative diseases:

       _____

       _____

       _____

    c. Other chronic diseases:

       _____

       _____

       _____

    d. Episodic illnesses:

       _____

       _____

       _____

**Exercise and Activity**

*Exercise* is physical activity for the purpose of conditioning the body, improving health, and maintaining fitness, or it may be used as a therapeutic measure.

21. *Activity tolerance* is _____

    _____.

The best program of physical activity includes a combination of exercises that produce different physiological and psychological benefits.

22. There are three categories of exercises. Briefly explain and give an example of each.

    a. Isotonic contraction:

       _____

       _____

       _____

    b. Isometric contraction:

       _____

       _____

       _____

    c. Resistive isometric:

       _____

       _____

       _____

## Nursing Knowledge Base

**Developmental Changes**

23. The greatest change and impact on the maturational process is observed _____

    _____.

24. Identify the descriptive characteristics of body alignment and mobility for the following age groups.

    a. Infants:

       _____

       _____

    b. Toddlers:

       _____

       _____

    c. Adolescents:

       _____

       _____

    d. Young to middle-aged adults:

       _____

       _____

    e. Older adults:

       _____

       _____

**Behavioural Aspects**

25. Patients are more likely to incorporate an exercise program into their daily life if this choice is

_____ and _____.

**Environmental Issues**

26. Explain the exercise and activity issues related to the following sites.

    a. Work sites:

    _____

    _____

    b. Schools:

    _____

    _____

    c. Community:

    _____

    _____

**Cultural and Ethnic Influences**

27. The nurse must consider what motivates and what is deemed appropriate and enjoyable when developing a physical fitness program for culturally diverse populations. Briefly describe a comprehensive fitness program that would be suitable for an ethnocultural group with which you interact.

    _____

    _____

    _____

    _____

    _____

    _____

**Family and Social Support**

28. Briefly explain how a family may be a motivational tool in regard to physical fitness.

    _____

    _____

    _____

    _____

## Nursing Process

## Assessment

**Body Alignment**

29. Briefly explain how the assessment of body alignment and posture is carried out.

    a. Standing:

    _____

    _____

    b. Sitting:

    _____

    _____

    c. Recumbent:

    _____

    _____

**Mobility**

30. There are three components to assess in regard to mobility. Explain each.

    a. *Range of motion*:

    _____

    _____

    b. *Gait*:

    _____

    _____

    c. *Exercise*:

    _____

    _____

**Activity Tolerance**

31. Identify three factors that affect activity tolerance.

    a. _____

    b. _____

    c. _____

## Nursing Diagnosis

32. Assessment of the patient's _____,

_____, _____, and _____
provides clusters of data or defining characteristics that can lead you to a nursing diagnosis.

33. Give five examples of nursing diagnoses related to exercise and activity.

    a. _____

    b. _____

    c. _____

    d. _____

    e. _____

## Planning

34. The plan should include consideration of

    a. _____

    b. _____

    c. _____

    d. _____

    e. _____

## Implementation

### Health Promotion

35. List the three recommendations for adult exercise.

    a. _____

    b. _____

    c. _____

36. Explain how to calculate the patient's maximum heart rate.

    _____

    _____

    _____

    _____

37. An exercise program should include the following. Explain each.

    a. Aerobic exercise:

    _____

    _____

    b. Stretching and flexibility exercises:

    _____

    _____

    c. Resistance training:

    _____

    _____

### Acute Care

Patients in acute care often have reduced activity tolerance or are immobile to varying degrees. Promoting activity and preventing the effects of immobility are paramount.

38. It is essential for nurses to utilize_____

    _____.

39. Briefly explain proper lifting technique.

    _____

    _____

The musculoskeletal system can be maintained by encouraging the use of stretching and isometric-type exercises.

40. Briefly explain the technique of stretching exercises.

    _____

    _____

    _____

    _____

41. Explain how you would help a patient to maintain or improve joint mobility.

    _____

    _____

    _____

    _____

42. Explain how walking affects joint mobility.

    _____

    _____

    _____

    _____

43. Explain how you would assist the patient to walk.

    _____

    _____

    _____

    _____

    _____

**Restorative and Continuing Care**

44. Explain how the nurse would implement a plan of care to increase activity and exercise in the following specific disease conditions.

   a. Coronary heart disease:

   _____

   _____

   _____

   b. Hypertension:

   _____

   _____

   _____

   c. Chronic obstructive pulmonary disease:

   _____

   _____

   _____

   d. Diabetes mellitus:

   _____

   _____

   _____

## Evaluation

**Patient Care**

Measure the effectiveness of nursing interventions by the success in meeting the patient's expected outcomes and goals of care.

45. Comparisons are made with baseline measures that include _____, _____, _____, _____, and _____.

**Patient Expectations**

You need to know your patient's expectations concerning activity and exercise.

## Review Questions

Select the appropriate answer, and cite the rationale for choosing that particular answer.

1. Which of the following is true of body mechanics?
   a. The narrower the base of support, the greater your stability.
   b. The higher the centre of gravity, the greater your stability.
   c. When friction is reduced between the object to be moved and the surface on which it is moved, less force is required to move it.
   d. Rolling, turning, or pivoting requires more work than lifting.

   Answer: _____ Rationale: _____

   _____

   _____

2. White, shiny, flexible bands of fibrous tissue binding joints together and connecting various bones and cartilage types are known as:
   a. Muscles
   b. Ligaments
   c. Joints
   d. Tendons

   Answer: _____ Rationale: _____

   _____

   _____

3. The nurse would expect all of the following physiological effects of exercise on the body systems except
   a. Decreased cardiac output
   b. Increased respiratory rate and depth
   c. Increased muscle tone, size, and strength
   d. Change in metabolic rate

   Answer: _____ Rationale: _____

   _____

   _____

4. Which of the following is a possible nursing diagnosis related to activity and exercise?
   a. Altered thought processes
   b. Altered oral mucous membrane
   c. Relocation stress syndrome
   d. Impaired gas exchange

   Answer: _____ Rationale: _____

   _____

   _____

## Critical Thinking Model for Nursing Care Plan for Activity Intolerance

Imagine that you are Eric, the nurse in the Care Plan on pages 782–783 of your text. Complete the *planning* phase of the critical thinking model by writing your answers in the appropriate boxes of the model shown. Think about the following:

- In developing Mrs. Wertenberger's plan of care, what knowledge did Eric apply?

- In what way might Eric's previous experience assist in developing a plan of care for Mrs. Wertenberger?

- When developing a plan of care, what intellectual or professional standards were applied to Mrs. Wertenberger?

- What critical thinking attitudes might have been applied in developing Mrs. Wertenberger's plan?

- How will Eric accomplish his goals?

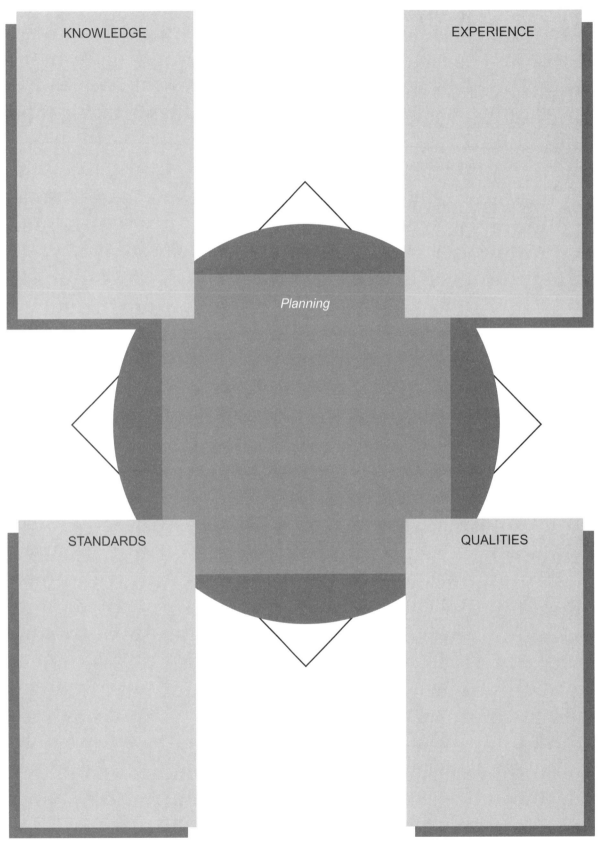

KNOWLEDGE

EXPERIENCE

*Planning*

STANDARDS

QUALITIES

CHAPTER 35   Critical Thinking Model for Nursing Care Plan for *Activity Intolerance*
See answers on Evolve site.

# 36

# Safety

*Preliminary Reading*

Chapter 36, pages 790–824

*Comprehensive Understanding*

1. Briefly define *safety*.

   _____

   _____

## Scientific Knowledge Base

**Environmental Safety**

2. A patient's environment includes _____

   _____.

3. List six characteristics of a safe environment.

   a. _____

   b. _____

   c. _____

   d. _____

   e. _____

   f. _____

**Basic Needs**

4. Give an example of the four basic physiological needs that influence a person's safety.

   a. Oxygen:

      _____

      _____

   b. Nutrition:

      _____

      _____

   c. Temperature:

      _____

      _____

   d. Humidity:

      _____

      _____

**Physical Hazards**

5. Physical hazards in the community and health care settings place patients at risk for accidental injury and death. List five physical hazards that contribute to accidental injury.

   a. _____

   b. _____

   c. _____

   d. _____

   e. _____

6. A *poison* is _____.

**Transmission of Pathogens**

7. Define *pathogen*.

   _____

   _____

8. Identify the most effective method for limiting the transmission of pathogens.

   _____

   _____

   _____

9. Define *immunization*.

_____

_____

10. Describe the two types of immunity.

   a. Active:

   _____

   _____

   b. Passive:

   _____

   _____

11. Describe how the following viruses are transmitted:

   a. Human immunodeficiency virus

   _____

   _____

   b. Hepatitis B

   _____

   _____

   c. Hepatitis C

   _____

   _____

**Pollution**

A healthy environment is free from pollution.

12. A *pollutant* is

_____

_____.

13. Define the following types of pollution.

   a. *Air pollution*:

   _____

   _____

   b. *Land pollution*:

   _____

   _____

   c. *Water pollution*:

   _____

   _____

   d. *Noise pollution*:

   _____

   _____

**Terrorism**

If a terrorist health threat were to occur in Canada, Health Canada would work with provincial, territorial, and local health officials to address the situation. Hospitals make up one of several components of a community's emergency response plan.

## Nursing Knowledge Base

14. In addition to being knowledgeable about the environment, to minimize threats to patient safety, nurses must be familiar with

   a. _____

   b. _____

   c. _____

   d. _____

   e. _____

**Risks at Developmental Stages**

15. Identify at least three threats to safety in the following developmental stages.

   a. Infant, toddler, preschooler:

   _____

   _____

   b. School-age:

   _____

   _____

   c. Adolescent:

   _____

   _____

   d. Adult:

   _____

   _____

   e. Older adult:

   _____

   _____

**Individual Risk Factors**

16. Explain how the following risk factors threaten safety.

   a. Lifestyle:

   _____

   _____

b. Impaired mobility:

_____

_____

c. Sensory or communication impairment:

_____

_____

d. Lack of safety awareness:

_____

_____

### Risks in the Health Care Agency

#### Workplace Risks

Various forms of chemicals used in health care settings are a source of environmental risk for both the patient and the health care worker.

17. Discuss the importance of *WHMIS*.

_____

_____

_____

_____

#### Risks to Patient Safety

18. List the four major risks to patient safety in the health care environment.

a. _____

b. _____

c. _____

d. _____

## Safety and the Nursing Process

## Assessment

To conduct a thorough patient assessment, consider possible threats to the patient's safety, including the patient's immediate environment, as well as any individual risk factors.

### Health History

By conducting a health history, you gather data about the patient's level of wellness to determine if any underlying conditions exist that pose threats to safety.

19. Identify the specific assessments you need to make in the following settings.

a. The patient's home:

_____

_____

### Health Care Environment

Discuss assessment of hazards in a health care environment:

_____

_____

20. Explain the following health care environment risks.

a. Risk for falls:

_____

_____

b. Risk for medical errors:

_____

_____

### Patient Expectations

Patients usually do not purposefully put themselves in jeopardy. When patients are uninformed or inexperienced, threats to their safety can occur. Patients must always be consulted on ways to reduce hazards in their environment.

## Nursing Process

## Nursing Diagnosis

21. Identify four actual or potential nursing diagnoses for safety risks.

a. _____

b. _____

c. _____

d. _____

## Planning

### Goals and Outcomes

22. Identify three common goals that focus on the patient's need for safety.

a. _____

b. _____

c. _____

### Setting Priorities

23. Planning also involves understanding the patient's _____. You and the patient _____ within the home and health care environment.

## Implementation

Nursing interventions are directed toward ensuring a patient's safety in all settings and include health promotion, developmental interventions, environmental interventions, and limiting specific risks to patient safety.

### Health Promotion

24. Distinguish between passive and active strategies for health promotion.

_____

_____

### Developmental Interventions

25. Identify at least four interventions for each of the following developmental age groups.

a. Infant, toddler, preschooler:

_____

_____

b. School-age:

_____

_____

c. Adolescent:

_____

_____

d. Adult:

_____

_____

e. Older adult:

_____

_____

### Environmental Interventions

26. Describe four fire-containment guidelines outlined in the mnemonic RACE.

a. _____

b. _____

c. _____

d. _____

27. List eight measures to prevent falls in the health care setting.

a. _____

b. _____

c. _____

d. _____

e. _____

f. _____

g. _____

h. _____

#### Restraints

28. A *restraint* is _____. The use of any type of restraint involves a psychological adjustment for the Patient and family.

29. A *physical restraint* is

_____

_____.

30. The immobility imposed by restraining a patient can lead to the following complications.

a. Physical:

_____

_____

b. Psychological:

_____

_____

For legal purposes, know the agency's policy and procedures for the appropriate use and monitoring of physical restraints.

31. Use of restraints must meet the following objectives.

a. _____

b. _____

c. _____

d. _____

32. Distinguish between the following fall prevention devices:

a. *Ambularm*:

_____

_____

b. *Bed-Check* alarm:

_____

_____

c. Posey Bed Enclosure

_____

_____

33. A *chemical restraint* is defined as

_____

_____ .

**Side Rails**

34. Explain the use of side rails.

_____

_____

**Electrical Hazards**

35. List five teaching strategies for prevention of electrical shocks.

a. _____

b. _____

c. _____

d. _____

e. _____

**Seizures**

36. *Seizure precautions* are nursing interventions during and after a seizure and include _____

_____ .

**Radiation**

Radiation is a health hazard in the health care setting from radiation and radioactive materials that are used in the diagnosis and treatment of patients. Additionally, the community can be at risk for radiation exposure if there has been incorrect disposal and transportation of radioactive waste products.

## Evaluation

**Patient Care**

37. The nurse continually assesses the patient's and family's need for additional support services

such as _____, _____,

_____, and _____.

**Patient Expectations**

38. The expected outcomes include a _____

and _____ environment.

## *Review Questions*

Select the appropriate answer, and cite the rationale for choosing that particular answer.

1. Which of the following would most threaten an individual's safety?
   a. 70% humidity
   b. Carbon dioxide
   c. Unrefrigerated fresh vegetables
   d. Lack of a clean water supply

   Answer:_____ Rationale: _____

   _____

   _____

2. The developmental stage that carries the highest risk of an injury from a fall is
   a. Preschool
   b. School-age
   c. Adulthood
   d. Older adulthood

   Answer:_____ Rationale: _____

   _____

   _____

3. Mrs. Gupta falls asleep while smoking in bed and drops the burning cigarette on her blanket. When she awakens, her bed is on fire, and she quickly calls the nurse. On observing the fire, the nurse should immediately
   a. Report the fire
   b. Attempt to extinguish the fire
   c. Assist Mrs. Gupta to a safe place
   d. Close all windows and doors to contain the fire

   Answer:_____ Rationale: _____

   _____

   _____

4. Sixteen-year-old Simon is admitted to an adolescent unit with a diagnosis of substance abuse. The nurse examines Simon and finds that he has bloodshot eyes, slurred speech, and an unstable gait. He smells of alcohol and is unable to answer questions appropriately. The appropriate nursing diagnosis would be
   a. Self-care deficit related to alcohol abuse
   b. Altered thought processes related to sensory overload
   c. Knowledge deficit related to alcohol abuse
   d. High risk for injury related to impaired sensory perception

Answer:_____ Rationale: _____
_____
_____

5. If a patient receives an electric shock, your first action should be to
   a. Assess the patient's airway, breathing, and circulation (pulse)
   b. Assess the patient for thermal injury
   c. Notify the physician
   d. Notify the maintenance department

Answer:_____ Rationale: _____
_____
_____

## Critical Thinking Model for Nursing Care Plan for Risk for Injury

Imagine that you are Mr. Key, the nurse in the Care Plan on pages 800–801 of your text. Complete the *assessment* phase of the critical thinking model by writing your answers in the appropriate boxes of the model shown. Think about the following:

• In developing Ms. Cohen's plan of care, what knowledge did Mr. Key apply?

• In what way might Mr. Key's previous experience assist in this case?

• What intellectual or professional standards were applied to Ms. Cohen's case?

• What critical thinking attitudes might have been applied in this case?

• As you review your assessment, what key areas did you cover?

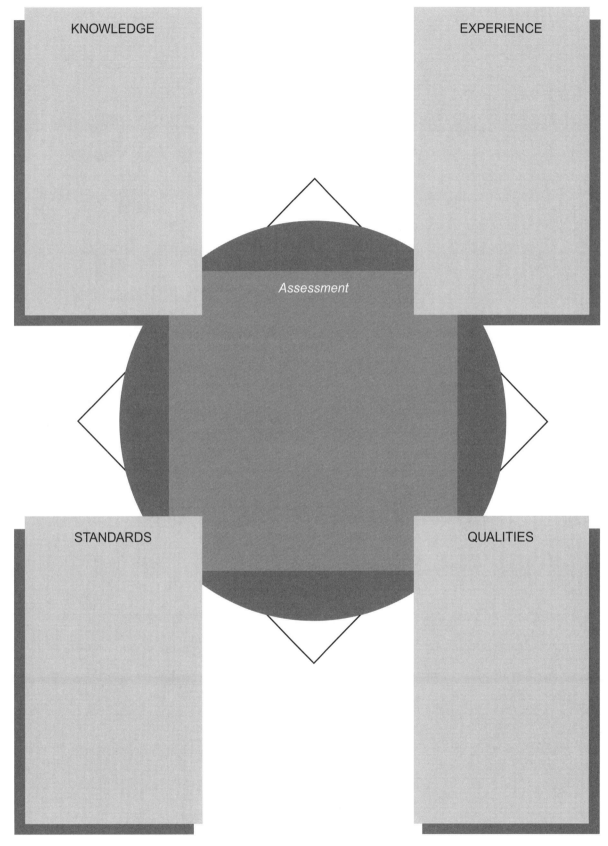

KNOWLEDGE

EXPERIENCE

*Assessment*

STANDARDS

QUALITIES

CHAPTER 36    Critical Thinking Model for Nursing Care Plan for *Risk for Injury*
See answers on Evolve site.

# 37

# Hygiene

## Preliminary Reading

Chapter 37, pages 825–876

## Comprehensive Understanding

Personal hygiene affects an individual's comfort, safety, and physical and psychological well-being. Individuals who are well are capable of meeting their own hygiene needs, but those who are ill or have disabilities may require various levels of assistance.

Hygiene care requires close contact with the patient; therapeutic communication skills should be used to build and promote a caring therapeutic relationship and to assist you in providing the patient with teaching regarding hygiene care.

### Scientific Knowledge Base

Proper hygiene care requires an understanding of the anatomy and physiology of the integument, oral cavity, eyes, ears, nose, hands, feet, and nails. Good hygiene techniques assist in promoting the normal structure and function of body tissues.

### The Skin

1. Identify the functions of the skin.

   _____

   _____

   _____

2. The skin has three primary layers:

   a. _____

   b. _____

   c. _____

3. Bacteria commonly reside on the outer layer of skin (the *epidermis*). These resident bacteria are normal flora; they do not _____ but instead _____ of disease-causing microorganisms.

The skin can provide crucial information regarding a patient's health status and provide important information regarding the functioning of other systems and organs.

### The Feet, Hands, and Nails

The feet, hands, and nails often require special attention to prevent infection.

4. Define the following terms.

   a. *Cuticle*:

   _____

   _____

   b. *Lunula*:

   _____

   _____

   c. Nail bed:

   _____

   _____

### The Oral Cavity

The oral cavity extends from the lips to the anterior pillars of the tonsils. It is the structure for taste, mastication, and speech articulation.

5. The *buccal mucosa* (oral mucosa) are normally

   _____ and _____.

6. The mouth also contains three pairs of salivary glands that start the digestive process by releasing enzymes that

   a. _____

   b. _____

   c. _____

Salivary secretion can be decreased by medications and disease processes.

7. Teeth are organs of chewing, or _____, and are designed to _____.

8. Regular oral hygiene is necessary to maintain the integrity of tooth surfaces and to prevent _____.

## The Hair

9. Identify the factors that can affect the hair's characteristics.

   _____

   _____

## The Eyes, Ears, and Nose

Cleansing of the sensitive sensory tissues should be done in a way to prevent injury and patient discomfort.

## Nursing Knowledge Base

No two individuals perform hygiene in the same manner, and it is important to individualize care from knowledge about the patient's unique hygiene practices and preferences.

10. Briefly explain each of the following factors influencing hygiene habits.

    a. Social practices:

       _____

       _____

       _____

    b. Personal preferences:

       _____

       _____

       _____

    c. Body image:

       _____

       _____

       _____

   d. Socioeconomic status:

      _____

      _____

      _____

   e. Health beliefs and motivation:

      _____

      _____

      _____

   f. Cultural variables:

      _____

      _____

      _____

   g. Physical condition:

      _____

      _____

      _____

## Critical Thinking

Hygiene care is so important for patients to feel comfortable, refreshed, and renewed; you should avoid making hygiene care a simple routine. Instead, integrate knowledge from nursing and other disciplines, previous experiences, and information gathered from patients.

## The Nursing Process

### Assessment

Important considerations include assessment of the patient's ability to perform self-care, usual hygiene practices and preferences, with special attention to balance, coordination, strength, range of motion, and activity tolerance.

#### Physical Examination

Nurses utilize the skills of inspection and palpation; look for alterations in the integrity and function of tissues.

#### The Skin

11. When inspecting the skin, the nurse thoroughly examines:

    a. _____

    b. _____

    c. _____

d. _____

e. _____

f. _____

12. Common skin problems can affect how hygiene is administered. Describe the hygiene provided for the following.

    a. Dry skin:

    _____

    _____

    b. Acne:

    _____

    _____

    c. Skin rashes:

    _____

    _____

    d. Contact dermatitis:

    _____

    _____

    e. Psoriasis:

    _____

    _____

    f. Abrasion:

    _____

    _____

13. Briefly explain the six conditions that place patients at risk for impaired skin integrity.

    a. Immobilization:

    _____

    _____

    b. Reduced sensation:

    _____

    _____

    c. Nutrition and hydration alterations:

    _____

    _____

    d. Secretions and excretions on the skin:

    _____

    _____

e. Vascular insufficiency:

_____

_____

f. External devices:

_____

_____

**The Feet and Nails**

Assessment of the feet involves a thorough examination of all skin surfaces, including the soles of the feet and the areas between the toes.

14. Inspection of the feet for lesions includes noting areas of

    a. _____

    b. _____

    c. _____

15. Define *neuropathy*.

    _____

    _____

    _____

16. Describe a nursing assessment for neuropathy.

    _____

    _____

17. Identify the characteristics of the following foot and nail problems.

    a. Calluses:

    _____

    _____

    b. Corns:

    _____

    _____

    c. Plantar warts:

    _____

    _____

    d. Athlete's foot:

    _____

    _____

    e. Ingrown nails:

    _____

    _____

f. Ram's horn nails:

_____

_____

g. Paronychia:

_____

_____

h. Foot odour:

_____

_____

**The Oral Cavity**

18. The nurse inspects all areas of the oral cavity for

a. _____

b. _____

c. _____

d. _____

19. Define the following terms.

a. *Halitosis*:

_____

_____

b. *Stomatitis*:

_____

_____

**The Hair**

20. Describe the characteristics of the following hair and scalp conditions.

a. Dandruff:

_____

_____

b. Ticks:

_____

_____

c. Pediculosis capitis:

_____

_____

d. Pediculosis corporis:

_____

_____

e. Pediculosis pubis:

_____

_____

f. Alopecia:

_____

_____

**The Eyes, Ears, and Nose**

21. Identify the normal assessment findings for the following.

a. Eyes:

_____

_____

_____

b. Ears:

_____

_____

_____

c. Nose:

_____

_____

_____

**Developmental Changes**

**The Skin**

22. For each developmental stage, briefly describe normal conditions that create a high risk for impaired skin integrity.

a. Neonate:

_____

_____

_____

b. Toddler:

_____

_____

_____

c. Adolescent:

_____

_____

_____

d. Older adult:

_____

_____

_____

**The Feet and Nails**

23. Identify the common foot problems of the older adult.

_____

_____

_____

_____

**The Oral Cavity**

24. Identify the factors associated with aging that can result in poor oral care.

_____

_____

_____

_____

**The Eyes, Ears, and Nose**

As patients age, they are also at risk for changes in visual clarity and visual field losses.

25. Older adults experience the following auditory changes as the result of aging.

a. _____

b. _____

c. _____

Changes in smell seem to be more common in older adults. These changes may also affect taste and patients' appetites.

**Self-Care Ability**

26. Identify the factors that are assessed to determine a patient's ability to perform routine hygiene.

_____

_____

_____

_____

When a patient has self-care limitations, part of the assessment is to determine whether family or friends are available to assist.

**Hygiene Practices**

Asking the patient to assist or teach how to perform preferred grooming practices gives the patient a greater sense of independence and helps you to avoid causing the patient discomfort or injury.

**Cultural Factors**

27. Explain how culture affects a patient's hygiene needs.

_____

_____

_____

_____

**Patients at Risk for Hygiene Problems**

28. Provide examples of patients at risk for the following.

a. Oral problems:

_____

_____

_____

b. Skin problems:

_____

_____

_____

c. Foot problems:

_____

_____

_____

d. Eye care problems:

_____

_____

_____

**Special Considerations in Hygiene Assessment**

29. Explain how footwear may predispose a patient to foot and nail problems.

_____

_____

_____

_____

## Nursing Diagnosis

30. List four possible nursing diagnoses that apply to patients in need of hygiene care.

    a. _____

    b. _____

    c. _____

    d. _____

## Planning

During planning, you synthesize information from multiple resources.

### Goals and Outcomes

31. When providing for patient hygiene, you care for a variety of patients with different self-care abilities and needs. List three possible outcomes.

    a. _____

    b. _____

    c. _____

### Setting Priorities

The patient's condition influences the plan for delivering hygiene.

## Implementation

32. The use of _____ helps to _____ and promote _____ while you perform each hygiene measure.

### Health Promotion

33. List four guidelines for educating patients about hygiene care.

    a. _____

    b. _____

    c. _____

    d. _____

### Acute and Restorative Care

34. Compare and contrast the four types of scheduled care in acute and long-term settings.

    a. _____

    b. _____

    c. _____

    d. _____

### Bathing and Skin Care

The extent of patients' baths and the methods used for bathing depend on their physical abilities, health problems, and the degree of hygiene required.

35. A complete bed bath is _____.

36. A partial bed bath involves _____.

37. Identify guidelines the nurse should follow when assisting or providing a patient with any type of bath.

    _____
    _____
    _____
    _____
    _____
    _____
    _____

### Perineal Care

38. Define *perineal care*, and identify the patients at risk for skin breakdown in the perineal area.

    _____
    _____
    _____
    _____

### Back Rub

39. A back rub promotes

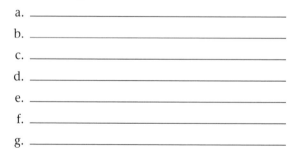

    a. _____

    b. _____

    c. _____

    d. _____

    e. _____

    f. _____

    g. _____

### Foot and Nail Care

40. List at least eight guidelines to include when advising patients with peripheral neuropathy or vascular insufficiency about foot care.

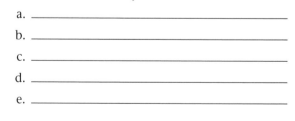

    a. _____

    b. _____

    c. _____

    d. _____

    e. _____

f. _____

g. _____

h. _____

**Oral Hygiene**

41. Oral hygiene helps to maintain _____

_____.

42. Briefly explain the following interventions in relation to oral hygiene.

a. Diet:

_____

_____

_____

b. Brushing and flossing:

_____

_____

_____

c. Oral care for patients with special needs:

_____

_____

_____

d. Denture care:

_____

_____

_____

**Hair and Scalp Care**

43. Briefly describe the rationales for the following.

a. Brushing and combing:

_____

_____

b. Shampooing:

_____

_____

c. Shaving:

_____

_____

d. Moustache and beard care:

_____

_____

**Care of the Eyes, Ears, and Nose**

Care focuses on preventing infection and maintaining normal sensory function.

**Basic Eye Care**

44. Describe basic eye care for a patient.

_____

_____

_____

_____

**Eyeglasses**

45. Describe the correct procedure for cleaning eyeglasses.

_____

_____

_____

_____

**Contact Lenses**

46. Briefly describe proper contact lens care technique.

_____

_____

_____

_____

**Artificial Eyes**

47. Describe each of the following techniques necessary in caring for an artificial eye.

a. Removal:

_____

_____

b. Cleansing:

_____

_____

c. Reinsertion:

_____

_____

d. Storage:

_____

_____

**Ear Care**

48. Describe the procedure for removing cerumen from the ear.

   _____

   _____

   _____

   _____

**Hearing Aid Care**

49. Describe the following types of hearing aids.

   a. In-the-canal:

   _____

   _____

   _____

   b. In-the-ear:

   _____

   _____

   _____

   c. Behind-the-ear:

   _____

   _____

   _____

**Nasal Care**

50. Describe three interventions used to remove secretions from the nose.

   a. _____

   b. _____

   c. _____

**Patient's Room Environment**

**Maintaining Comfort**

51. Identify four factors the nurse can control to create a more comfortable environment.

   a. _____

   b. _____

   c. _____

   d. _____

**Room Equipment**

52. A typical hospital room contains the following basic pieces of furniture:

   a. _____

   b. _____

   c. _____

   d. _____

**Beds**

53. A patient's bed must be frequently inspected to ensure that the linens are _____, _____, and _____.

54. Identify the factors a nurse considers when making a patient's bed.

   _____

   _____

   _____

   _____

   _____

   _____

## Evaluation

**Patient Care**

Evaluation of hygiene measures occurs both before, during, and after each particular skill.

   The standards for evaluation are the expected outcomes established in the planning stage of the patient's care.

**Patient Expectations**

The patient's expectations are important guidelines in determining patient satisfaction.

## Review Questions

Select the appropriate answer, and cite the rationale for choosing that particular answer.

1. Mr. Ng is a 19-year-old patient in the rehabilitation unit. He is completely paralyzed below the neck. The most appropriate bath for Mr. Ng is a
   a. Partial bed bath
   b. Complete bed bath
   c. Sitz bath
   d. Tepid bath

Answer:_____ Rationale: _____

_____

_____

2. All of the following will help maintain skin integrity in the older adult except
   a. Environmental air that is cold and dry
   b. Use of warm water and mild cleansing agents for bathing

c. Bathing every other day
d. Drinking 8 to 10 glasses of water a day

Answer:_____ Rationale: _____
_____
_____

3. When preparing to give complete morning care to a patient, what would the nurse do first?
   a. Gather the necessary equipment and supplies.
   b. Remove the patient's gown or pyjamas while maintaining privacy.
   c. Assess the patient's preferences for bathing practices.
   d. Lower the side rails, and assist the patient to assume a comfortable position.

Answer:_____ Rationale: _____
_____
_____

4. Mrs. Veech has diabetes. Which intervention should be included in her teaching plan regarding foot care?
   a. Use a pumice stone to smooth corns and calluses.
   b. File toenails straight across and square.
   c. Apply powder to dry areas along the feet and between the toes.
   d. Wear elastic stockings to improve circulation.

Answer:_____ Rationale: _____
_____
_____

5. Assessment of the hair and scalp reveals that a patient has pediculosis capitis. An appropriate intervention would be
   a. Shave hair off the affected area
   b. Place oil on the hair and scalp until all of the lice are dead
   c. Use a medicated shampoo, and repeat 7 to 10 days later
   d. Shampoo with regular shampoo, and dry with the hair dryer set at the hottest setting

Answer:_____ Rationale: _____
_____
_____

## Critical Thinking Model for Nursing Care Plan for Ineffective Tissue Perfusion, Improper Foot Care and Hygiene

Imagine that you are the nurse in the Care Plan on pages 839–840 of your text. Complete the *planning* phase of the critical thinking model by writing your answers in the appropriate boxes of the model shown. Think about the following:

- In developing Mr. James's plan of care, what knowledge did you apply?
- In what way might your previous experience assist in developing a plan of care for Mr. James?
- When developing a plan of care, what intellectual and professional standards were applied?
- What critical thinking attitudes might have been applied in developing Mr. James's plan of care?
- How will you accomplish the goals?

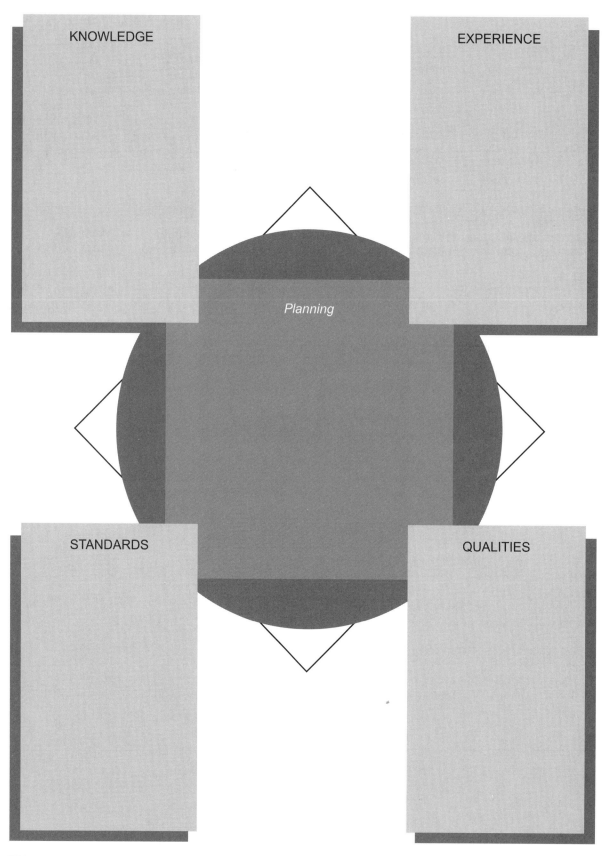

CHAPTER 37   Critical Thinking Model for Nursing Care Plan for *Ineffective Tissue Perfusion, Improper Foot Care, and Hygiene*
See answers on Evolve site.

# 38

# Cardiopulmonary Functioning and Oxygenation

## Preliminary Reading

Chapter 38, pages 877–935

## Comprehensive Understanding

The cardiac and respiratory systems function to supply the body's oxygen demands.

### Scientific Knowledge Base

**Cardiovascular Physiology**

1. Cardiopulmonary physiology involves delivery

   of _____ to the right side of the heart and to the pulmonary circulation, and

   _____ from the lungs to the left side of the heart and the tissues.

2. The cardiac system delivers _____,

   _____, and other _____

   to the tissues, and removes the _____

   through the _____, _____,

   and the _____.

**Structure and Function**

3. The right ventricle pumps blood through the

   _____. The left ventricle pumps

   blood to the _____.

**Myocardial Pump**

4. The four chambers of the heart fill with blood

   during _____ and empty during

   _____.

5. Describe the Frank-Starling law of the heart.

   _____

   _____

   _____

   _____

**Myocardial Blood Flow**

6. Briefly describe the flow of blood through the heart.

   _____

   _____

   _____

   _____

7. Describe the following types of circulation.

   a. Coronary artery:

   _____

   _____

   _____

   b. Systemic:

   _____

   _____

   _____

**Blood Flow Regulation**

8. Describe the following terms related to blood flow regulation.

   a. *Cardiac output:*

   _____

   _____

   b. *Cardiac index:*

   _____

   _____

   c. *Stroke volume:*

   _____

   _____

   d. *Preload:*

   _____

   _____

   e. *Afterload:*

   _____

   _____

   f. *Myocardial contractility:*

   _____

   _____

**Conduction System**

The rhythmic relaxation and contraction of the atria and ventricles depend on continuous, organized transmission of electrical impulses.

9. Describe how the following affect the conduction system of the heart.

   a. Sympathetic nerve fibres:

   _____

   _____

   _____

   _____

   b. Parasympathetic nerve fibres:

   _____

   _____

   _____

   _____

10. Diagram and label the electrical conduction system of the heart in the box below.

11. Diagram and label the components of the electrocardiogram (ECG) waveform for normal sinus rhythm in the box below.

**Respiratory Physiology**

12. The three steps in the process of oxygenation are _____, _____, and _____.

[blank box]

**Structure and Function**

13. The _____, _____, _____, and _____ are essential for ventilation, perfusion, and exchange of respiratory gases.

14. Define *ventilation*.

_____

_____

_____

**Work of Breathing**

Breathing is the effort required for expanding and contracting the lungs.

15. _____ is an _____ process, stimulated by chemical receptors in the

aorta. _____ is a _____ process that depends on the elastic-recoil properties of the lungs, requiring little or no muscle work.

16. Define the following terms related to the work of breathing.

a. Surfactant:

_____

_____

_____

b. Accessory muscles:

_____

_____

_____

c. Compliance:

_____

_____

_____

d. Airway resistance:

_____

_____

_____

### Lung Volumes and Capacities

17. Spirometry is used to _____.

18. Variations in lung volumes may be associated with health states such as _____, _____, _____, or _____ and _____ conditions of the lungs.

19. The amount of _____, _____, and _____ can affect pressures and volumes within the lungs.

### Pulmonary Circulation

20. Briefly describe the pulmonary circulation.

_____

_____

_____

_____

_____

21. Identify the normal distribution of pressures within the pulmonary circulation.

_____

_____

_____

_____

### Respiratory Gas Exchange

22. Respiratory gases are exchanged in the _____ and the _____ of the body tissues.

23. Define *diffusion*.

_____

_____

24. How can the rate of diffusion be affected?

_____

_____

_____

_____

### Oxygen Transport

25. List four factors required for oxygen transport and delivery.

a. _____

b. _____

c. _____

d. _____

### Carbon Dioxide Transport

26. Describe the breakdown of carbon dioxide as it is diffused into the red blood cells.

_____

_____

_____

_____

_____

### Regulation of Respiration

27. Explain the two regulators that control the process of respiration.

a. Neural:

_____

_____

b. Chemical:

_____

_____

### Factors Affecting Oxygenation

28. List the four factors that influence oxygenation.

a. _____

b. _____

c. _____

d. _____

**Physiological Factors**

29. Explain the following factors that affect the body's ability to meet oxygen demands. Give examples of each.

    a. Decreased oxygen-carrying capacity:

    _____
    _____
    _____

    b. Decreased inspired oxygen concentration:

    _____
    _____
    _____

    c. Hypovolemia:

    _____
    _____
    _____

    d. Increased metabolic rate:

    _____
    _____
    _____

**Conditions Affecting Chest Wall Movement**

30. Explain how the following conditions affect chest wall movement.

    a. Pregnancy:

    _____
    _____
    _____

    b. Obesity:

    _____
    _____
    _____

    c. Musculoskeletal abnormalities:

    _____
    _____
    _____

    d. Trauma:

    _____
    _____
    _____

    e. Neuromuscular diseases:

    _____
    _____
    _____

    f. Central nervous system alterations:

    _____
    _____
    _____

    g. Influences of chronic disease:

    _____
    _____
    _____

**Alterations in Cardiac Functioning**

31. Illnesses and conditions that affect _____,

    _____, _____, _____,

    and _____ cause alterations in cardiac functioning.

**Disturbances in Conduction**

32. Define *dysrhythmias.*

    _____
    _____
    _____
    _____

33. Briefly describe the following dysrhythmias.

    a. Sinus tachycardia:

    _____
    _____

    b. Sinus bradycardia:

    _____
    _____

    c. *Atrial fibrillation*:

    _____
    _____

    d. *Ventricular tachycardia*:

    _____
    _____

    e. *Ventricular fibrillation*:

    _____
    _____

f. *Asystole*:

_____

_____

**Altered Cardiac Output**

34. Failure of the myocardium to eject sufficient volume to the systemic and pulmonary circulations can result in left-sided and right-sided heart failure. Complete the grid below.

| Type of Heart Failure | Clinical Findings |
|---|---|
| Left-sided | |
| Right-sided | |

**Impaired Valvular Function**

35. Define each of the following.

a. Valvular heart disease:

_____

_____

_____

b. Stenosis:

_____

_____

_____

c. Regurgitation:

_____

_____

_____

d. Myocardial ischemia:

_____

_____

_____

e. Angina pectoris:

_____

_____

_____

f. Myocardial infarction:

_____

_____

_____

36. Describe the chest pain associated with myocardial infarction.

_____

_____

_____

_____

**Acute Coronary Syndrome**

37. Briefly explain acute coronary syndrome.

_____

_____

_____

_____

**Alterations in Respiratory Functioning**

38. The three primary alterations in respiratory function are _____, _____, and _____.

39. Complete the grid below to identify the causes, signs, and symptoms of alterations in respiratory functioning.

| Alterations | Causes | Signs and Symptoms |
|---|---|---|
| Hyperventilation | | |
| Hypoventilation | | |
| Hypoxia | | |

40. Define the following terms.

   a. *Atelectasis*:

   _____

   _____

   _____

   b. *Cyanosis*:

   _____

   _____

   _____

## Nursing Knowledge Base

**Developmental Factors**

41. Identify at least one physiological factor influencing tissue oxygenation for each developmental level listed.

   a. Infants and toddlers:

   _____

   _____

   b. School-age children and adolescents:

   _____

   _____

   c. Young and middle-aged adults:

   _____

   _____

   d. Older adults:

   _____

   _____

**Lifestyle Risk Factors**

42. Briefly describe how the following lifestyle factors influence respiratory function.

   a. Poor nutrition:

   _____

   _____

   _____

   b. Inadequate exercise:

   _____

   _____

   _____

   c. Smoking:

   _____

   _____

   _____

   d. Substance abuse:

   _____

   _____

   _____

   e. Stress:

   _____

   _____

   _____

**Environmental Factors**

43. List four occupational pollutants.

   a. _____

   b. _____

   c. _____

   d. _____

**Nursing Process**

**Assessment**

44. Briefly describe health history for

   a. Cardiac function:

   _____
   _____
   _____

   b. Respiratory function:

   _____
   _____
   _____

45. Define the following terms.

   a. Fatigue:

   _____
   _____
   _____

   b. *Dyspnea*:

   _____
   _____
   _____

   c. *Orthopnea*:

   _____
   _____
   _____

   d. Cough:

   _____
   _____
   _____

   e. Productive cough:

   _____
   _____
   _____

   f. *Hemoptysis*:

   _____
   _____
   _____

   g. *Wheezing*:

   _____
   _____

46. Briefly explain why special considerations are necessary for older patients during the physical examination.

   _____
   _____
   _____

47. Briefly explain the following techniques used during the physical examination to assess tissue oxygenation.

   a. Inspection:

   _____
   _____
   _____

   b. Palpation:

   _____
   _____
   _____

   c. Percussion:

   _____
   _____
   _____

   d. Auscultation:

   _____
   _____
   _____

**Diagnostic Tests**

48. Describe the following tests that determine myocardial contraction and blood flow.

   a. Echocardiography:

   _____
   _____

   b. Scintigraphy:

   _____
   _____

   c. Cardiac catheterization and angiography:

   _____
   _____

49. Describe the following diagnostic tests used to determine the adequacy of the cardiac conduction system.

    a. Electrocardiogram:

    _____

    _____

    b. Holter monitor:

    _____

    _____

    c. ECG exercise stress test:

    _____

    _____

    d. Thallium stress test:

    _____

    _____

50. Describe the following tests used to measure the adequacy of ventilation and oxygenation.

    a. Pulse oximetry:

    _____

    _____

    b. Arterial blood gases:

    _____

    _____

    c. Pulmonary function tests:

    _____

    _____

    d. Chest X-ray examination:

    _____

    _____

    e. Computed tomography scan:

    _____

    _____

    f. Ventilation/perfusion (nuclear medicine) lung scan:

    _____

    _____

51. Describe the following tests used to determine abnormal cells or infection in the respiratory tract.

    a. Sputum tests:

    _____

    _____

    b. Tracheal aspiration via endotracheal tube in intubated patients:

    _____

    _____

    c. Bronchoscopy:

    _____

    _____

    d. Thoracentesis:

    _____

    _____

    e. Nasopharyngeal aspirate or swab:

    _____

    _____

## Nursing Diagnosis

Patients with an altered level of oxygenation can have nursing diagnoses that are primarily from a cardiovascular or pulmonary origin.

## Planning

### Goals and Outcomes

52. List four goals appropriate for a patient with actual or potential oxygenation needs.

    a. _____

    b. _____

    c. _____

    d. _____

## Implementation

### Health Promotion

53. Describe the purpose of the influenza and pneumococcal vaccines, and explain for whom the vaccines are recommended.

_____

_____

_____

_____

_____

### Healthy Lifestyle Behaviour

54. Identify some healthy lifestyle behaviours that decrease the risk of cardiopulmonary disease.

_____

_____

_____

_____

### Acute Care

55. Nursing interventions for the patient with acute pulmonary illnesses are directed toward

_____, _____, and _____.

### Dyspnea Management

56. List four treatment modalities appropriate for a patient with dyspnea.

a. _____

b. _____

c. _____

d. _____

### Airway Maintenance

The airway is patent when the trachea, bronchi, and large airways are free from obstructions.

### Mobilization of Pulmonary Secretions

57. Nursing interventions that promote mobilization of pulmonary secretions include the following. Briefly explain each one.

a. _Humidification_:

_____

_____

_____

b. _Nebulization_:

_____

_____

_____

c. _Chest physiotherapy (CPT)_:

_____

_____

_____

58. Briefly describe the three activities involved in CPT.

a. Chest percussion:

_____

_____

_____

b. Vibration:

_____

_____

_____

c. Postural drainage:

_____

_____

_____

### Suctioning Techniques

Suctioning is necessary when a patient is unable to clear respiratory tract secretions with coughing.

59. Briefly explain the following types of suctioning techniques.

a. Oropharyngeal and nasopharyngeal:

_____

_____

_____

b. Orotracheal and nasotracheal:

_____

_____

_____

c. Tracheal:

_____

_____

_____

**Maintenance and Promotion of Lung Expansion**

60. Nursing interventions that maintain or promote lung expansion include the following noninvasive techniques. Briefly explain each.

    a. Positioning:

    _____
    _____
    _____
    _____

    b. Incentive spirometry:

    _____
    _____
    _____
    _____

**Chest Tubes**

61. Identify the three reasons for inserting chest tubes.

    a. _____
    b. _____
    c. _____

62. Define the following.

    a. *Pneumothorax*:

    _____
    _____
    _____

    b. *Hemothorax*:

    _____
    _____
    _____

63. Discuss the two types of drainage devices used with chest tubes.

    a. _____
    b. _____

**Special Considerations**

64. Identify five special considerations the nurse needs to address when dealing with chest tubes.

    a. _____
    b. _____
    c. _____
    d. _____
    e. _____

**Maintenance and Promotion of Oxygenation**

Promotion of lung expansion, mobilization of secretions, and maintenance of a patent airway assist the patient in meeting oxygenation needs.

65. Identify the goal of oxygen therapy.

    _____
    _____
    _____

**Safety Precautions**

66. List five safety measures to institute when a patient receives oxygen.

    a. _____
    b. _____
    c. _____
    d. _____
    e. _____

**Methods of Oxygen Delivery**

67. Describe the following methods of oxygen delivery, and identify the usual flow rates.

    a. *Nasal cannula*:

    _____
    _____

    b. Face mask:

    _____
    _____

    c. Partial-rebreathing mask and the non-rebreathing mask:

    _____
    _____

    d. Venturi mask:

    _____
    _____

**Home Oxygen Therapy**

68. Identify the indications for a patient to receive home oxygen therapy.

    _____
    _____
    _____
    _____

69. Identify the teaching required by the patient for use of home oxygen therapy.

_____

_____

_____

_____

**Restoration of Cardiopulmonary Functioning**

If a patient's hypoxia is severe and prolonged, cardiac arrest may result. Permanent heart, brain, and other tissue damage occur within 4 to 6 minutes.

**Cardiopulmonary Resuscitation (CPR)**

70. List the sequence of steps for CPR.

    a. _____

    b. _____

    c. _____

**Restorative and Continuing Care**

71. Cardiopulmonary rehabilitation is

_____.

**Hydration**

Maintenance of adequate systemic hydration keeps mucociliary clearance normal.

**Coughing Techniques**

72. Coughing is effective for maintaining a patent airway. List four coughing techniques.

    a. _____

    b. _____

    c. _____

    d. _____

**Respiratory Muscle Training**

Respiratory muscle training improves muscle strength and endurance, resulting in improved activity tolerance.

**Breathing Exercises**

73. Briefly explain the following breathing exercises used to improve ventilation and oxygenation.

    a. *Pursed-lip breathing*:

_____

_____

_____

    b. *Diaphragmatic breathing*:

_____

_____

_____

## Evaluation

**Patient Care**

The nurse evaluates the actual care provided to the patient by the health care team based on the expected outcomes.

The patient is the only person who can evaluate his or her degree of breathlessness.

74. The evaluation of _____ and _____ are done by comparing the patient's _____ with the goals and _____ of the nursing care plan.

**Patient Expectations**

Evaluate the care from the patient's perspective.

Working closely with the patient will enable the nurse to redefine those patient expectations that can be realistically met within the limitations of the patient's condition and treatment.

## *Review Questions*

Select the appropriate answer, and cite the rationale for choosing that particular answer.

1. Ventilation, perfusion, and exchange of gases are the major purposes of
    a. Respiration
    b. Circulation
    c. Aerobic metabolism
    d. Anaerobic metabolism

Answer: _____ Rationale: _____

_____

_____

2. Afterload refers to
   a. The amount of blood ejected from the left ventricle each minute
   b. The amount of blood ejected from the left ventricle with each contraction
   c. The resistance to left ventricle ejection
   d. The amount of blood in the left ventricle

Answer: _____ Rationale: _____
_____
_____

3. The movement of gases into and out of the lungs depends on the
   a. 50% oxygen content in the atmospheric air
   b. Pressure gradient between the atmosphere and the alveoli
   c. Use of accessory muscles of respiration during expiration
   d. Amount of carbon dioxide dissolved in the fluid of the alveoli

Answer: _____ Rationale: _____
_____
_____

4. The patient's ECG shows a regular rhythm with a rate of 140-160 beats per minute. The P-wave and QRS complex are normal. This is referred to as
   a. Sinus tachycardia
   b. Sinus dysrhythmia
   c. Supraventricular tachycardia
   d. Premature ventricular contractions

Answer: _____ Rationale: _____
_____
_____

5. Mr. Isaac comes to the emergency department complaining of difficulty breathing. An objective finding associated with his dyspnea might be
   a. Statements about a sense of impending doom
   b. Complaints of shortness of breath
   c. Feelings of heaviness in the chest
   d. Use of accessory muscles of respiration

Answer: _____ Rationale: _____
_____
_____

6. The use of chest physiotherapy to mobilize pulmonary secretions involves the use of:
   a. Hydration
   b. Percussion
   c. Nebulization
   d. Humidification

Answer: _____ Rationale: _____
_____
_____

## Critical Thinking Model for Nursing Care Plan for Ineffective Airway Clearance/Retained Secretions

Imagine that you are the student nurse in the Care Plan on page 898 of your text. Complete the assessment phase of the critical thinking model by writing your answers in the appropriate boxes of the model shown. Think about the following:

- What knowledge base was applied to Mr. Edwards?

- In what way might your previous experience apply in this case?

- What intellectual or professional standards were applied to Mr. Edwards?

- What critical thinking attitudes did you use in assessing Mr. Edwards?

- As you review your assessment, what key areas did you cover?

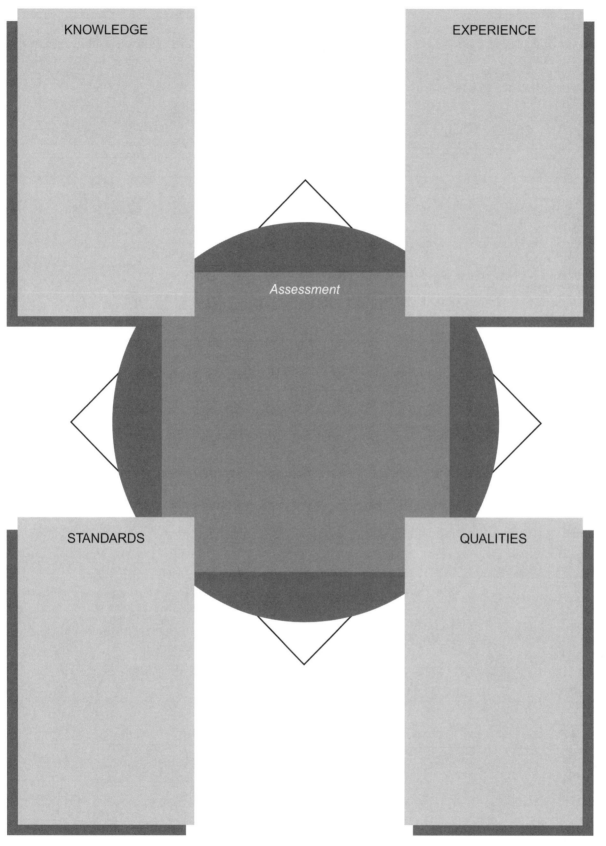

KNOWLEDGE

EXPERIENCE

Assessment

STANDARDS

QUALITIES

CHAPTER 38   Critical Thinking Model for Nursing Care Plan for *Ineffective Airway Clearance/Retained Secretions*
See answers on Evolve site.

# 39

# Fluid, Electrolyte, and Acid-Base Balances

## Preliminary Reading

Chapter 39, pages 936–991

## Comprehensive Understanding

Fluid, electrolyte, and acid–base balances within the body are essential for normal body function.

### Scientific Knowledge Base

1. _____ is the largest single component of the body, 60% of the average adult's weight.

### Distribution of Body Fluids

2. Body fluids are distributed in two distinct compartments. Briefly explain each one.

   a. *Extracellular fluid (ECF)*:

   _____
   _____

   b. *Intracellular fluid (ICF)*:

   _____
   _____

3. ECFs are divided into three smaller compartments. Explain each.

   a. *Interstitial fluid*:

   _____
   _____

   b. *Intravascular fluid*:

   _____
   _____

   c. *Transcellular fluid*:

   _____
   _____

### Composition of Body Fluids

4. Define *electrolytes*.

   _____
   _____
   _____

5. Define the following terms related to the composition of body fluids.

   a. *Cations*:

   _____
   _____

   b. *Anions*:

   _____
   _____

   c. mmol/L:

   _____
   _____

   d. *Solute*:

   _____
   _____

   e. *Solvent*:

   _____
   _____

f. Minerals:

_____

_____

## Movement of Body Fluids

Fluids and electrolytes constantly shift between compartments to facilitate body processes.

6. List and briefly describe the four factors responsible for the movement of body fluids.

a. _____

b. _____

c. _____

d. _____

## Osmosis

7. Define the following terms related to osmosis.

a. *Osmotic pressure*:

_____

_____

b. *Colloid osmotic pressure or oncotic pressure*:

_____

_____

8. Define *hydrostatic pressure*.

_____

_____

_____

## Carrier-Mediated Transport

9. *Carrier-mediated transport* moves molecules across the plasma membrane. Give two examples of carrier-mediated transport.

a. _____

b. _____

## Regulation of Body Fluids

10. Body fluids are regulated by _____, _____, and _____. This balance is termed _____.

## Fluid Output Regulation

11. Fluid output occurs through four organs. List and explain each one.

a. _____

b. _____

c. _____

d. _____

## Fluid Intake Regulation

12. Briefly describe the physiological stimuli triggering the thirst mechanism.

_____

_____

_____

_____

## Hormonal Regulation

13. For each hormone in the grid below, identify the stimuli for its release and its influence on fluid and electrolyte balance.

| Hormone | Stimuli | Action |
|---|---|---|
| *Antidiuretic hormone* | | |
| *Aldosterone* | | |

## Regulation of Electrolytes

For normal cell function and human well-being, the body maintains a normal balance of electrolytes in the ECF and ICF despite changes in intake and loss.

14. The major cations within the body fluids include _____, _____, _____, and _____.

15. The major anions are _____, _____, and _____.

16. Give the normal values, function, and regulatory mechanisms for the major body electrolytes in the following grid.

| Electrolyte | Normal Value | Function | Regulatory Mechanism |
| --- | --- | --- | --- |
| Sodium | | | |
| Potassium | | | |
| Calcium | | | |
| Magnesium | | | |
| Chloride | | | |
| Bicarbonate | | | |
| Phosphate | | | |

**Regulation of Acid–Base Balance**

Acid–base balance exists when the rate at which the body produces and gains acids or bases, through cellular metabolism and gastrointestinal (GI) absorption, equals the rate at which acids or bases are excreted.

17. A _____ is a substance or a group of substances, such as _____, _____ and _____ that can absorb or release hydrogen ions to stabilize pH. Whereas the _____ act immediately, the response by the _____ may take minutes, and the response in the _____ much longer.

The four main types of buffer systems are protein; hemoglobin; carbonic acid and bicarbonate; and phosphate.

**Regulatory Mechanisms**

When the ability of buffer systems is exceeded, acid–base homeostasis is regulated by the lungs and the kidneys.

18. Describe how the following organs adapt to acid–base regulation.

a. Kidneys:

_____

_____

b. Lungs:

_____

_____

**Disturbances in Electrolyte, Fluid, and Acid–Base Balance**

Disturbances in electrolyte, fluid, or acid–base balance seldom occur alone and can disrupt normal body processes.

19. For each electrolyte disturbance, identify the diagnostic laboratory finding, and list at least four characteristic signs and symptoms in the grid below.

| Imbalance | Lab Findings | Signs and Symptoms |
|---|---|---|
| Hyponatremia | | |
| Hypernatremia | | |
| Hypokalemia | | |
| Hyperkalemia | | |
| Hypocalcemia | | |
| Hypercalcemia | | |
| Hypomagnesemia | | |
| Hypermagnesemia | | |

20. The basic types of fluid imbalances are
_____ and _____.

**Fluid Disturbances**

21. *Isotonic* deficit and excess exist when
_____.

22. Osmolar imbalances are _____.

**Acid–Base Balance**

23. Briefly explain the following components of the acid–base balance.

   a. pH:
   _____
   _____

   b. PaCO$_2$:
   _____
   _____

   c. PaO$_2$:
   _____
   _____

   d. Oxygen saturation:
   _____
   _____

   e. *Base excess*:
   _____
   _____

   f. Bicarbonate:
   _____
   _____

24. Complete the grid below giving the causes and signs and symptoms of the listed fluid disturbances.

| Fluid Disturbances | Causes | Signs and Symptoms |
|---|---|---|
| *Fluid volume deficit* | | |
| *Fluid volume excess* | | |
| Hyperosmolar imbalance | | |
| Hypo-osmolar imbalance | | |

**Types of Acid–Base Imbalances**

25. The four primary types of acid–base imbalances are listed in the following grid. For each acid–base imbalance, identify the diagnostic laboratory finding, and list the characteristic signs and symptoms.

| Acid-Base Imbalance | Causes | Signs and Symptoms |
|---|---|---|
| *Respiratory acidosis* | | |
| *Respiratory alkalosis* | | |
| *Metabolic acidosis* | | |
| *Metabolic alkalosis* | | |

## Knowledge Base of Nursing Practice

26. List five major risk factors that can affect fluid and electrolyte imbalances. Give two examples of each.

   a. _____

   b. _____

   c. _____

   d. _____

   e. _____

## Assessment

**Health History**

**Age**

27. Briefly describe the fluid changes that are associated with aging and development.

   a. Infants:

   _____

   _____

   b. Children:

   _____

   _____

   c. Adolescents:

   _____

   _____

   d. Older adults:

   _____

   _____

**Environmental Factors**

28. Briefly explain how the following affect fluid, electrolyte, and acid–base imbalances.

   a. Environmental factors:

   _____

   _____

   _____

b. Diet:

_____

_____

_____

c. Lifestyle factors:

_____

_____

_____

d. Medication:

_____

_____

_____

**Prior Medical History**

**Acute Illness**

29. Explain how the following acute illnesses affect fluid, electrolyte, and acid–base balances.

a. Surgery:

_____

_____

_____

b. Burns:

_____

_____

_____

c. Respiratory disorders:

_____

_____

_____

d. GI disturbances:

_____

_____

_____

e. Head injury:

_____

_____

_____

**Chronic Illness**

30. Describe how the following chronic illnesses affect fluid, electrolyte, and acid–base imbalances.

a. Cancer:

_____

_____

_____

b. Cardiovascular disease:

_____

_____

_____

c. Renal disorders:

_____

_____

_____

d. GI disorders:

_____

_____

_____

e. HIV/AIDS:

_____

_____

_____

**Physical Assessment**

A thorough physical examination is necessary because fluid and electrolyte imbalances or acid–base disturbances can affect all body systems.

31. Indicate the possible fluid, electrolyte, or acid–base imbalances associated with each physical finding.

a. Weight loss of 5% to 10%:

_____

_____

b. Irritability:

_____

_____

c. Lethargy:

_____

_____

d. Periorbital edema:

_____

_____

e. Sticky, dry mucous membranes:

_____

_____

f. Distended neck veins:

_____

_____

g. Dysrhythmias:

_____

_____

h. Weak pulse:

_____

_____

i. Low blood pressure:

_____

_____

j. Third heart sound:

_____

_____

k. Increased respiratory rate:

_____

_____

l. Crackles:

_____

_____

m. Anorexia:

_____

_____

n. Abdominal cramps:

_____

_____

o. Poor skin turgor:

_____

_____

p. Oliguria or anuria:

_____

_____

q. Increased specific gravity:

_____

_____

r. Muscle cramps, tetany:

_____

_____

s. Hypertonicity of muscles on palpation:

_____

_____

t. Decreased or absent deep-tendon reflexes:

_____

_____

u. Increased body temperature:

_____

_____

v. Distended abdomen:

_____

_____

w. Cold, clammy skin:

_____

_____

x. Edema (dependent body parts):

_____

_____

**Measuring Fluid Intake and Output**

32. When implementing specific measures to increase or decrease fluid, three interventions are necessary. Explain each one.

a. Daily weights:

_____

_____

_____

b. Intake:

_____

_____

_____

c. Output:

_____

_____

_____

Recording intake and output is essential for obtaining an accurate database. This information helps maintain an ongoing evaluation of the patient's hydration status to prevent severe imbalances.

### Arterial Blood Gases

To determine arterial blood gas levels, a sample of blood from an artery must be taken to assess the patient's acid–base status and the adequacy of ventilation and oxygenation.

## Nursing Diagnosis

33. List five potential or actual nursing diagnoses for a patient with fluid, electrolyte, or acid–base imbalances.

    a. _____

    b. _____

    c. _____

    d. _____

    e. _____

## Planning

### Goals and Outcomes

34. List three goals that are appropriate for a patient with a fluid, electrolyte, or acid–base imbalance.

    a. _____

    b. _____

    c. _____

### Setting Priorities

The patient's clinical condition will determine which diagnosis takes the greatest priority. Many nursing diagnoses in the area of fluid, electrolyte, and acid–base balances are of highest priority because the consequences for the patient can be serious or even life-threatening.

## Implementation

### Health Promotion

35. Identify some common risk factors for imbalances for which the caregiver may implement appropriate preventive measures.

    _____

    _____

    _____

    _____

### Acute Care

### Enteral Replacement of Fluids

36. List and briefly describe the enteral replacement of fluids.

    a. _____

    b. _____

### Restriction of Fluids

37. Briefly explain the need for a restricted fluid intake and how the nurse would implement the restriction.

    _____

    _____

    _____

    _____

    _____

### Interventions for Acid–Base Imbalances

Nursing interventions to promote acid–base balance support prescribed medical therapies and are aimed at reversing the acid–base imbalance.

### Parenteral Replacement of Fluids and Electrolytes

Fluid and electrolytes may be replaced through infusion directly into the blood rather than via the digestive system.

38. List the three methods of parenteral fluid replacement.

    a. _____

    b. _____

    c. _____

### Vascular Access Devices

39. Vascular access devices are

    _____.

40. Discuss the difference between peripheral vascular access devices and central vascular access devices.

    _____

    _____

    _____

41. Total parenteral nutrition is

    _____.

Administration of Intravenous Therapy

42. Identify the primary goal of intravenous (IV) fluid administration.

_____
_____
_____
_____

43. Define the following types of electrolyte solutions.

a. Isotonic:

_____
_____

b. Hypertonic:

_____
_____

c. Hypotonic:

_____
_____

Venipuncture Site

44. List three groups of patients for whom venipunctures may be difficult.

a. _____
b. _____
c. _____

Complications of Intravenous Therapy

48. Complete the grid below describing complications of IV therapy.

| Complication | Assessment Finding | Nursing Action |
| --- | --- | --- |
| Infiltration | | |
| Phlebitis | | |
| Bleeding | | |

Discontinuing Intravenous Infusions

49. Briefly summarize the procedure for discontinuing IV infusions.

_____
_____
_____
_____

Regulating the Infusion Flow Rate

45. List two major purposes of infusion pumps.

a. _____
b. _____

46. List four factors that may affect IV flow rates.

a. _____
b. _____
c. _____
d. _____

Maintaining the System

47. After the IV line is in place and the flow rate is regulated, you must maintain the system. Line maintenance is achieved by _____, _____, and _____.

Blood Replacement

50. List three objectives for blood transfusion.

a. _____
b. _____
c. _____

**Blood Groups and Types**

51. Complete the grid below describing the major blood groups.

|  | **A** | **B** | **O** | **AB** |
|---|---|---|---|---|
| Antigens present |  |  |  |  |
| Antibodies present |  |  |  |  |

52. Define a *transfusion reaction*.

_____

_____

_____

**Autologous Transfusion**

53. Define *autologous transfusion* (auto-transfusion).

_____

_____

_____

_____

**Blood Transfusions**

54. Identify the five nursing interventions associated with blood transfusions and give the rationale for each.

a. _____

b. _____

c. _____

d. _____

e. _____

**Transfusion Reactions**

A *transfusion reaction* is a systemic response by the body to incompatible blood.

55. Discuss causes of transfusion reactions.

_____

_____

_____

56. Identify types of transfusion reactions and their causes.

a. _____

b. _____

c. _____

d. _____

e. _____

f. _____

57. List the steps the nurse should follow if a transfusion reaction is suspected.

a. _____

b. _____

c. _____

d. _____

e. _____

f. _____

g. _____

h. _____

**Restorative Care**

58. Older adults and patients with chronic illnesses require special considerations to prevent complications from developing. Briefly summarize the following.

a. Home IV therapy:

_____

_____

_____

b. Nutritional support:

_____

_____

_____

c. Medication safety:

_____

_____

_____

# Evaluation

**Patient Care**

The nurse evaluates the actual care delivered by the health care team based on the expected outcomes.

The nurse will perform evaluative measures and determine if changes have occurred since the last patient assessment. The patient's level of progress determines whether the nurse needs to continue or revise the care plan.

### Patient Expectations

Nurses routinely review with their patient their success in meeting expectations of care.

Often the patient's level of satisfaction with care also depends on the nurse's success in involving friends and family.

## *Review Questions*

Select the appropriate answer, and cite the rationale for choosing that particular answer.

1. The body fluids composing the interstitial fluid and blood plasma are:
   a. Intracellular
   b. Extracellular
   c. Hypotonic
   d. Hypertonic

   Answer: _____ Rationale: _____
   _____
   _____

2. Which of the following statements is true with regard to the lungs' regulation of acid–base balance?
   a. The lungs serve a minor role in the physiological buffering of $H^+$ ions.
   b. It takes several days for the lungs to restore pH to a normal level.
   c. The lungs correct imbalances by altering the rate and depth of respiration.
   d. The lungs maintain normal pH by either retaining or excreting bicarbonate.

   Answer: _____ Rationale: _____
   _____
   _____

3. Mrs. Singh's arterial blood gas results are as follows: pH 7.32; $PaCO_2$ 52 mm Hg; $PaO_2$ 78 mm Hg; $HCO_3^-$ 24 mmol/L. Mrs. Singh has
   a. Respiratory acidosis
   b. Respiratory alkalosis
   c. Metabolic acidosis
   d. Metabolic alkalosis

   Answer: _____ Rationale: _____
   _____
   _____

4. Mr. Frank is an 82-year-old patient who has had a 3-day history of vomiting and diarrhea. Which symptom would you expect to find on a physical examination?
   a. Neck vein distension
   b. Crackles in the lungs
   c. Tachycardia
   d. Hypertension

   Answer: _____ Rationale: _____
   _____
   _____

5. Which of the following is most likely to result in respiratory alkalosis?
   a. Fad dieting
   b. Hyperventilation
   c. Chronic alcoholism
   d. Steroid use

   Answer: _____ Rationale: _____
   _____
   _____

## *Critical Thinking Model for Nursing Care Plan for Fluid, Electrolyte, and Acid–Base Balances*

Imagine that you are the student nurse in the Care Plan on pages 956–957 of your text. Complete the *planning* phase of the critical thinking model by writing your answers in the appropriate boxes of the model shown. Think about the following:

* When developing a plan of care, what intellectual and professional standards did you apply?

* In developing Mrs. Topping's plan of care, what knowledge did you apply?

* In what way might your previous experience assist you in developing a plan of care for Mrs. Topping?

* What critical thinking attitudes might have been applied in developing Mrs. Topping's care?

* How will you accomplish your goals?

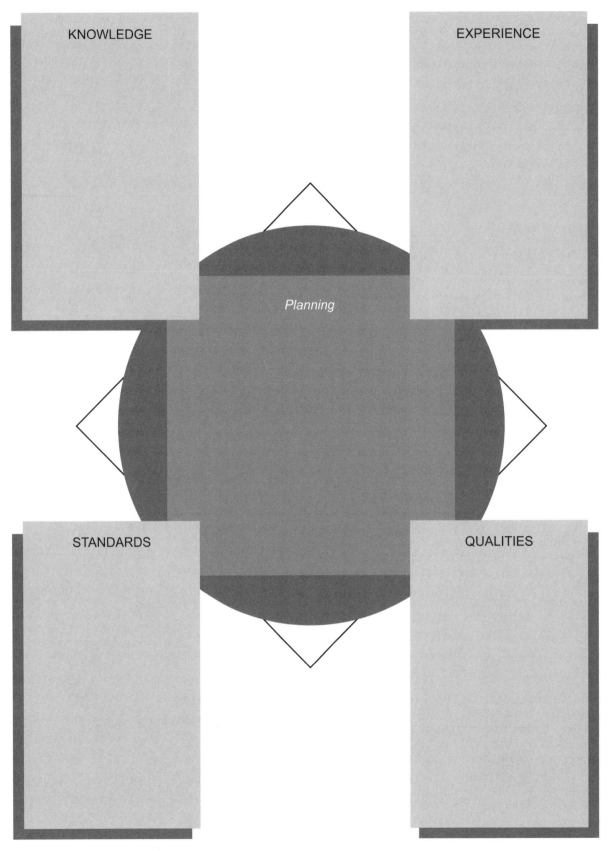

KNOWLEDGE

EXPERIENCE

Planning

STANDARDS

QUALITIES

CHAPTER 39   Critical Thinking Model for Nursing Care Plan for *Fluid, Electrolyte, and Acid-Base Balances*
See answers on Evolve site.

# 40

# Sleep

*Preliminary Reading*

Chapter 40, pages 992–1016

## *Comprehensive Understanding*

Sleep is a basic necessity of life and is as important as air, food, and water.

## Scientific Knowledge Base

### Definition of Sleep

1. Define *sleep*.

    _____

    _____

    _____

### Physiology of Sleep

2. *Sleep* is a cyclical physiological process that alternates with longer periods of wakefulness.
Sleep physiology is controlled by

    a. _____

    b. _____

    c. _____

### Circadian Rhythms

3. Define c*ircadian rhythm*.

    _____

    _____

    _____

4. List four factors that affect circadian rhythms:

    a. _____

    b. _____

    c. _____

    d. _____

5. Define *biological clocks*.

    _____

    _____

### Sleep Regulation

6. Sleep involves a sequence of physiological states maintained by highly integrated central nervous system activity that is associated with changes in the systems listed below:

    a. _____

    b. _____

    c. _____

    d. _____

    e. _____

    f. _____

    g. _____

7. Summarize the function of the reticular activating system.

    _____

    _____

    _____

    _____

Whether a person remains awake or falls asleep depends on a balance of impulses received from higher centres, peripheral sensory receptors, and the limbic system.

8. Describe what the area of the brain called the *bulbar synchronizing region* (BSR) is responsible for.

_____

_____

_____

**Stages of Sleep**

9. Explain the two stages of sleep.

   a. NREM sleep:

   _____

   _____

   b. REM sleep:

   _____

   _____

**Sleep Cycle**

10. Describe the characteristics of the following cycles of sleep.

   a. Stage 1:

   _____

   _____

   b. Stage 2:

   _____

   _____

   c. Stage 3:

   _____

   _____

   d. Stage 4:

   _____

   _____

   e. REM:

   _____

   _____

**Functions of Sleep**

11. Explain briefly the functions of sleep.

_____

_____

_____

_____

**Dreams**

Dreaming is defined as a mental activity that occurs while individuals are asleep.

12. Differentiate between dreams occurring in

   a. NREM sleep:

   _____

   _____

   b. REM sleep:

   _____

   _____

**Physical Illness**

13. Explain how the following conditions affect sleep.

   a. Illness:

   _____

   b. Respiratory disease:

   _____

   c. Cardiovascular disease:

   _____

   _____

   d. Musculoskeletal disorders:

   _____

   e. Nocturia:

   _____

   _____

**Sleep Disorders**

Sleep disorders are conditions that interfere with nighttime sleep. Increasingly, evidence suggests sleep disorders are related to serious medical conditions.

14. Briefly describe the following categories of sleep disorders.

   a. *Hypersomnias*:

   _____

   _____

   b. *Parasomnias*:

   _____

   _____

**Insomnia**

15. Define *insomnia*.

_____

_____

Insomnia is the second most commonly expressed complaint reported in clinical practice after pain. Insomnia is more common in women, and its incidence increases with advancing age.

16. Discuss the condition that is associated with insomnia.

_____

_____

**Sleep Apnea**

17. Define *sleep apnea*.

_____

_____

18. Define the following types of apnea.

   a. Central sleep apnea:

   _____

   _____

   _____

   b. Obstructive sleep apnea (OSA):

   _____

   _____

   _____

19. Discuss the symptoms of OSA.

_____

_____

_____

20. The risk factors for developing OSA are

   a. _____
   b. _____
   c. _____
   d. _____
   e. _____
   f. _____
   g. _____

21. Briefly explain excessive daytime sleepiness.

_____

_____

_____

_____

22. Define *narcolepsy*.

_____

_____

_____

23. Define *cataplexy*.

_____

_____

_____

**Narcolepsy**

24. Identify the developmental stage in which narcolepsy symptoms first develop.

_____

_____

_____

There is no known cure for narcolepsy, and therefore, treatment is targeted at symptom management.

25. Identify the following treatment modalities for a patient with narcolepsy.

   a. Pharmacological:

   _____

   _____

   b. Nonpharmacological:

   _____

   _____

**Parasomnias**

Parasomnias are undesirable sleep problems that occur while falling asleep, between sleep phases, or during transitions from sleep to wakefulness.

26. Explain the following parasomnias.

   a. Somnambulism:

   _____

   b. Nocturnal enuresis:

   _____

   c. Bruxism:

   _____

**Shift Work**

Shift work sleep disorder is a common sleep disorder experienced by individuals who work outside the traditional 9-to-5 workday.

27. The most common problems reported by shift

workers are _____, _____,

and _____, resulting from imposing

a sleep–wake schedule that is _____.

**Sleep Deprivation**

28. Sleep deprivation is _____

_____.

Physicians and nurses are particularly prone to sleep deprivation because of their long work schedules and rotating shifts.

# Nursing Knowledge Base

**Sleep and Rest**

29. Define *rest*.

_____

_____

_____

_____

**Normal Sleep Requirements and Patterns**

30. Discuss the normal sleep patterns for the various developmental stages listed here.

a. Neonates:

_____

_____

b. Infants:

_____

_____

c. Toddlers:

_____

_____

d. Preschoolers:

_____

_____

e. School-age children:

_____

_____

f. Adolescents:

_____

_____

g. Young adults:

_____

_____

h. Middle-aged adults:

_____

_____

i. Older adults:

_____

_____

**Factors Affecting Sleep**

31. Sleepiness and sleep deprivation are common side effects of medications. Describe how each of the following affects sleep, and give an example.

a. Drugs and substances:

_____

_____

_____

b. Lifestyle:

_____

_____

_____

**Usual Sleep Patterns**

32. List three alterations in routine that can disrupt sleep patterns.

a. _____

b. _____

c. _____

**Emotional Stress**

33. Explain how emotional stress affects sleep.

_____

_____

_____

**Environment**

34. List and briefly describe three environmental factors that affect sleep.

a. _____

b. _____

c. _____

**Exercise and Fatigue**

35. Explain how exercise promotes sleep.

_____

_____

_____

_____

**Food and Caloric Intake**

36. List and briefly describe five foods that affect sleep and why.

a. _____

b. _____

c. _____

d. _____

e. _____

## Nursing Process

## Assessment

Sleep and restfulness are subjective experiences. Assessment is aimed at understanding the characteristics of a sleep problem and the patient's sleep habits.

**Sleep Assessment**

**Sources for Sleep Assessment**

37. Identify three sources for sleep assessment.

a. _____

b. _____

c. _____

**Tools for Sleep Assessment**

Methods for assessing sleep quality are the use of a visual analogue scale or a numerical scale with a 0 to 10 sleep rating.

**Sleep History**

38. List seven components of a sleep history.

a. _____

b. _____

c. _____

d. _____

e. _____

f. _____

g. _____

**Description of Sleeping Problems**

39. List and briefly describe the six areas to assess with a patient when asking about the nature of a sleeping problem.

a. _____

b. _____

c. _____

d. _____

e. _____

f. _____

40. Identify the information recorded in a sleep–wake diary.

_____

_____

_____

_____

41. Briefly explain how the following factors interfere with sleep.

a. Physical and psychological illness:

_____

_____

_____

b. Current life events:

_____

_____

_____

c. Bedtime routines:

_____

_____

_____

d. Bedroom environment:

_____

_____

_____

**Behaviours of Sleep Deprivation**

42. List four behaviours a patient may manifest with sleep deprivation.

a. _____

b. _____

c. _____

d. _____

### Patient Expectations

When a patient experiences a poor night's sleep, a vicious cycle of anticipatory anxiety may begin.

## Nursing Diagnosis

It is important that your assessment identifies the probable cause of or factors related to the sleep disturbance.

## Planning

### Goals and Outcomes

An effective plan includes outcomes that focus on the goal of improving the quantity and quality of sleep in the home over a realistic period of time.

43. List four goals appropriate for a patient needing rest or sleep.

   a. _____

   b. _____

   c. _____

   d. _____

## Implementation

Nursing interventions designed to improve the quality of a person's sleep are largely focused on health promotion.

### Health Promotion

44. Many factors affect the ability to gain adequate rest and sleep. Briefly give examples of each of the following.

   a. Environmental controls:

   _____

   _____

   b. Promoting bedtime routines:

   _____

   _____

   c. Promoting safety:

   _____

   _____

d. Promoting comfort:

   _____

   _____

e. Periods of rest and sleep:

   _____

   _____

f. Stress reduction:

   _____

   _____

g. Bedtime snacks:

   _____

   _____

h. Pharmacological approaches:

   _____

   _____

### Acute Care

45. For each of the following situations, give two examples of nursing measures that will promote sleep.

   a. Environmental controls:

      i. _____

      ii. _____

   b. Promoting comfort:

      i. _____

      ii. _____

   c. Establishing periods of rest and sleep:

      i. _____

      ii. _____

   d. Promoting safety:

      i. _____

      ii. _____

   e. Stress reduction:

      i. _____

      ii. _____

### Restorative or Continuing Care

46. Give an example of the following interventions that are implemented in the restorative environment.

   a. Promoting comfort:

      _____

      _____

b. Controlling physiological disturbances:

_____

_____

c. Pharmacological approaches:

_____

_____

**Pharmacological Approaches**

47. Briefly describe the effect of benzodiazepines in promoting sleep.

_____

_____

_____

_____

48. Identify three types of patients who should not use benzodiazepines.

a. _____

b. _____

c. _____

49. The regular use of sleep medication can lead to

_____.

## Evaluation

Each patient has a unique need for sleep and rest, and only the patient will know whether sleep problems have improved, and which interventions or therapies are most successful in promoting sleep.

50. Identify some subtle behaviours a patient may exhibit that indicate sleep satisfaction.

_____

_____

_____

## Review Questions

Select the appropriate answer, and cite the rationale for choosing that particular answer.

1. The 24-hour day–night cycle is known as the
   a. Circadian rhythm
   b. Infradium rhythm
   c. Ultradian rhythm
   d. Non-REM rhythm

Answer: _____ Rationale: _____

_____

_____

2. Which of the following substances will promote normal sleep patterns?
   a. L-tryptophan
   b. Beta-adrenergic blockers
   c. Alcohol
   d. Narcotics

Answer: _____ Rationale: _____

_____

_____

3. All of the following are symptoms of sleep deprivation, *except*
   a. Hyperactivity
   b. Irritability
   c. Rise in body temperature
   d. Decreased motivation

Answer: _____ Rationale: _____

_____

_____

4. Mrs. Phan complains of difficulty falling asleep, awakening earlier than desired, and not feeling rested. She attributes these problems to leg pain that is secondary to her arthritis. What would be the appropriate nursing diagnosis for her?
   a. Sleep pattern disturbances related to arthritis
   b. Fatigue related to leg pain
   c. Knowledge deficit related to sleep hygiene measures
   d. Sleep pattern disturbances related to chronic leg pain

Answer: _____ Rationale: _____

_____

_____

5. A nursing care plan for a patient with sleep problems has been implemented. All of the following would be expected outcomes *except*
   a. Patient reports no episodes of awakening during the night.
   b. Patient falls asleep within 1 hour of going to bed.
   c. Patient reports satisfaction with amount of sleep.
   d. Patient rates sleep as an 8 or above on the visual analogue scale.

Answer: _____ Rationale: _____

_____

_____

## *Critical Thinking Model for Nursing Care Plan for Disturbed Sleep Pattern*

Imagine that you are the nurse in the Care Plan on pages 1007–1009 of your text. Complete the *evaluation* phase of the critical thinking model by writing your answers in the appropriate boxes of the model shown. Think about the following:

- What knowledge did you apply in evaluating Andree's care?

- In what way might your previous experience influence your evaluation of Andree's care?

- During evaluation, what intellectual and professional standards were applied to Andree's care?

- In what way do critical thinking attitudes play a role in how you approach the evaluation of Julie's care plan?

- How might you evaluate Andree's care plan?

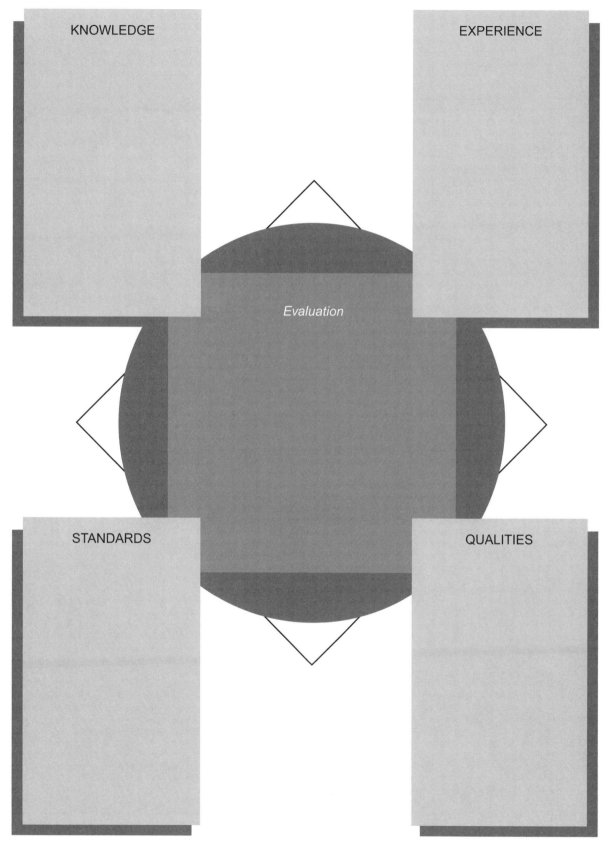

KNOWLEDGE

EXPERIENCE

*Evaluation*

STANDARDS

QUALITIES

CHAPTER 40   Critical Thinking Model for Nursing Care Plan for *Disturbed Sleep Pattern*
See answers on Evolve site.

# 41

# Pain Assessment and Management

## Preliminary Reading

Chapter 41, pages 1017–1049

## Comprehensive Understanding

1. Define *pain*.

———————————————————
———————————————————
———————————————————

Pain is a highly personal experience that can only be accurately described by the individual experiencing it.

Pain and pain management options are viewed within the context of comfort; providing comfort is central to nursing.

The relief from pain is considered a basic human right.

### Scientific Knowledge Base

**Nature of Pain**

The nature of the stimulus for pain can be physical, psychological, or a combination of both.

**Physiology of Pain**

2. Explain the four processes of nociceptive pain.

   a. *Transduction*:

   ———————————————————
   ———————————————————

   b. *Transmission*:

   ———————————————————
   ———————————————————

   c. *Perception*:

   ———————————————————
   ———————————————————

   d. *Modulation*:

   ———————————————————
   ———————————————————

3. Explain the two types of neuroregulators.

   a. Neurotransmitters:

   ———————————————————
   ———————————————————

   b. Neuromodulators:

   ———————————————————
   ———————————————————

4. Identify the neurophysiological function of the following neuroregulators.

   a. Substance P:

   ———————————————————
   ———————————————————

   b. Prostaglandins:

   ———————————————————
   ———————————————————

   c. Serotonin:

   ———————————————————
   ———————————————————

   d. Endorphins:

   ———————————————————
   ———————————————————

e. Bradykinin:

_____

_____

**Gate-Control Theory of Pain**

5. Explain the gate-control theory of pain.

_____

_____

_____

_____

**Physiological Responses**

6. List some physiological responses to pain.

a. Sympathetic stimulation:

(i) _____

(ii) _____

(iii) _____

(iv) _____

(v) _____

(vi) _____

(vii) _____

(viii) _____

b. Parasympathetic stimulation:

(i) _____

(ii) _____

(iii) _____

(iv) _____

(v) _____

**Behavioural Responses**

7. Identify four behavioural changes that characterize a patient experiencing pain.

a. _____

b. _____

c. _____

d. _____

**Types of Pain**

**Acute Pain**

8. List four characteristics of *acute pain.*

a. _____

b. _____

c. _____

d. _____

**Chronic Pain**

9. Define *chronic pain.*

_____

_____

_____

_____

10. Chronic pain may be _____ or

_____.

11. Discuss the impact of chronic noncancer pain.

_____

_____

_____

**Cancer Pain**

Many individuals with cancer pain live in community settings, and pain relief is often provided by their families. Accessing community resources may be difficult for these families, and the stress of caring for a loved one with cancer pain can affect the health of family caregivers.

**Pain by Inferred Pathology Process**

12. Nociceptive pain is subdivided into _____ and _____ pain. Neuropathic pain arises from _____.

**Breakthrough Pain**

13. Define *breakthrough pain.*

_____

_____

_____

## Nursing Knowledge Base

**Knowledge, Attitudes, and Beliefs**

14. Identify common biases and misconceptions about pain.

_____

_____

_____

_____

**Factors Influencing Pain**

**Physiological Factors**

**Age**

15. Explain the developmental differences of the following patients' reaction to pain.

   a. Young children:

   _____

   _____

   b. Toddlers and preschoolers:

   _____

   _____

   c. Older adults:

   _____

   _____

16. Identify five misconceptions about pain in older patients.

   a. _____

   b. _____

   c. _____

   d. _____

   e. _____

**Fatigue**

17. Fatigue heightens the perception of pain. Explain.

   _____

   _____

   _____

**Neurological Function**

18. Explain how a patient's neurological function can influence pain.

   _____

   _____

   _____

   _____

**Social Factors**

19. Discuss how each of the following influences pain.

   a. Attention:

   _____

   _____

   _____

   b. Previous experience:

   _____

   _____

   _____

   c. Family and social support:

   _____

   _____

   _____

   d. Spiritual factors:

   _____

   _____

   _____

**Psychological Factors**

20. Explain how the following psychological factors affect pain.

   a. Anxiety:

   _____

   _____

   _____

   b. Meaning of pain:

   _____

   _____

   _____

**Cultural Factors**

21. Explain how cultural factors affect pain.

   _____

   _____

   _____

   _____

## Nursing Process and Pain

22. Pain management extends beyond pain relief; it encompasses the patient's _____ and ability to _____, and _____.

## Assessment

Pain assessment is the basis of all pain management, and pain is often referred to as the fifth vital sign.

23. Monitor the patient's pain consistently along

    with _____, _____, and

    _____, especially if the pain is not well controlled.

24. Assessment of chronic pain should focus

    on _____, _____, and

    _____ dimensions of the pain and on its history and context.

25. Explain what is meant by the pain assessment and management approach "ABCDE."

    A: _____

    B: _____

    C: _____

    D: _____

    E: _____

### Expression of Pain

Cognitively impaired patients might require simple assessment approaches involving close observation of behaviour changes, especially movement.

### Characteristics of Pain

26. Briefly explain the common characteristics of pain.

    a. Onset and duration:

       _____

       _____

       _____

    b. Location:

       _____

       _____

       _____

    c. Intensity:

       _____

       _____

       _____

27. Describe the following descriptive scales for measuring the severity of pain.

    a. Numerical rating scale:

       _____

       _____

    b. Verbal descriptor scale:

       _____

       _____

    c. Visual analogue scale:

       _____

       _____

    d. FACES scale:

       _____

       _____

### Quality

28. Identify some terms a patient can use to describe the quality of his or her pain.

    _____

    _____

    _____

    _____

### Pain Pattern

It is important to assess for factors that precipitate or aggravate pain. This will help to plan effective interventions.

### Relief Measures

29. Identify some measures a patient may use to relieve pain.

    _____

    _____

    _____

    _____

### Contributing Symptoms

30. Identify some contributing symptoms that may aggravate pain.

    _____

    _____

    _____

    _____

**Effects of Pain**

31. Pain is a _____, _____ and _____ stressor that _____.

**Behavioural Effects**

32. Give examples of the following behavioural indicators of pain.

    a. Vocalizations:

    _____
    _____

    b. Facial expressions:

    _____
    _____

    c. Body movement:

    _____
    _____

    d. Social interaction:

    _____
    _____

**Influence on Activities of Daily Living**

33. Explain how pain can influence activities of daily living in regard to the following:

    a. Sleep:

    _____
    _____

    b. Hygiene:

    _____
    _____

    c. Sexual relations:

    _____
    _____

    d. Employment:

    _____
    _____

    e. Social activities:

    _____
    _____

## Nursing Diagnosis

The nursing diagnosis focuses on the nature of the pain so that the nurse can identify the best interventions for relieving pain and minimizing its effect on the patient's lifestyle and function.

34. List five potential or actual nursing diagnoses related to a patient in pain.

    a. _____
    b. _____
    c. _____
    d. _____
    e. _____

## Planning

Patients in pain frequently have interrelated problems. As one problem worsens, others also change.

**Goals and Outcomes**

35. List the patient outcomes appropriate for the patient experiencing pain.

    a. _____
    b. _____
    c. _____

**Setting Priorities**

Your priorities will change as the patient's pain experience changes.

## Implementation

**Health Promotion**

Provide patients and their families with education and information about pain; it will help to reduce anxiety, and it increases a patient's sense of control.

36. Describe how you would teach a child about a painful procedure.

    _____
    _____
    _____
    _____

**Nonpharmacological Pain-Relief Interventions**

37. Discuss the goals of the following pain-relief interventions:

   a. Cognitive-behavioural interventions:

   _____

   _____

   b. Physical interventions:

   _____

   _____

**Relaxation and Guided Imagery**

38. Briefly explain how *relaxation* lessens pain.

   _____

   _____

   _____

   _____

39. Briefly explain how the nurse would lead a patient through guided imagery.

   _____

   _____

   _____

   _____

40. Briefly explain how the nurse would guide a patient through progressive relaxation exercises.

   _____

   _____

   _____

   _____

**Distraction**

41. Define *distraction*, and list one disadvantage and one advantage of using distraction to alleviate perception of pain.

   _____

   _____

   _____

42. Describe the effects of using music as a distraction to decrease pain.

   _____

   _____

   _____

   _____

43. Define the following pain-relief measures and the rationale for their use.

   a. *Biofeedback*:

   _____

   _____

   b. *Acupuncture*:

   _____

   _____

   c. *Cutaneous stimulation*:

   _____

   _____

   d. *Herbal supplements*:

   _____

   _____

   e. Reducing pain perception:

   _____

   _____

44. What is TENS, and how is it believed to reduce pain?

   _____

   _____

   _____

**Acute Care**

**Acute Pain Management**

The key to pain relief's success is the ongoing evaluation of interventions.

**Pharmacological Pain-Relief Interventions**

The ideal analgesic has yet to be developed, but many opioid and nonopioid pain-relieving medications are available.

*Analgesics*

Analgesics are the most common method of pain relief.

45. Identify the three types of analgesics.

   a. _____

   b. _____

   c. _____

46. Discuss the importance of around-the-clock dosing.

_____

_____

_____

_____

47. Describe four major principles for analgesic administration.

a. _____

b. _____

c. _____

d. _____

**Patient-Controlled Analgesia**

48. Explain the benefits of patient-controlled analgesia.

_____

_____

_____

_____

*Local and Regional Anaesthetics and Analgesics*

49. Describe what a local anaesthetic is, how it may be applied, and possible side effects.

_____

_____

50. Describe what a regional anaesthetic is and list three types.

_____

_____

_____

_____

51. Explain an advantage of *epidural analgesia* and how it is administered.

_____

_____

_____

_____

*Nursing Implications*

52. Describe six goals of nursing care for a patient with epidural infusions. Explain one intervention for each goal.

a. _____

b. _____

c. _____

d. _____

e. _____

f. _____

**Invasive Interventions for Pain Relief**

53. When pain is severe, invasive interventions may give relief when more conservative treatment is neither tolerated nor effective. List three invasive interventions used to relieve pain.

a. _____

b. _____

c. _____

**Procedure Pain Management**

Premedicating patients before painful procedures may assist them to cooperate and may help to reduce the experience of pain.

**Cancer Pain Management**

54. Identify the three-step approach to cancer pain management recommended by the World Health Organisation (1990).

a. _____

b. _____

c. _____

55. Identify patients who are candidates for continuous infusions.

a. _____

b. _____

c. _____

56. Discuss the guidelines for safe administration of morphine sulphate via ambulatory infusion pumps.

_____

_____

_____

**Barriers to Effective Pain Management**

57. Multiple barriers prevent effective pain management. Identify four barriers for the following categories.

   a. Barriers for patients:

   _____

   _____

   _____

   _____

   b. Barriers for health care providers:

   _____

   _____

   _____

   _____

   c. Barriers for the health care system:

   _____

   _____

   _____

   _____

**Restorative and Continuing Care**

**Pain Clinics, Palliative Care, and Hospices**

58. Briefly discuss the following terms:

   a. Palliative care

   _____

   _____

   b. Hospice care

   _____

   _____

# Evaluation

**Patient Care**

If a patient continues to have discomfort after an intervention, a different approach may be needed. For example, if an analgesic provides only partial relief, the nurse may add relaxation exercises or guided-imagery exercises.

Pain assessment and responses to intervention should be accurately and thoroughly documented so that they can be communicated to others caring for the patient.

**Patient Perceptions**

The patient, if able, is the best judge of whether pain-relief measures work.

The family often is another valuable resource, particularly in the case of the patient with cancer who may not be able to express discomfort during the latter stages of terminal illness.

## *Review Questions*

Select the appropriate answer, and cite the rationale for choosing that particular answer.

1. Pain is a protective mechanism warning of tissue injury and is largely a(n)
   a. Symptom of a severe illness or disease
   b. Subjective experience
   c. Objective experience
   d. Acute symptom of short duration

   Answer: _____ Rationale: _____

   _____

   _____

2. A substance that can cause analgesia when it attaches to opiate receptors in the brain is
   a. Substance P
   b. Serotonin
   c. Prostaglandin
   d. Endorphin

   Answer: _____ Rationale: _____

   _____

   _____

3. To adequately assess the quality of a patient's pain, which question would be appropriate?
   a. "Tell me what your pain feels like."
   b. "Is your pain a crushing sensation?"
   c. "How long have you had this pain?"
   d. "Is it a sharp pain or a dull pain?"

   Answer: _____ Rationale: _____

   _____

   _____

4. The use of patient distraction in pain control is based on the principle that
   a. Small C fibres transmit impulses via the spinothalamic tract
   b. The reticular formation can send inhibitory signals to gating mechanisms
   c. Large A fibres compete with pain impulses to close gates to painful stimuli
   d. Transmission of pain impulses from the spinal cord to the cerebral cortex can be inhibited

Answer: _____ Rationale: _____
_____
_____

5. Teaching a child about painful procedures is best achieved by
   a. Early warnings of the anticipated pain
   b. Storytelling about the upcoming procedure
   c. Relevant play and language directed toward procedure activities
   d. Avoiding explanations until the pain is experienced

Answer: _____ Rationale: _____
_____
_____

## Critical Thinking Model for Nursing Care Plan for Acute Pain

Imagine that you are the student nurse in the Care Plan on pages 1034–1035 of your text. Complete the *assessment* phase of the critical thinking model by writing your answers in the appropriate boxes of the model shown. Think about the following:

• What knowledge base is applied to Mrs. Mays?

• In what way might previous experience assist you in this case?

• What intellectual and professional standards were applied to the care of Mrs. Mays?

• What critical thinking attitudes did you use in assessing Mrs. Mays?

• As you review your assessment, what key areas did you cover?

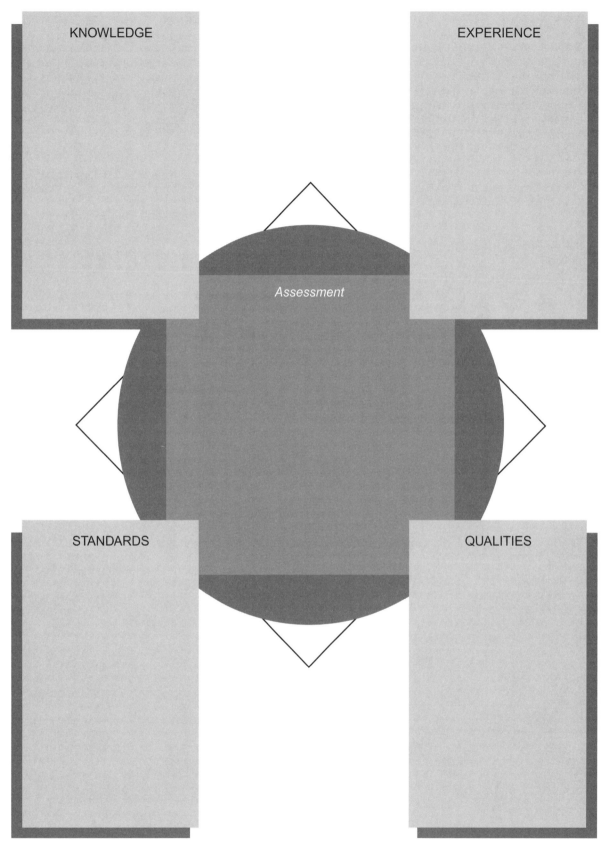

KNOWLEDGE

EXPERIENCE

Assessment

STANDARDS

QUALITIES

CHAPTER 41   Critical Thinking Model for Nursing Care Plan for *Acute Pain*
See answers on Evolve site.

# 42

# Nutrition

## *Preliminary Reading*

Chapter 42, pages 1050–1111

## *Comprehensive Understanding*

### Scientific Knowledge Base

**Nutrients: The Biochemical Units of Nutrition**

The body requires fuel to provide energy for the chemical reactions that enable cellular growth and repair, organ function, and body movement.

1. Define the following terms.

   a. *Basal metabolic rate*:

   _____

   _____

   _____

   b. *Resting energy expenditure*:

   _____

   _____

   _____

   c. *Nutrients*:

   _____

   _____

   _____

   d. *Nutrient density*:

   _____

   _____

   _____

2. List the six categories of nutrients.

   a. _____

   b. _____

   c. _____

   d. _____

   e. _____

   f. _____

3. Foods may also be described as _____, _____, or _____.

**Carbohydrates**

4. Each gram of *carbohydrate* produces _____ kilocalories (kcal).

5. Identify the three classes of carbohydrates.

   a. _____

   b. _____

   c. _____

**Proteins**

6. Proteins are essential for _____ of body tissue in _____, _____, and _____.

7. The simplest form of protein is the _____.

8. Explain the two types of amino acids.

   a. *Essential amino acids*:

   _____

   _____

   b. *Nonessential amino acids*:

   _____

   _____

9. Define the following terms.

　　a. Incomplete protein:

　　　　_____

　　　　_____

　　b. Complete protein:

　　　　_____

　　　　_____

　　c. Complementary proteins:

　　　　_____

　　　　_____

10. Protein is the only major nutrient that contains

　　_____ and is the only source of

　　_____ for the body.

11. *Nitrogen balance* is _____

　　_____.

**Fats**

12. Fats (*lipids*) are the most calorically dense nutri-

　　ent, providing _____ kcal/g.

13. Describe the composition of the following forms
of fats.

　　a. *Triglycerides*:

　　　　_____

　　　　_____

　　b. *Fatty acids*:

　　　　_____

　　　　_____

14. Define the following types of fatty acids, and
give an example of each.

　　a. *Saturated fatty acids*:

　　　　_____

　　　　_____

　　b. *Unsaturated fatty acids*:

　　　　_____

　　　　_____

　　c. *Monounsaturated fatty acids*:

　　　　_____

　　　　_____

　　d. *Polyunsaturated fatty acids*:

　　　　_____

　　　　_____

　　e. *Trans fatty acids*:

　　　　_____

　　　　_____

15. Define cholesterol, and identify two sources of
cholesterol.

　　_____

　　_____

　　_____

　　_____

**Water**

16. Water makes up _____ of total body
weight.

17. _____ have the greatest percentage of

　　total body weight as water, and _____
have the least.

18. Fluid needs are met by ingesting _____

　　and _____, and by water produced

　　during _____.

19. Identify the role of water in the body.

　　_____

　　_____

　　_____

　　_____

**Vitamins**

20. *Vitamins* are _____.

21. Identify the *fat-soluble vitamins*.

　　a. _____

　　b. _____

　　c. _____

　　d. _____

22. Identify the *water-soluble vitamins*:

　　a. _____

　　b. _____

23. Define *hypervitaminosis*.

_____
_____
_____
_____

**Minerals**

24. *Minerals* are _____.

25. Minerals are classified as _____ when the daily requirement is 100 mg or more, and as _____ or _____ when fewer than 100 mg are needed daily.

**Anatomy and Physiology of the Digestive System**

**Digestion**

Digestion of food consists of the mechanical breakdown and chemical reactions by which food is reduced to its simplest form.

26. *Enzymes* are _____.

27. Explain the mechanical, chemical, and hormonal activities of digestion:

_____
_____

28. The major portion of digestion occurs in the _____.

29. Define the following terms.

   a. *Peristalsis*:

   _____
   _____

   b. *Chyme*:

   _____
   _____

**Absorption**

30. The primary absorption site of nutrients is the _____.

31. The main source of water absorption is via the _____.

32. In addition to water, electrolytes and minerals are absorbed, and bacteria in the colon synthesize vitamins _____ and some _____.

**Metabolism and Storage of Nutrients**

33. *Metabolism* refers to _____.

34. Describe the two types of metabolism.

   a. *Anabolism*:

   _____
   _____

   b. *Catabolism*:

   _____
   _____

35. Nutrient metabolism consists of three main processes. Explain each one.

   a. *Glycogenolysis*:

   _____
   _____

   b. *Glycogenesis*:

   _____
   _____

   c. *Gluconeogenesis*:

   _____
   _____

36. Glycogen is synthesized from _____.

37. The body's major form of reserved energy is _____, which is stored as _____.

**Elimination**

38. Feces contain _____.

**Dietary Guidelines**

**Dietary Reference Intakes**

39. Explain *dietary reference intakes*.

_____
_____
_____
_____

40. Define the four components to the dietary reference intakes.

   a. _____
   b. _____
   c. _____
   d. _____

**Food Guidelines**

41. Using the space below, diagram and label *Canada's Food Guide*.

[box]

42. List five dietary guidelines identified in *Eating Well With Canada's Food Guide*.

   a. _____

     _____

   b. _____

     _____

   c. _____

     _____

   d. _____

     _____

   e. _____

     _____

43. List the nutritional recommendations identified in *Eating Well With Canada's Food Guide*.

   a. _____

     _____

   b. _____

     _____

   c. _____

     _____

   d. _____

     _____

   e. _____

     _____

   f. _____

     _____

   g. _____

     _____

   h. _____

     _____

## Nursing Knowledge Base

### Nutrition During Human Growth and Development

**Infants Through School-Age Children**

44. An energy intake of approximately _____ kcal/kg is needed in the first half of infancy, and

    _____ kcal/kg is needed in the second half.

45. A full-term newborn is able to digest and absorb

    _____, _____, and _____.

46. Infants need _____ mL/kg per day of fluid.

**Breastfeeding**

47. List at least four benefits for breastfeeding an infant.

    a. _____

    b. _____

    c. _____

    d. _____

**Formula**

48. Explain why the following should not be used in infant formula.

    a. Cow's milk:

    _____

    _____

    b. Honey:

    _____

    _____

**Introduction to Solid Food**

49. The addition of solid foods to an infant's diet should be governed by the infant's

    a. _____

    b. _____

    c. _____

    d. _____

    e. _____

    f. _____

50. When should dental visits begin?

    _____

    _____

    _____

51. What practice puts children at risk for developing early-childhood tooth decay? Why?

    _____

    _____

    _____

    _____

    _____

52. What is the role of parents in ensuring the dental health of their young child?

    _____

    _____

    _____

    _____

53. The toddler needs _____ kilocalories, but an increased amount of _____ in relation to body weight.

54. Identify examples of foods that have been implicated in the choking deaths of toddlers and preschoolers.

    _____

    _____

    _____

    _____

55. School-age children's diets should be assessed

    for _____.

56. Explain some reasons for the increase in childhood obesity.

    _____

    _____

    _____

    _____

**Adolescents**

57. Identify the common nutritional deficiencies in the following adolescent population groups.

    a. Girls:

    _____

    _____

    _____

b. Boys:

_____

_____

_____

c. Those who eat fast food:

_____

_____

_____

d. Athletes:

_____

_____

_____

e. Pregnant adolescent girls aged 14 to 18:

_____

_____

_____

58. Identify the diagnostic criteria for the following eating disorders.

a. *Anorexia nervosa*:

_____

_____

b. *Bulimia nervosa*:

_____

_____

**Young and Middle-Aged Adults**

59. Obesity may become a problem because of _____.

60. Adult women who use oral contraceptives need extra _____.

**Pregnancy**

61. The energy requirements of pregnancy are re-lated to _____ and _____.

62. During pregnancy, supplementation is usually recommended along with dietary modification to increase intake of the following:

a. _____

b. _____

c. _____

**Lactation**

63. During lactation, there is an increased need for vitamins _____ and _____.

**Older Adults**

64. List four factors that influence the nutritional status of the older adult.

a. _____

b. _____

c. _____

d. _____

**Alternative Food Patterns**

**Vegetarian Diet**

65. What knowledge is necessary to implement a healthy vegetarian diet?

_____

_____

_____

_____

## Nursing Process and Nutrition

Close daily contact with patients and their families enables nurses to make observations about their physical status, food intake, weight changes, and responses to therapy.

## Assessment

66. Define the following terms.

a. *Nutritional screening*:

_____

_____

_____

b. *Nutritional assessment*:

_____

_____

_____

c. *Anthropometry*:

_____

_____

_____

d. *Ideal body weight*:

_____
_____
_____

e. *Body mass index*:

_____
_____
_____

67. Describe how to obtain a *waist circumference* measurement.

_____
_____
_____
_____

**Laboratory and Biochemical Tests**

68. Identify the common laboratory tests used to study the nutritional status of a patient.

_____
_____
_____
_____

**Dietary History and Health History**

69. List 12 components of a dietary history, and provide a sample question for each.

a. _____
b. _____
c. _____
d. _____
e. _____
f. _____
g. _____
h. _____
i. _____
j. _____
k. _____
l. _____

**Clinical Observation and Physical Examination**

70. For each assessment area, list at least two signs of good and poor nutrition.

a. General appearance:

_____
_____

b. General vitality:

_____
_____

c. Weight:

_____
_____

d. Hair:

_____
_____

e. Skin:

_____
_____

f. Mouth, oral membranes:

_____
_____

g. GI function:

_____
_____

h. Cardiovascular function:

_____
_____

i. Nervous system function:

_____
_____

j. Muscles:

_____
_____

71. Define the following terms:

a. *Aspiration*:

_____
_____
_____

b. *Dysphagia*:

_____
_____
_____

72. Describe the steps involved in an in-depth assessment for aspiration risk.

_____
_____
_____
_____

73. Identify the warning signs of dysphagia.

_____
_____
_____
_____
_____

## Nursing Diagnosis

74. List three potential or actual nursing diagnoses for altered nutritional status.

a. _____
b. _____
c. _____

## Planning

The planning for enhanced, optimal nutritional status requires a higher level of care than simply correcting problems. Information from multiple sources must be synthesized to devise an individualized approach to care that is relevant to the patient's needs.

### Goals and Outcomes

75. Provide an example of a goal and associated outcomes appropriate for a patient with nutritional problems.

Goal:_____

Outcomes:_____

a. _____
b. _____
c. _____
d. _____

## Implementation

### Health Promotion/Illness Prevention

76. Nurses are in a key position to educate patients about_____.

77. Describe the relationship between income and healthy eating.

_____
_____
_____
_____
_____

78. List two examples of interventions to counter the threat to nutrition and health from lack of purchasing power.

a. Individual level:

_____
_____

b. Collective level:

_____
_____

79. Patient education about food safety and reducing the risk of foodborne illnesses includes the following instructions:

a. _____
b. _____
c. _____
d. _____
e. _____
f. _____
g. _____
h. _____
i. _____
j. _____

**Acute Care**

80. List three factors that can cause *anorexia* (loss of appetite) in acute care settings.

   a. _____

   b. _____

   c. _____

81. Identify factors that put patients at nutritional risk during hospitalizations.

   _____

   _____

   _____

   _____

   _____

82. Describe the following therapeutic diets.

   a. Clear liquid:

   _____

   _____

   b. Thickened liquid:

   _____

   _____

   c. Full liquid:

   _____

   _____

   d. Puréed:

   _____

   _____

   e. Mechanical soft:

   _____

   _____

   f. Soft or low residue:

   _____

   _____

   g. High fibre:

   _____

   _____

   h. Low sodium:

   _____

   _____

   i. Low cholesterol:

   _____

   _____

   j. Diabetic:

   _____

   _____

   k. Regular:

   _____

   _____

**Promoting Appetite**

83. List five ways in which you can promote appetite.

   a. _____

   b. _____

   c. _____

   d. _____

   e. _____

**Assisting Patients With Feeding**

84. List eight nursing interventions to assist dysphagic patients with feeding.

   a. _____

   b. _____

   c. _____

   d. _____

   e. _____

   f. _____

   g. _____

   h. _____

85. List six nursing measures to help patients retain comfort and a sense of independence in relation to their food intake.

   a. _____

   b. _____

   c. _____

   d. _____

   e. _____

   f. _____

## Evaluation

**Patient Care**

**Patient Expectations**

86. Patients expect competent and accurate care. You must _____ if outcomes of nutritional therapies are unsuccessful.

## Self-Monitoring of Blood Glucose

87. By providing a real-time blood glucose reading, self-monitoring of blood glucose enables the patient to make self-management decisions regarding diet, exercise, and medication _____.

88. The frequency of monitoring blood sugar depends on

    a. _____

    b. _____

    c. _____

    d. _____

## Enteral Tube Feeding

89. Briefly describe enteral nutrition.

**Preventing Complications**

90. Risks of complications associated with enteral feedings are increased with

    a. _____

    b. _____

    c. _____

    d. _____

    e. _____

91. Discuss the major complications of enteral nutrition.

## Large-Bore Tube and Nasogastric or Orogastric Suctioning

92. Discuss gastric decompression.

## Parenteral Nutrition

93. Define parental nutrition.

    _____

**Preventing Complications**

94. Discuss 10 complications of parenteral nutrition.

    _____

## *Review Questions*

Select the appropriate answer, and cite the rationale for choosing that particular answer.

1. Which nutrient is the body's preferred energy source?
   a. Protein
   b. Fat
   c. Carbohydrate
   d. Vitamins

   Answer: _____ Rationale: _____
   _____
   _____

2. Positive nitrogen balance would occur in which condition?
   a. Infection
   b. Starvation
   c. Burn injury
   d. Wound healing

   Answer: _____ Rationale: _____
   _____
   _____

3. Mrs. Schultz is talking with you about the dietary needs of her 23-month-old daughter, Anita. Which of the following responses would be appropriate?
   a. "Use skim milk to cut down on the fat in Anita's diet."
   b. "Anita should be drinking at least 720 mL of milk per day."
   c. "Anita needs fewer calories in relation to her body weight now than she did as an infant."
   d. "Anita needs less protein in her diet now because she isn't growing as fast."

   Answer: _____ Rationale: _____
   _____
   _____

4. All of the following patients are at risk for alteration in nutrition, *except*
   a. Patient J, who is 86 years old, lives alone, and
      has poorly fitting dentures
   b. Patient K, who has been on nothing-by-mouth
      status for 7 days following bowel surgery and
      is receiving intravenous fluids
   c. Patient L, whose weight is 10% above his
      ideal body weight
   d. Patient M, a 17-year-old girl who weighs 40 kg
      and frequently complains about her baby fat

Answer: _____ Rationale: _____
_____
_____

5. To help counter childhood obesity, you should
   recommend which of the following for 9- to
   11-year-olds?
   a. Consume two to three servings of fruit and
      vegetables daily.
   b. Consume two to three servings of milk products
      daily.
   c. Eliminate all fat from the daily diet.
   d. Reduce the hours spent in front of the
      television.

Answer: _____ Rationale: _____
_____
_____

6. The current diet of Aboriginal peoples is high in
   which of the following?
   a. Calcium
   b. Fibre
   c. Fat and sugar
   d. Fruits and vegetables

Answer: _____ Rationale: _____
_____
_____

## Critical Thinking Model for Nursing Care Plan for Imbalanced Nutrition: Less Than Body Requirements

Imagine that you are Belinda, the nurse in the Care Plan on pages 1075–1076 of your text. Complete the *planning* phase of the critical thinking model by writing your answers in the appropriate boxes of the model shown. Think about the following:

- In developing Mrs. Cooper's plan of care, what knowledge did Belinda apply?

- In what ways might Belinda's previous experience assist in developing Mrs. Cooper's plan of care?

- When developing a plan of care for Mrs. Cooper, what intellectual and professional standards were applied?

- What critical thinking attitudes might have been applied in developing Mrs. Cooper's plan of care?

- How will Belinda accomplish these goals?

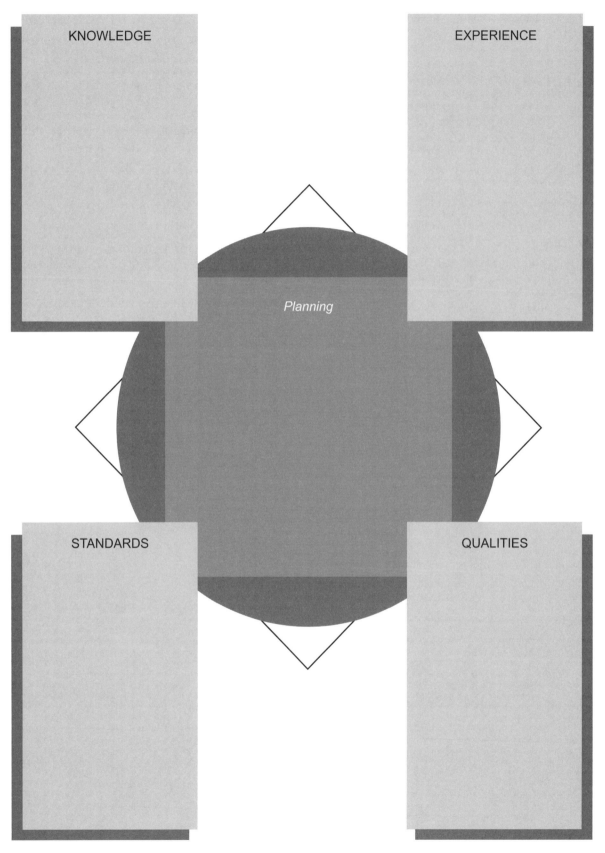

CHAPTER 42    Critical Thinking Model for Nursing Care Plan for *Imbalanced Nutrition: Less Than Body Requirements*
See answers on Evolve site.

# 43

# Urinary Elimination

## *Preliminary Reading*

Chapter 43, pages 1112–1158

## *Comprehensive Understanding*

### Scientific Knowledge Base

1. Summarize the function of each of the following organs in the urinary system.

   a. Kidneys:

   _____

   _____

   b. Ureters:

   _____

   _____

   c. Bladder:

   _____

   _____

   d. Urethra:

   _____

   _____

2. Define the following terms related to urine elimination.

   a. *Nephron*:

   _____

   _____

   b. *Proteinuria*:

   _____

   _____

   c. *Erythropoietin*:

   _____

   _____

   d. *Renin*:

   _____

   _____

   e. *Micturition*:

   _____

   _____

   f. *Urethral meatus*:

   _____

   _____

The ability of the urethra to maintain adequate closure is critical to continence.

3. Briefly describe the *urethral closure mechanism*.

   _____

   _____

   _____

### Act of Urination

4. Number the steps describing the normal act of micturition in sequential order.

   _____ The *detrusor muscle* contracts.

   _____ Urine volume stretches the bladder walls, sending impulses to the micturition centre in the spinal cord.

   _____ The urethral sphincter relaxes.

   _____ Impulses travel from the pontine micturition centre.

   _____ The bladder empties.

**Factors Influencing Urination**

Pathophysiological conditions may be acute and reversible (urinary tract infection, or UTI), whereas others may be chronic and irreversible (slow, progressive development of renal dysfunction).

**Disease Conditions**

5. Discuss how each of the following can affect urinary elimination.

   a. Cerebral vascular accident:

   _____

   _____

   b. Multiple sclerosis:

   _____

   _____

   c. Diabetes mellitus:

   _____

   _____

   d. Parkinson's disease:

   _____

   _____

   e. Alzheimer's disease:

   _____

   _____

   f. Rheumatoid arthritis:

   _____

   _____

6. Disease processes that primarily affect renal function (changes in urine volume or quality) are generally categorized as follows. Briefly explain each.

   a. Prerenal:

   _____

   _____

   b. Renal:

   _____

   _____

   c. Postrenal:

   _____

   _____

7. Define *oliguria*.

   _____

   _____

8. Define *anuria*.

   _____

   _____

9. List the characteristic signs of the *uremic syndrome*.

   _____

   _____

   _____

**Renal Replacement Therapies**

10. Briefly describe the two methods of dialysis.

    a. *Peritoneal dialysis*:

    _____

    _____

    _____

    b. *Hemodialysis*:

    _____

    _____

    _____

11. Identify some indications for dialysis.

    _____

    _____

    _____

    _____

**Fluid Balance**

The kidneys maintain a sensitive balance between retention and excretion of fluids.

12. Define *polyuria*.

    _____

    _____

13. Explain how the following affect the balance of urine excreted.

    a. Caffeine drinks:

    _____

    _____

    b. Alcohol:

    _____

    _____

c. Febrile conditions:

_____

_____

d. Peripheral edema:

_____

_____

**Medications**

14. List three types of medications that affect urination, and describe their major effect.

a. _____

b. _____

c. _____

**Diagnostic Examination**

15. Explain what a cystoscopy is and how it may affect urination.

_____

_____

_____

_____

**Surgical Procedures**

16. Briefly explain how the stress of surgery affects urine output.

_____

_____

_____

_____

17. Briefly explain how anaesthetics and narcotic analgesics affect urine output.

_____

_____

_____

_____

**Psychological Factors**

18. _____ and _____ may cause a sense of urgency and increased_____.

_____ also may prevent a person from being able to _____; as a result, the urge to void may return _____.

**Common Alterations in Urinary Elimination**

19. Most patients with urinary problems have disturbances in the act of micturition that involve a failure to store urine, a failure to empty urine, or both. List the four most common alterations in urinary elimination.

a. _____

b. _____

c. _____

d. _____

**Urinary Tract Infections**

20. Although several microorganisms may cause UTIs, _____ is the most frequent causative pathogen.

21. Describe two host defence mechanisms specific to each of the following.

a. Both females and males:

_____

_____

b. Females:

_____

_____

c. Males:

_____

_____

22. List four risk factors for UTI in women.

a. _____

b. _____

c. _____

d. _____

23. Identify the most common cause of UTIs.

_____

_____

_____

**Signs and Symptoms**

24. List six signs or symptoms of UTIs.

a. _____

b. _____

c. _____

d. _____

e. _____

f. _____

25. Define the following terms related to UTIs.

a. *Pyelonephritis*:

_____

_____

b. *Bacteriuria*:

_____

_____

26. Explain why residual urine is a risk factor for UTIs.

_____

_____

_____.

27. Define *urinary incontinence*.

_____

_____.

28. Briefly describe the major types of urinary incontinence.

a. Transient:

_____

_____

b. Urge:

_____

_____

c. Urinary frequency:

_____

_____

d. Stress:

_____

_____

e. Mixed:

_____

_____

f. Functional:

_____

_____

g. Overflow:

_____

_____

h. Reflex:

_____

_____

i. Total:

_____

_____

**Overactive Bladder Syndrome**

29. Explain the term *overactive bladder*.

_____

_____

_____

_____

**Nocturia**

Nocturia has been defined as waking at night to void. It is associated with aging and an overactive bladder, as well as with an enlarged prostate in men.

**Urinary Retention**

30. Define *urinary retention*.

_____

_____

_____

31. List five signs of urinary retention.

a. _____

b. _____

c. _____

d. _____

e. _____

**Urinary Diversions**

32. Identify three indications for urinary diversions.

a. _____

b. _____

c. _____

33. Briefly describe the following urinary diversions.

    a. Ileal loop or conduit:

    _____
    _____
    _____

    b. *Ureterostomy*:

    _____
    _____
    _____

    c. *Nephrostomy*:

    _____
    _____
    _____

## Nursing Knowledge Base

You need to know concepts other than anatomy and physiology, as well as an understanding of concepts such as infection control, hygiene measures, growth and development, and psychosocial influences.

### Infection Control and Hygiene

34. Hospital-acquired UTIs are often related to

    _____, _____, or _____.

### Growth and Development

35. Briefly summarize the developmental changes that may influence urination.

    _____
    _____
    _____
    _____
    _____

### Psychosocial and Cultural Considerations

36. Identify the psychosocial and cultural factors that may influence urination.

    _____
    _____
    _____
    _____
    _____

## Nursing Process and Alterations in Urinary Function

### Assessment

To identify a urinary elimination problem obtain information by collecting a health history, performing a focused physical assessment, assessing the patient's urine, and reviewing information from diagnostic tests and examinations.

### Health History

37. List three factors to be explored when completing a health history related to urinary elimination.

    a. _____

    b. _____

    c. _____

38. List five topics that should be included in a *urinary diary*.

    a. _____

    b. _____

    c. _____

    d. _____

    e. _____

### Factors Affecting Urination

39. Describe the following symptoms of urinary alterations.

    a. Incontinence:

    _____
    _____

    b. Urgency:

    _____
    _____

    c. Dysuria:

    _____
    _____

    d. Frequency:

    _____
    _____

e. Hesitancy:

_____

_____

f. Polyuria:

_____

_____

g. Oliguria:

_____

_____

h. Nocturia:

_____

_____

i. Dribbling:

_____

_____

j. Hematuria:

_____

_____

k. Retention:

_____

_____

l. Elevated postvoid residual urine:

_____

_____

## Physical Assessment

40. Briefly explain the four structures assessed in a physical exam to determine the presence and severity of urinary problems.

a. _____

b. _____

c. _____

d. _____

## Assessment of Urine

41. Assessment of urine involves _____ and _____.

## Characteristics of Urine

42. Describe the following characteristics of urine.

a. Colour:

_____

_____

_____

b. Clarity:

_____

_____

_____

c. Odour:

_____

_____

_____

## Urine Testing

43. Describe the following types of urine specimens collected for testing.

a. Random:

_____

_____

b. Clean-voided or midstream:

_____

_____

c. Sterile:

_____

_____

d. Timed:

_____

_____

## Common Urine Tests

44. Common urine tests include the following. Briefly explain each.

a. *Urinalysis*:

_____

_____

_____

b. *Specific gravity*:

_____

_____

_____

c. *Urine culture*:

_____

_____

_____

_____

**Diagnostic Examinations**

45. Briefly explain the following types of diagnostic examinations, and give the nursing implications for each.

a. Abdominal roentgenogram:

_____

_____

b. Computerized axial tomography scan:

_____

_____

c. Intravenous pyelogram:

_____

_____

d. Renal scan:

_____

_____

e. Ultrasonography:

_____

_____

46. List the three types of invasive diagnostic examinations and the nursing implications.

a. _____

b. _____

c. _____

## Nursing Diagnosis

47. List six potential or actual nursing diagnoses related to urinary elimination.

a. _____

b. _____

c. _____

d. _____

e. _____

f. _____

## Planning

**Goals and Outcomes**

48. List two examples of goals appropriate for a patient with a urinary elimination problem.

_____

_____

_____

_____

## Implementation

**Health Promotion**

49. Identify five health topics that the primary health provider should teach on bladder health:

a. _____

b. _____

c. _____

d. _____

e. _____

**Promoting Regular Micturition**

50. Maintaining regular patterns of urinary elimination can help prevent many urination problems. You should reinforce the importance of

voiding regularly every _____ to

_____ hours during the day.

**Stimulating Micturition Reflex**

51. List three techniques that may be used to stimulate the micturition reflex.

a. _____

b. _____

c. _____

**Maintaining Adequate Fluid Intake**

52. Maintaining an adequate fluid intake of

_____ to _____mL promotes continence because concentrated urine can irritate the bladder mucosa.

**Avoiding Food and Fluids That Can Irritate the Bladder Mucosa**

53. List several food substances that can be irritating to the bladder mucosa.

_____

_____

_____

_____

**Promoting Complete Bladder Emptying**

Normally, a small amount of urine remains in the bladder after voiding; however, urinary incontinence may occur when too much residual urine is in the bladder or when the urinary sphincters are too weak to maintain closure pressure.

**Preventing Infection**

54. One of the most important considerations for a patient with alterations in urinary elimination is the need to prevent infection of the urinary system. List three preventative measures:

    a. _____

    b. _____

    c. _____

**Acute Care**

**Maintaining Elimination Habits**

55. Briefly explain how you can help the hospitalized patient to maintain normal elimination habits.

    _____
    _____
    _____
    _____
    _____

**Medications**

56. List and explain three types of medications that can be used to treat incontinence or retention.

    a. _____

    b. _____

    c. _____

**Catheterization**

57. List three indications for each of the following.

    a. Short-term catheterization:

    _____
    _____

    b. Long-term catheterization:

    _____
    _____

    c. Intermittent catheterization:

    _____
    _____

**Types of Catheterization**

58. Briefly describe the following types of catheters.

    a. Straight:

    _____
    _____

    b. Coudé:

    _____
    _____

    c. Foley:

    _____
    _____

**Catheter Insertion**

For urethral catheterization of any type, a physician's order is required. You must use the strict aseptic technique.

**Routine Catheter Care**

59. Explain the following nursing measures taken to maintain patient comfort, prevent infection, and maintain an unobstructed flow of urine in catheterized patients.

    a. Perineal hygiene:

    _____
    _____
    _____

    b. Catheter care:

    _____
    _____
    _____

    c. Fluid intake:

    _____
    _____
    _____

**Preventing Infection**

The most important strategy in preventing the onset of infection is performing hand hygiene between patients.

## Catheter Irrigations and Instillations

60. Briefly describe catheter irrigations and instillations.

_____

_____

_____

_____

_____

## Removal of In-Dwelling Catheter

61. Name two benefits of removing an in-dwelling catheter.

a. _____

b. _____

## Alternatives to Urethral Catheterization

62. Briefly explain the two alternatives for urinary catheterization, and give the nursing implications for each.

a. Suprapubic catheterization:

_____

_____

_____

b. Condom catheterization:

_____

_____

_____

## Maintenance of Skin Integrity

63. List the nursing measures used to maintain skin integrity when urine comes in contact with the skin.

a. _____

b. _____

c. _____

d. _____

## Promotion of Comfort

64. List comfort measures for a patient with the following sources of discomfort.

a. Inflamed tissues near urethral meatus:

_____

_____

_____

b. Painful distension:

_____

_____

_____

## Conservative Therapies to Restore Bladder Control and Promote Continence

65. List measures the nurse can teach the incontinent patient to gain control over elimination.

a. _____

b. _____

c. _____

d. _____

e. _____

f. _____

g. _____

h. _____

i. _____

j. _____

66. Conservative therapies should be the first line of treatment because they are _____, have _____, and _____.

## Lifestyle Modification

67. Describe three lifestyle modifications that can improve symptoms of urinary incontinence.

a. _____

b. _____

c. _____

## Pelvic Floor Muscle Exercises

68. Define *pelvic floor muscle (PFM) exercises* (Kegel exercises), and list the types of incontinence for which they are generally indicated.

_____

_____

_____

_____

_____

**Bladder Training**

69. Describe a regimen of bladder training and the patients most likely to benefit.

_____

_____

_____

_____

_____

**Habit Retraining and Prompted Voiding**

70. Describe the behavioural therapies most appropriate for patients with cognitive impairment, physical impairment, or both.

a. _____

b. _____

## Evaluation

**Patient Care**

The patient is the best source of evaluation of outcomes and responses to nursing care; however, the nurse also evaluates interventions through comparisons with baseline data.

71. You should evaluate for changes in the

_____, _____, and _____.

**Patient Expectations**

You need to confirm whether the patient's expectations have been met to his or her full satisfaction.

You can also assist the patient in redefining unrealistic goals when an impairment is not likely to be altered as completely as the patient might like.

## Review Questions

Select the appropriate answer, and cite the rationale for choosing that particular answer.

1. All of the following factors will influence the production of urine, *except*
   a. Poor PFM tone
   b. Acute renal disease
   c. Febrile conditions
   d. Diuretic medications

Answer: _____ Rationale: _____

_____

_____

2. Mrs. Rantz complains of a small amount of leaking urine when she coughs or laughs. This is known as
   a. Transient incontinence
   b. Stress incontinence
   c. Urge incontinence
   d. Reflex incontinence

Answer: _____ Rationale: _____

_____

_____

3. Ms. Worobetz has a UTI. Which of the following symptoms would you expect her to exhibit?
   a. Proteinuria
   b. Oliguria
   c. Dysuria
   d. Polyuria

Answer: _____ Rationale: _____

_____

_____

4. The nurse is working with a patient who is having an intravenous pyelogram. Which of the following complaints by the patient is an abnormal response?
   a. Shortness of breath and audible wheezing
   b. Feeling dizzy and warm with obvious facial flushing
   c. Thirst and feeling "worn out"
   d. Frequent, loose stools

Answer: _____ Rationale: _____

_____

_____

5. A postsurgical patient who has recently had her in-dwelling catheter removed complains of feeling the urge to void every 20 to 30 minutes but is only voiding small amounts. Which of the following behavioural therapies would be most appropriate?
   a. Habit retraining
   b. Prompted voiding
   c. PFM exercise
   d. Bladder training

Answer: _____ Rationale: _____

_____

_____

## Critical Thinking Model for Nursing Care Plan for Functional Urinary Incontinence

Imagine that you are Kay, the home care nurse in the Care Plan on pages 1131–1133 of your text. Complete the *assessment* phase of the critical thinking model by writing your answers in the appropriate boxes of the model shown. Think about the following:

- What knowledge base was applied to the care of Mrs. Grayson?

- In what ways might Kay's previous experience assist in this case?

- What intellectual or professional standards were applied to Mrs. Grayson?

- What critical thinking attitudes did you utilize in assessing Mrs. Grayson?

- As you review the assessment, what key areas did Kay cover?

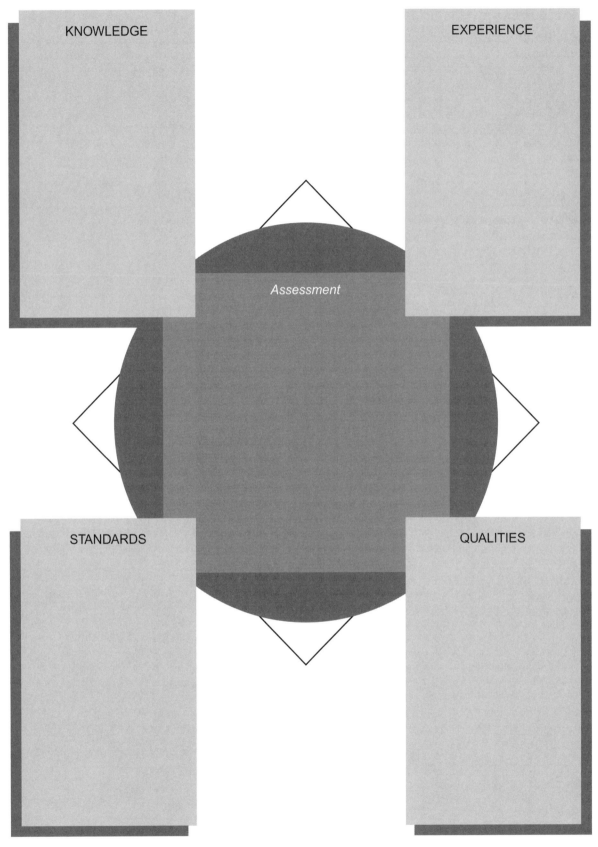

CHAPTER 43   Critical Thinking Model for Nursing Care Plan for *Functional Urinary Incontinence*
See answers on Evolve site.

# 44

# Bowel Elimination

*Preliminary Reading*

Chapter 44, pages 1159–1195

*Comprehensive Understanding*

## Scientific Knowledge Base

The gastrointestinal (GI) tract is a series of hollow, multilayered, muscular organs that are lined with mucous membranes.

1. Summarize the functions of the following:

   a. Mouth:

   _____

   _____

   _____

   b. Esophagus:

   _____

   _____

   _____

   c. Stomach:

   _____

   _____

   _____

   d. Small intestine:

   _____

   _____

   _____

   e. Large intestine:

   _____

   _____

   _____

2. Define the following terms and identify the portion of the GI tract to which they relate.

   a. *Masticate*:

   _____

   _____

   b. *Bolus*:

   _____

   _____

   c. *Peristalsis*:

   _____

   _____

   d. *Chyme*:

   _____

   _____

   e. *Flatus*:

   _____

   _____

   f. *Feces*:

   _____

   _____

# Nursing Knowledge Base

## Process of Defecation

3. Indicate with numbers the correct sequence of mechanisms involved in normal defecation.

_____ Abdominal muscles contract, increasing intrarectal pressure.

_____ The external sphincter relaxes.

_____ The internal sphincter relaxes, and awareness of the need to defecate occurs.

_____ Movement in the left colon occurs, moving stool toward the anus.

4. Describe the *Valsalva manoeuvre* and the risk it poses to certain patients.

_____
_____
_____
_____

5. Describe how the squatting position facilitates defecation.

_____
_____
_____
_____

### Promotion of Normal Defecation

Several interventions can stimulate the defecation reflex, affect the character of feces, or increase peristalsis to help patients evacuate bowel contents normally and without discomfort.

6. List three interventions to facilitate defecation when using a bedpan.

a. _____
b. _____
c. _____

7. Explain how the following can assist the patient to evacuate his or her bowels.

a. Sitting position:

_____
_____
_____

b. Positioning on the bedpan:

_____
_____
_____

8. Explain the proper technique for positioning a patient on a bedpan.

_____
_____
_____
_____

## Factors Affecting Normal Bowel Elimination

### Diet

9. Identify the mechanisms that cause high-fibre diets to promote elimination.

_____
_____
_____
_____

10. List three types of foods that are considered high in fibre (bulk).

a. _____
b. _____
c. _____

11. Define *lactose intolerance*.

_____
_____
_____
_____

### Fluid Intake

12. Summarize how an inadequate intake of fluids can affect the character of feces.

_____
_____
_____
_____
_____

### Physical Activity

13. Physical activity _____ peristalsis; immobilization _____ peristalsis.

14. Weakened abdominal and pelvic floor muscles impair the ability to _____ and to _____.

**Personal Bowel Elimination Habits**

15. List four personal elimination habits that influence bowel function.

    a. _____

    b. _____

    c. _____

    d. _____

**Privacy**

The patient's privacy must be maintained during bowel elimination.

## Nursing Process and Bowel Elimination

## Assessment

**Health History**

What a patient defines as "normal" may differ from factors and conditions that typically promote normal bowel elimination. You can determine the patient's problems by first identifying the normal and abnormal patterns and habits, and then understanding the patient's perception of normal and abnormal regarding bowel elimination.

16. List 16 factors affecting elimination that need to be included in a health history for patients with altered elimination status.

    a. _____

    b. _____

    c. _____

    d. _____

    e. _____

    f. _____

    g. _____

    h. _____

    i. _____

    j. _____

    k. _____

    l. _____

    m. _____

    n. _____

    o. _____

    p. _____

**Physical Assessment**

17. Summarize the following steps for assessing the abdomen.

    a. Inspection:

    _____

    _____

    b. Percussion:

    _____

    _____

    c. Auscultation:

    _____

    _____

    d. Palpation:

    _____

    _____

18. Summarize the assessment of the rectum.

    _____

    _____

    _____

    _____

**Factors Related to Altered Patterns of Bowel Elimination**

**Age-Related Changes**

19. List five changes that occur in the GI system of the older adult that impair normal digestion and elimination.

    a. _____

    b. _____

    c. _____

    d. _____

    e. _____

**Infectious Disease**

20. Microbial agents, including viruses, bacteria, and protozoa, can infect the GI tract. These infections can cause diarrhea and inflammatory or ulcerative changes in the small or large intestine. Most infections are spread by the _____ through _____ or _____.

21. List four infection control procedures to be taken with the Norwalk virus.

    a. _____

    b. _____

    c. _____

    d. _____

**Irritable Bowel Syndrome**

22. Management of irritable bowel syndrome is _____, based on the patient's most troublesome symptoms.

**Diabetes**

23. Patients with diabetes frequently report problems with constipation and/or diarrhea due to _____.

**Pain**

24. List conditions that may result in painful defecation.

    a. _____

    b. _____

    c. _____

    d. _____

**Pelvic Floor Trauma**

25. Identify the common problems related to defecation that occur during pregnancy, and explain why they occur.

    _____

    _____

    _____

    _____

**Acute Illness, Surgery, and Anaesthesia**

26. Summarize the effects of anaesthetic agents and peristalsis on defecation.

    _____

    _____

    _____

    _____

**Enteral Feeding**

27. Discuss the etiology of diarrhea and constipation in patients receiving their nutrition through enteral feedings.

    _____

    _____

    _____

    _____

**Medications That Affect Elimination**

28. Describe the effect on elimination of each of the following medications.

    a. Opioids:

       _____

       _____

    b. Anticholinergics:

       _____

       _____

    c. Antibiotics:

       _____

       _____

    d. Nonsteroidal anti-inflammatory drugs:

       _____

       _____

    e. Histamines:

       _____

       _____

    f. Iron:

       _____

       _____

    g. Calcium carbonate:

       _____

       _____

**Laboratory Tests**

**Fecal Specimens**

29. Briefly describe the appropriate technique for collecting a fecal specimen.

    _____

    _____

    _____

    _____

    _____

30. Define *fecal occult blood test.*

_____

_____

_____

**Fecal Characteristics**

31. Describe the normal fecal characteristics.

a. Colour:

_____

_____

b. Odour:

_____

_____

c. Consistency:

_____

_____

d. Frequency:

_____

_____

e. Amount:

_____

_____

f. Shape:

_____

_____

g. Constituents:

_____

_____

32. Indicate the possible cause for each of the following abnormal fecal characteristics.

a. White or clay colour:

_____

_____

b. Black and tarry (melena):

_____

_____

c. Liquid consistency:

_____

_____

d. Narrow, pencil-shaped:

_____

_____

**Diagnostic Examinations**

**Diagnostic Tests**

33. List three types of diagnostic tests for visualization of GI structures.

a. _____

b. _____

c. _____

## Nursing Diagnosis

34. List five potential or actual nursing diagnoses for a patient with alterations in bowel elimination.

a. _____

b. _____

c. _____

d. _____

e. _____

**Common Bowel Elimination Problems**

35. List five factors that place a patient at risk for elimination problems.

a. _____

b. _____

c. _____

d. _____

e. _____

**Constipation**

36. Define *constipation.*

_____

_____

_____

_____

_____

37. List and briefly describe four causes of constipation.

a. _____

b. _____

c. _____

d. _____

38. List three groups of patients in whom constipation could pose a significant health hazard.

    a. _____

    b. _____

    c. _____

**Impaction**

39. Define *fecal impaction*.

    _____

    _____

    _____

    _____

40. List four signs and symptoms of fecal impaction.

    a. _____

    b. _____

    c. _____

    d. _____

**Diarrhea**

41. Define *diarrhea*.

    _____

    _____

42. List four conditions that cause diarrhea.

    a. _____

    b. _____

    c. _____

    d. _____

43. Name the major complications associated with diarrhea.

    _____

    _____

    _____

**Incontinence**

44. Define *fecal incontinence*.

    _____

    _____

**Flatulence**

45. Flatulence results from _____.

    It is a common cause of _____,

    _____, and _____.

**Hemorrhoids**

46. Define *hemorrhoids*.

    _____

    _____

    _____

    _____

47. List four conditions that cause hemorrhoids.

    a. _____

    b. _____

    c. _____

    d. _____

# Planning

**Goals and Outcomes**

48. List an example of a goal and five associated outcomes appropriate for patients with elimination problems.

    a. _____

    b. _____

    c. _____

    d. _____

    e. _____

# Implementation

Defecation patterns vary among individuals. For this reason, you and your patient must work together closely to plan effective interventions.

Teach the patient and the patient's family about proper diet, adequate fluid intake, and factors that stimulate or slow peristalsis, such as emotional stress.

**Patient Expectations**

Patients expect a knowledgeable nurse who can teach them methods of promoting and maintaining a normal bowel elimination pattern.

**Management of Bowel Elimination**

**Maintenance of Proper Fluid and Food Intake**

Daily fluid intake should be between 1500 and 2000 mL of noncaffeinated beverages. Dietary fibre intake should be from 25 to 30 g/day.

49. Identify four interventions to reduce the risk of constipation:

    a. _____

    b. _____

    c. _____

    d. _____

### Promotion of Regular Exercise

Walking, riding a stationary bicycle, or swimming stimulates peristalsis. Patients who are sedentary at work are most in need of regular exercise.

### Bowel Retraining

50. Briefly explain *bowel retraining*.

    _____

    _____

    _____

    _____

51. Describe two nursing interventions that promote comfort for patients who experience the following:

    a. Hemorrhoids:

    _____

    _____

    b. Risks to skin integrity:

    _____

    _____

### Medications

52. Identify the primary action of the following medications.

    a. Cathartics:

    _____

    _____

    b. Laxatives:

    _____

    _____

    c. Antidiarrheals:

    _____

    _____

### Enemas

53. The primary reason for an enema is

    _____.

54. Briefly describe the following types of enemas.

    a. Tap water:

    _____

    _____

    _____

    b. Normal saline:

    _____

    _____

    _____

    c. Hypertonic solution:

    _____

    _____

    _____

    d. Soapsuds:

    _____

    _____

    e. Oil retention:

    _____

    _____

    _____

    f. Carminative:

    _____

    _____

    _____

### Enema Administration

55. Explain the physician's order "Give enemas until clear."

    _____

    _____

    _____

    _____

56. List four complications of digital removal of stool.

    a. _____

    b. _____

    c. _____

    d. _____

**Surgical Management of Bowel Elimination**

57. List four reasons to insert a nasogastric tube for decompression.

    a. _____

    b. _____

    c. _____

    d. _____

58. Explain how the Salem sump tube works.

    _____

    _____

    _____

    _____

**Bowel Diversions**

59. Define the following.

    a. *Stoma*:

       _____

       _____

    b. *Ileostomy*:

       _____

       _____

    c. *Colostomy*:

       _____

       _____

The location of the ostomy determines the consistency of the stool.

60. Briefly explain each of the following types of colostomy construction.

    a. Loop colostomy:

       _____

       _____

       _____

    b. End colostomy:

       _____

       _____

    c. Double-barrel colostomy:

       _____

       _____

       _____

61. Briefly describe the Kock continent ileostomy.

    _____

    _____

    _____

**Psychological Considerations**

62. Identify a major psychological concern of a patient with an ostomy.

    _____

    _____

    _____

    _____

**Care of Ostomies**

63. Define *effluent*.

    _____

    _____

**Pouching Ostomies**

64. List nine factors to consider when selecting a pouching system for a patient.

    a. _____

    b. _____

    c. _____

    d. _____

    e. _____

    f. _____

    g. _____

    h. _____

    i. _____

**Nutritional Considerations for Patients With Ostomies**

65. Summarize the nutritional considerations for patients with ostomies.

    _____

    _____

    _____

    _____

    _____

## Evaluation

### Patient Care

The effectiveness of care depends on success in meeting the goals and expected outcomes of care.

The patient is the only one who is able to determine if the bowel elimination problems have been relieved and which therapies were the most effective.

### Patient Expectations

The patient will relate a feeling of comfort and freedom from pain as elimination needs are met within the limits of the patient's condition and treatment.

## Review Questions

Select the appropriate answer, and cite the rationale for choosing that particular answer.

1. Most nutrients and electrolytes are absorbed in the
   a. Esophagus
   b. Small intestine
   c. Colon
   d. Stomach

   Answer:_____ Rationale: _____
   _____
   _____

2. Regarding diagnostic examinations involving visualization of the lower GI structures, all of the following are true, *except*
   a. The patient must drink fluids immediately before the test
   b. The patient will probably receive a prescribed bowel preparation before the test
   c. The patient is not allowed to eat or drink before the test
   d. Changes in elimination may occur following the procedure until normal eating patterns resume

   Answer:_____ Rationale: _____
   _____
   _____

3. Mrs. Ahmed has secretory diarrhea. The first action to be taken would be to
   a. Administer Imodium
   b. Increase fluid intake with clear fluids
   c. Increase fluid intake with Gastrolyte
   d. Administer opiates, if prescribed

   Answer:_____ Rationale: _____
   _____
   _____

4. After positioning a patient on the bedpan, you should
   a. Leave the head of the bed flat
   b. Raise the head of the bed 30 degrees
   c. Raise the head of the bed to a 90-degree angle
   d. Raise the bed to the highest working level

   Answer:_____ Rationale: _____
   _____
   _____

5. The physician has ordered a cleansing enema for 7-year-old Michael. The nurse administers
   a. Tap water enema
   b. Low-volume hypertonic saline enema
   c. Normal saline enema
   d. Soapsuds solution enema

   Answer:_____ Rationale: _____
   _____
   _____

## Critical Thinking Model for Nursing Care Plan for Constipation

Imagine that you are Javier, the home care nurse in the Care Plan on pages 1177–1178 of your text. Complete the *planning* phase of the critical thinking model by writing your answers in the appropriate boxes of the model shown. Think about the following:

- In developing Larry's plan of care, what knowledge did Javier apply?

- In what way might Javier's previous experience assist in developing a plan of care for Larry?

- When developing a plan of care, what intellectual or professional standards were applied?

- What critical thinking attitudes might have been applied in developing a plan for Larry?

- How will Javier accomplish the goals?

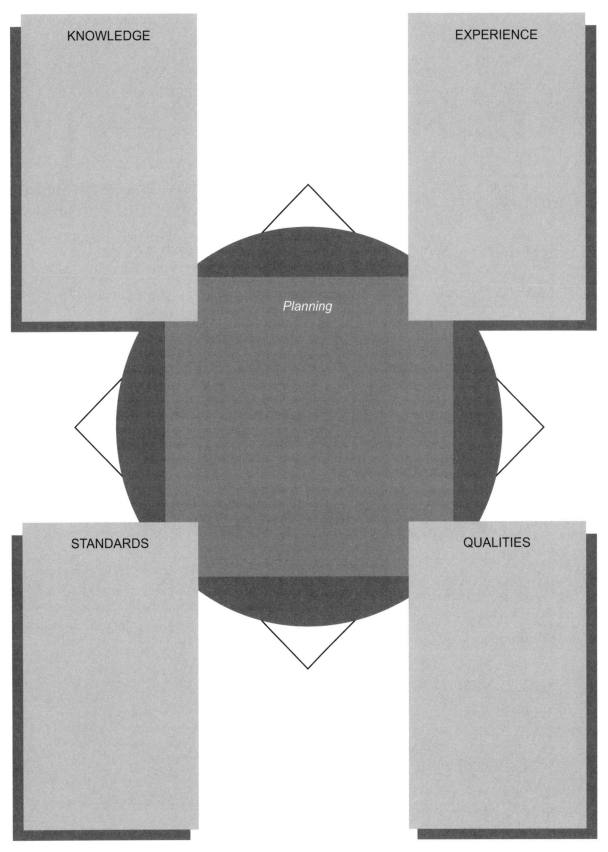

KNOWLEDGE

EXPERIENCE

Planning

STANDARDS

QUALITIES

CHAPTER 44    Critical Thinking Model for Nursing Care Plan for *Constipation*
See answers on Evolve site.

# 45

# Mobility and Immobility

## *Preliminary Reading*

Chapter 45, pages 1195–1249

## *Comprehensive Understanding*

1. *Mobility* refers to _____.

## Scientific Knowledge Base

**Physiology and Principles of Body Mechanics**

2. Define the following:

   a. *Body mechanics*:

     _____
     _____
     _____

   b. *Body alignment or posture*:

     _____
     _____
     _____

3. Balance is required for _____, for _____, and for _____.

4. The ability to balance can be compromised by many situations, such as _____.

**Gravity and Friction**

5. Define *friction*.

    _____
    _____

6. List two techniques that minimize friction.

   a. _____
   b. _____

**Regulation of Movement**

7. List three systems responsible for coordinating body movements.

   a. _____
   b. _____
   c. _____

**Pathological Influences on Mobility**

8. Briefly explain how the following pathological conditions affect mobility.

   a. Postural abnormalities:

     _____
     _____
     _____

   b. Impaired muscle development:

     _____
     _____
     _____

   c. Damage to the central nervous system:

     _____
     _____
     _____

   d. Direct trauma to the musculoskeletal system:

     _____
     _____
     _____

9. Describe *pathological fractures*.

   _____

   _____

## Nursing Knowledge Base

**Mobility–Immobility**

10. *Mobility* refers to _____, and *immobility*

    refers to _____.

11. Define *bed rest*.

    _____

    _____

    _____

12. *Impaired physical mobility* is defined as

    _____.

**Developmental Changes**

13. Identify the descriptive characteristics of body alignment and mobility related to the following developmental stages.

    a. Infants:

       _____

       _____

    b. Toddlers:

       _____

       _____

    c. Preschoolers:

       _____

       _____

    d. Adolescents:

       _____

       _____

    e. Adults:

       _____

       _____

    f. Older adults:

       _____

       _____

14. Briefly describe the hazards of immobility in hospitalized older adults.

    a. Musculoskeletal:

       _____

       _____

    b. Elimination:

       _____

       _____

    c. Nutrition:

       _____

       _____

    d. Psychosocial:

       _____

       _____

## Nursing Process for Impaired Body Alignment and Mobility

### Assessment

15. Briefly describe the four major areas for assessment of patient mobility.

    a. Range of motion:

       _____

       _____

       _____

    b. Body alignment:

       _____

       _____

    c. Gait:

       _____

       _____

       _____

    d. Exercise and activity tolerance:

       _____

       _____

       _____

**Immobility**

**Physiological Assessment**

16. Briefly describe the physiological hazards of immobility in relation to the following systems.

   a. Metabolic:

   _____

   _____

   b. Respiratory:

   _____

   _____

   c. Cardiovascular:

   _____

   _____

   d. Musculoskeletal:

   _____

   _____

   e. Elimination:

   _____

   _____

   f. Integumentary:

   _____

   _____

## Nursing Diagnosis

17. List six actual or potential nursing diagnoses related to an immobilized or partially immobilized patient.

   a. _____

   b. _____

   c. _____

   d. _____

   e. _____

   f. _____

## Planning

**Goals and Outcomes**

The goals and expected outcomes are developed to assist the patient in achieving his or her highest level of mobility.

**Setting Priorities**

18. The nurse plans therapies according to the severity of risks to the patient, and the plan is individualized according to the patient's _____, _____, and _____.

## Implementation

**Health Promotion**

19. Briefly explain the benefits of *exercise*.

   _____

   _____

   _____

   _____

**Acute Care**

20. Identify two nursing interventions to meet each of the following goals for the immobilized patient.

   a. Maintain optimal nutritional (metabolic) state:

   _____

   _____

   b. Promote expansion of the chest and lungs:

   _____

   _____

   c. Prevent stasis of pulmonary secretions:

   _____

   _____

   d. Maintain a patent airway:

   _____

   _____

   e. Reduce *orthostatic hypotension*:

   _____

   _____

   f. Reduce cardiac workload:

   _____

   _____

g. Prevent thrombus formation:

_____

_____

h. Maintain muscle strength and joint mobility:

_____

_____

i. Maintain normal elimination patterns:

_____

_____

j. Prevent pressure ulcers:

_____

_____

k. Maintain usual psychosocial state:

_____

_____

21. Identify two nursing interventions for the immobilized child.

a. _____

b. _____

**Positioning Devices and Techniques**

22. Describe the following positions:

a. Supported Fowler's:

_____

_____

b. Supine:

_____

_____

c. Prone:

_____

_____

d. Side-lying:

_____

_____

e. Sims':

_____

_____

**Transfer Techniques**

23. List some general guidelines to apply in any transfer procedure.

_____

_____

_____

_____

**Moving Patients**

Always enlist the patient's help to the fullest extent possible.

24. List four areas the nurse needs to consider in determining if assistance is required when moving a patient in bed.

a. _____

b. _____

c. _____

d. _____

**Transferring a Patient from a Bed to a Chair**

25. Discuss the purpose of a *transfer belt*.

_____

_____

_____

**Transferring a Patient from a Bed to a Stretcher**

To transfer a patient who is immobile from a bed to a stretcher or from a bed to another bed, use a friction-reducing device under the patient.

**Restorative Care**

26. The goal of restorative care for the immobile patient is to

_____.

27. Instrumental activities of daily living are

_____.

**Joint Mobility**

**Range-of-Motion Exercises**

28. Indicate the type of joint and range-of-motion exercises for the body parts listed in the table below.

| Body Part | Type of Joint | Type of Movement |
|---|---|---|
| Neck | | |
| Shoulder | | |
| Forearm | | |
| Wrist | | |
| Fingers and thumb | | |
| Hip | | |
| Knee | | |
| Ankle and foot | | |
| Toes | | |

**Walking**

**Helping a Patient Walk**

29. Identify the steps you should take to prepare to assist a patient to walk.

_____
_____
_____
_____
_____

30. Describe how you would assist patients with hemiplegia or hemiparesis in walking.

_____
_____
_____
_____
_____

Using Assistive Devices for Walking

31. The nurse, in collaboration with others, promotes activity and exercise by teaching the use of assistive devices most appropriate for a patient's condition. Briefly explain the appropriate use of the following.

    a. Walkers:

    _____
    _____
    _____

    b. Canes:

    _____
    _____
    _____

    c. Crutches:

    _____
    _____
    _____

32. Explain the following crutch gaits.

    a. Three-point:

    _____
    _____
    _____

    b. Two-point:

    _____
    _____
    _____

    c. Swing-through:

    _____
    _____
    _____

33. Explain how you would instruct the patient in each of the following.

    a. Crutch walking on stairs:

    _____
    _____
    _____

    b. Sitting in the chair with crutches:

    _____
    _____
    _____

## Evaluation

### Patient Care

To evaluate outcomes, the nurse measures the effectiveness of all interventions. The actual outcomes are compared with the outcomes selected during planning.

The optimal outcomes are the patient's ability to maintain or improve body alignment and joint mobility.

### Patient Expectations

Patient expectations evaluate care from the patient's perspective.

## Review Questions

Select the appropriate answer, and cite the rationale for choosing that particular answer.

1. The nurse would expect all of the following physiological effects of exercise on the body systems, *except*
   a. Decreased cardiac output
   b. Increased respiratory rate and depth
   c. Increased muscle tone, size, and strength
   d. Change in metabolic rate

   Answer: _____ Rationale: _____
   _____
   _____

2. Which of the following is a potential hazard for which you should assess when the patient is in the prone position?
   a. Unprotected pressure points at the sacrum and heels
   b. Internal rotation of the shoulder
   c. Increased cervical flexion
   d. Plantar flexion

   Answer: _____ Rationale: _____
   _____
   _____

3. Which of the following is a physiological effect of prolonged bed rest?
   a. A decrease in urinary excretion of nitrogen
   b. An increase in cardiac output
   c. A decrease in lean body mass
   d. A decrease in lung expansion

   Answer: _____ Rationale: _____
   _____
   _____

4. All of the following measures are used to assess for deep-vein thrombosis, *except*
    a. Measuring the circumference of each leg daily, placing the tape measure at the midpoint of the knee
    b. Observing the dorsal aspect of lower extremities for redness, warmth, and tenderness
    c. Asking the patient about the presence of calf pain
    d. Checking for a positive Homans' sign, if not contraindicated

Answer: _____ Rationale: _____
_____
_____

5. Which of the following is *not* true of the two-point gait with crutches?
    a. The patient requires at least partial weight bearing on each foot.
    b. The patient is required to bear all of the weight on one foot.
    c. The patient moves one crutch at the same time as the opposing leg.
    d. Crutch movements are similar to arm motion during normal walking.

Answer: _____ Rationale: _____
_____
_____

6. Which of the following is an appropriate intervention to maintain the respiratory system of the immobilized patient?
    a. Turn the patient every four hours.
    b. Maintain a maximum fluid intake of 1500 mL per day.
    c. Apply and maintain an abdominal binder.
    d. Encourage the use of an incentive spirometer.

Answer: _____ Rationale: _____
_____
_____

## Critical Thinking Model for Nursing Care Plan for Impaired Physical Mobility

Imagine that you are the student nurse in the Care Plan on pages 1214–1215 of your text. Complete the *evaluation* phase of the critical thinking model by writing your answers in the appropriate boxes of the model shown. Think about the following:

• What knowledge did you apply in evaluating Ms. Adams's care?

• In what way might your previous experience influence your evaluation of Ms. Adams?

• During evaluation, what intellectual and professional standards were applied to Ms. Adams's care?

• In what ways do critical thinking attitudes play a role in how you approach evaluation of Ms. Adams's care?

• How might you adjust Ms. Adams's care?

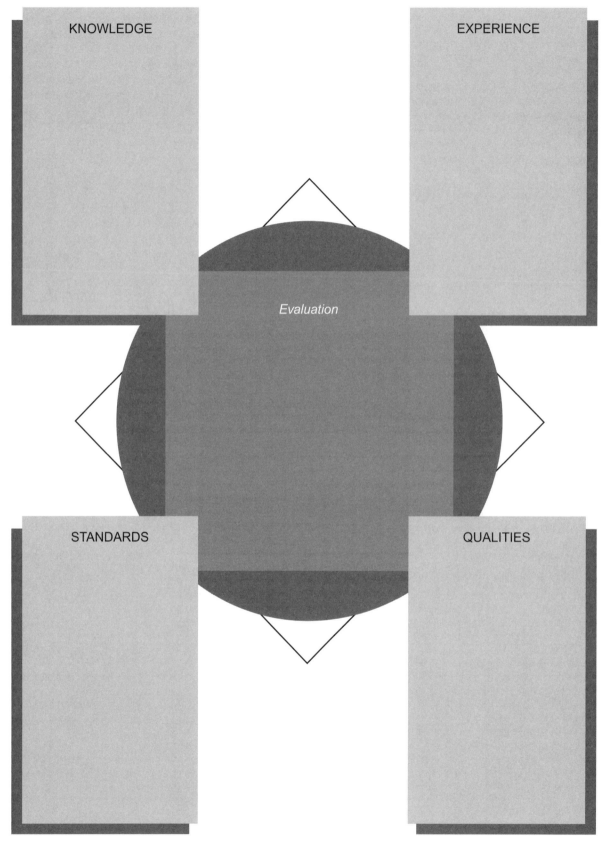

CHAPTER 45   Critical Thinking Model for Nursing Care Plan for *Impaired Physical Mobility*
See answers on Evolve site.

# 46

# Skin Integrity and Wound Care

## Preliminary Reading

Chapter 46, pages 1250–1300

## Comprehensive Understanding

### Scientific Knowledge Base

#### Skin

1. Describe the function of each of the following layers of skin.

   a. Epidermis:

   _____
   _____
   _____

   b. Dermis:

   _____
   _____
   _____

#### Pressure Ulcers

2. Define *pressure ulcer*.

   _____
   _____
   _____
   _____

#### Pathogenesis of Pressure Ulcers

3. Identify the pressure factors that contribute to pressure ulcer development.

   a. _____
   b. _____
   c. _____

4. Define the following.

   a. *Hyperemia* (erythema):

   _____
   _____

   b. *Blanching*:

   _____
   _____

5. Explain the difference between normal reactive hyperemia and abnormal reactive hyperemia. Indicate which of the two is a sign of deep tissue damage.

   _____
   _____
   _____
   _____

### Nursing Knowledge Base

#### Prediction and Prevention of Pressure Ulcers

Consistent, planned skin care interventions are critical to ensuring high-quality care. You need to take every opportunity to observe and assess your patients' skin for impaired skin integrity.

**Risk Factors for Pressure Ulcer Development**

6. Briefly explain how the following factors contribute to an increased risk for pressure ulcers.

   a. Impaired sensory perception:

   _____
   _____
   _____

   b. Impaired mobility:

   _____
   _____
   _____

   c. Altered level of consciousness:

   _____
   _____
   _____

   d. *Shear*:

   _____
   _____
   _____

   e. *Friction*:

   _____
   _____
   _____

   f. Moisture:

   _____
   _____
   _____

   g. Nutrition:

   _____
   _____
   _____

   h. Tissue perfusion:

   _____
   _____
   _____

   i. Infection:

   _____
   _____
   _____

   j. Pain:

   _____
   _____
   _____

   k. Age:

   _____
   _____
   _____

**Psychosocial Impact of Wounds**

7. Identify the factors that may affect the patient's perception of the wound.

   _____
   _____
   _____
   _____
   _____

## Nursing Process

## Assessment

Skin integrity is subject to change over time. Baseline and continual assessment data support critical information about the patient's skin integrity and the increased risk of pressure ulcer development.

**Skin**

8. Explain what factors should be considered in each of the four areas when assessing skin integrity:

   a. Sensation:

   _____
   _____

   b. Mobility:

   _____
   _____

   c. Continence:

   _____
   _____

   d. Presence of a wound:

   _____
   _____

**Risk Assessment**

Evidence exists that a program of prevention guided by consistent risk assessment simultaneously reduces the institutional incidence of pressure ulcers by as much as 60%.

**Braden Scale**

9. List the six categories of the Braden Scale used to predict for pressure ulcer risk.

   a. _____

   b. _____

   c. _____

   d. _____

   e. _____

   f. _____

**Classification of Pressure Ulcers**

10. A pressure ulcer is classified in stages according to its severity. Briefly describe the staging system devised by the National Pressure Ulcer Advisory Panel.

   a. Suspected deep tissue injury:

   _____

   _____

   _____

   b. Stage I:

   _____

   _____

   _____

   c. Stage II:

   _____

   _____

   _____

   d. Stage III:

   _____

   _____

   _____

   e. Stage IV:

   _____

   _____

   _____

   f. Unstageable:

   _____

   _____

   _____

**Wound Classification**

It is imperative that you understand that *all wounds are not created equal.* Understanding the etiology of a wound is important because the treatment for the wound varies depending on the underlying disease process. Some treatments are even harmful to certain wounds, so you always need to obtain a complete history, including the etiology of the wound.

**Process of Wound Healing**

11. Describe the physiological process involved with wound healing.

   a. *Primary intention*:

   _____

   _____

   b. *Secondary intention*:

   _____

   _____

   c. *Tertiary intention*:

   _____

   _____

**Wound Repair**

**Partial-Thickness Wound Repair**

12. Explain the three components involved in the healing of a partial-thickness wound.

   a. _____

   b. _____

   c. _____

**Full-Thickness Wound Repair**

13. Explain the three phases involved in the healing of a full-thickness wound.

   a. Inflammatory phase:

   _____

   _____

   _____

b. Proliferative phase:

_____

_____

_____

c. Remodelling:

_____

_____

_____

14. Briefly describe the etiology of and two main treatment points to consider for each type of wound listed below.

a. Skin tear:

_____

_____

_____

b. Venous ulcer:

_____

_____

_____

c. Arterial ulcer:

_____

_____

_____

d. Diabetic ulcer:

_____

_____

_____

e. Malignant or fungating wound:

_____

_____

_____

f. Acute or surgical wound:

_____

_____

_____

**Character of Wound Drainage**

15. Describe the four major types of wound drainage (*exudate*).

a. _____

b. _____

c. _____

d. _____

**Wound Cultures**

16. What is the purpose of obtaining a wound culture?

_____

_____

_____

_____

17. Describe the method of obtaining a wound culture.

_____

_____

_____

_____

**Complications of Wound Healing**

18. Briefly explain the following complications of wound healing.

a. *Hemorrhage*:

_____

_____

_____

b. *Infection*:

_____

_____

_____

c. *Dehiscence*:

_____

_____

_____

d. *Evisceration*:

_____

_____

_____

e. *Fistulas*:

_____

_____

_____

19. What are the characteristics of wound infection?

 a. _____

 b. _____

 c. _____

 d. _____

 e. _____

## Nursing Diagnosis

20. List three nursing diagnoses related to impaired skin integrity.

 a. _____

 b. _____

 c. _____

## Planning

21. List six possible goals for the patient at risk for pressure ulcers.

 a. _____

 b. _____

 c. _____

 d. _____

 e. _____

 f. _____

### Collaborative Care

22. Discuss the information that should be provided when a patient is discharged or moves to another care setting.

 _____
 _____
 _____

## Implementation: Preventing Skin Breakdown

23. Briefly explain the following nursing interventions for the prevention of pressure ulcers.

 a. Topical skin care:

 _____
 _____
 _____

 b. Positioning:

 _____
 _____
 _____

 c. Support surfaces (therapeutic beds and mattresses):

 _____
 _____
 _____

 d. Education:

 _____
 _____
 _____

 e. Management of pressure ulcers:

 _____
 _____
 _____

### Wound Management

Prevention of wound infection includes wound cleansing and removal of nonviable tissue (*debridement*).

24. List and explain the principles to follow when cleansing a wound or the area around a drain.

 _____
 _____
 _____

25. _____ is a common method of delivering the wound cleansing solution to the wound.

Studies have shown that an optimal effective range of irrigation pressures exists that ensures adequate removal of bacteria. To ensure an irrigation pressure within the correct range, use a 35-mL syringe with a 19-gauge angiocatheter or a single 100-mL saline squeeze bottle.

26. Describe the following methods of debridement.

 a. Mechanical:

 _____
 _____
 _____

b. Biological:

_____

_____

_____

c. Chemical:

_____

_____

_____

d. Autolytic:

_____

_____

_____

e. Surgical:

_____

_____

_____

**Nutritional Status**

27. List four recommendations for nutritional assessment and management of pressure ulcers in the malnourished patient.

a. _____

b. _____

c. _____

d. _____

**Protein Status**

28. Patients require a higher intake of the following to promote healing:

a. _____

b. _____

c. _____

**Dressings**

29. List the purposes for dressings.

a. _____

b. _____

c. _____

d. _____

e. _____

f. _____

g. _____

30. List the clinical guidelines to use when selecting the appropriate dressing.

a. _____

b. _____

c. _____

d. _____

e. _____

f. _____

31. Briefly describe the following types of dressings and their uses.

a. Woven gauze:

_____

_____

b. Transparent film:

_____

_____

c. Nonadherent contact layer:

_____

_____

d. Soft silicone:

_____

_____

e. Hydrocolloid:

_____

_____

f. Hydrogel:

_____

_____

g. Foam:

_____

_____

h. Calcium alginate:

_____

_____

i. Composite:

_____

_____

j. Topical treatment:

_____

_____

k. Hypertonic:

_____

_____

l. Cadexomer iodine:

_____

_____

m. Silver:

_____

_____

n. Honey

_____

_____

o. Negative-pressure wound therapy:

_____

_____

32. To prepare for a dressing change, you must know _____, _____, and _____.

### Clean or Sterile Technique

The RNAO guidelines (2011) recommend sterile dressings, good handwashing, and clean gloves changed between each of the patient's wounds or when soiled.

33. List the activities you would perform to prepare a patient for a dressing change.

a. _____

b. _____

c. _____

d. _____

e. _____

### Packing a Wound

34. The first step in packing a wound is to assess the _____, _____, and _____ of the wound.

35. Summarize the principles of packing a wound.

_____

_____

_____

_____

_____

_____

### Securing Dressings

36. A dressing may be secured by _____, _____, _____, or _____.

### Surgical or Traumatic Wound Considerations

37. Summarize the nursing responsibilities for *suture* care.

_____

_____

_____

_____

38. The manner in which the suture _____ and _____ the skin determines the _____.

39. Discuss the suture removal procedure.

_____

_____

_____

### Drainage Evacuation

40. Explain the purpose for drainage evacuation.

_____

_____

_____

_____

_____

### Bandages and Binders

41. Explain how bandages and binders applied over or around dressings provide extra protection and therapeutic benefits.

a. _____

b. _____

c. _____

d. _____

e. _____

f. _____

### Principles for Applying Bandages and Binders

42. List the nursing responsibilities when applying a bandage or binder.

a. _____

b. _____

c. _____

d. _____

Abdominal Binders

43. Describe the abdominal binder.

_____

_____

_____

_____

## Evaluation

You evaluate nursing interventions for reducing and treating pressure ulcers by determining the patient's response to nursing therapies and whether the patient achieved each goal.

44. The optimal outcomes are to _____, _____, and _____.

## *Review Questions*

Select the appropriate answer, and cite the rationale for choosing that particular answer.

1. Ischemia is defined as
   a. Increased tissue buildup during the healing process
   b. A reduction of blood flow to the tissues
   c. Decreased fluid to the tissues
   d. Increased irritability of nerves

Answer: _____ Rationale: _____

_____

_____

2. Mr. Prada is in a Fowler's position to improve his oxygenation status. You note that he frequently slides down in the bed and needs to be repositioned. Mr. Prada is at risk for developing a pressure ulcer on his coccyx because of
   a. Friction
   b. Shearing force
   c. Maceration
   d. Impaired peripheral circulation

Answer: _____ Rationale: _____

_____

_____

3. Which of the following is *not* a subscale on the Braden Scale for predicting pressure ulcer risk?
   a. Age
   b. Sensory perception
   c. Moisture
   d. Activity

Answer: _____ Rationale: _____

_____

_____

4. Which of the following patients has a nutritional risk for pressure ulcer development?
   a. Patient A has a serum albumin level of 37 g/L.
   b. Patient B has a lymphocyte count of 2000/mm³.
   c. Patient C has a body mass index of 17.
   d. Patient D has a body weight that is 5% greater than his ideal weight.

Answer: _____ Rationale: _____

_____

_____

5. Mrs. Tootoosis is an immobilized patient. Which of the following will *not* increase her risk of developing a pressure ulcer?
   a. She has unrelieved pressure to her hip of greater than 32 mm Hg.
   b. After being turned to her side, she displays normal reactive hyperemia on her coccyx that lasts for 5 minutes.
   c. She has low-intensity pressure over a long period to her heels as a result of elastic stockings.
   d. She is positioned so that she has an unequal distribution of body weight.

Answer: _____ Rationale: _____

_____

_____

6. Mr. Wong has a stage II ulcer of his right heel. What would be the most appropriate treatment for this ulcer?
   a. Apply a thick layer of enzymatic ointment to the ulcer and the surrounding skin.
   b. Apply a calcium alginate dressing, and change when strikethrough is noted.
   c. Apply a heat lamp to the area for 20 minutes twice daily.
   d. Apply a hydrocolloid dressing and change it as necessary.

Answer: _____ Rationale: _____

_____

_____

## Critical Thinking Model for Nursing Care Plan for Impaired Skin Integrity

Imagine that you are the student nurse in the Care Plan on page 1299 of your text. Complete the *assessment* phase of the critical thinking model by writing your answers in the appropriate boxes of the model shown. Think about the following:

• What knowledge base was applied to Mrs. Stein?

• In what way might your previous experience assist you in this case?

• What intellectual or professional standards were applied to Mrs. Stein?

• What critical thinking attitudes did you use in assessing Mrs. Stein?

• As you review your assessment, what key areas did you cover?

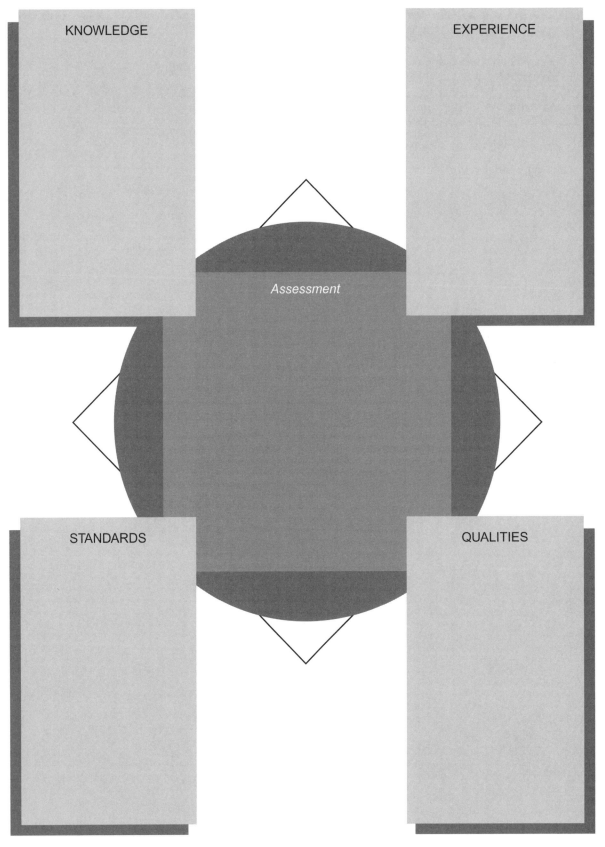

KNOWLEDGE

EXPERIENCE

Assessment

STANDARDS

QUALITIES

CHAPTER 46 Critical Thinking Model for Nursing Care Plan for *Impaired Skin Integrity*
See answers on Evolve site.

# 47

# Sensory Alterations

## Preliminary Reading

Chapter 47, pages 1301–1324

## Comprehensive Understanding

1. Define *stereognosis*.

   _____

   _____

   _____

### Scientific Knowledge Base

**Normal Sensation**

2. List and briefly explain the three functional components necessary for any sensory experience.

   a. _____

   _____

   _____

   b. _____

   _____

   _____

   c. _____

   _____

   _____

**Sensory Alterations**

3. The types of sensory alterations commonly seen

   by the nurse are _____, _____,

   and _____,

**Sensory Deficits**

4. Define *sensory deficit*.

   _____

   _____

   _____

   _____

5. For each of the following, describe a disease or condition that may cause it.

   a. Visual deficit:

   _____

   _____

   b. Hearing deficit:

   _____

   _____

   c. Balance deficit:

   _____

   _____

   d. Taste deficit:

   _____

   _____

**Sensory Deprivation**

6. List the three major types of sensory deprivation and give an example of each.

   a. _____

   b. _____

   c. _____

**Sensory Overload**

7. Define *sensory overload*.

_____

_____

_____

8. Identify the behavioural changes that are associated with sensory overload.

_____

_____

_____

_____

## Nursing Knowledge Base

**Factors Affecting Sensory Function**

9. Explain how and why the following factors affect sensory function.

a. Age:

_____

_____

_____

_____

b. Quality of stimuli:

_____

_____

_____

_____

c. Quantity of stimuli:

_____

_____

_____

_____

d. Social interaction:

_____

_____

_____

_____

e. Family factors:

_____

_____

_____

_____

f. Environmental factors:

_____

_____

_____

_____

## Nursing Process

### Assessment

10. The nurse collects a history that assesses the patient's current sensory status and the degree to which a sensory deficit affects the patient's

_____, _____, _____,

_____, and _____.

**Mental Status**

11. When assessing the patient's mental status, you need to evaluate each of the following. Give an example of each.

a. Physical appearance and behaviour:

_____

_____

b. Cognitive ability:

_____

_____

c. Emotional status:

_____

_____

12. Complete the grid that follows by describing at least one assessment technique for the identified sensory function and the behaviours for an adult and child that would indicate a sensory deficit.

| Sense | Assessment Technique | Child Behaviour | Adult Behaviour |
|---|---|---|---|
| Vision | | | |
| Hearing | | | |
| Touch | | | |
| Smell | | | |
| Taste | | | |
| Position sense | | | |

13. Give an example of an assessment for the following that might assist you in deciding if the patient has a sensory alteration.

   a. Ability to perform self-care:

   _____

   _____

   b. Health promotion habits:

   _____

   _____

   c. Hazards:

   _____

   _____

**Communication Methods**

To understand the nature of a communication problem, you must know whether a patient has trouble speaking, understanding, naming, reading, or writing. Patients with existing sensory deficits often develop alternative ways of communicating.

## Nursing Diagnosis

14. List six or more actual or potential nursing diagnoses that might apply to a patient with sensory alterations.

   a. _____

   b. _____

   c. _____

   d. _____

   e. _____

   f. _____

   g. _____

   h. _____

   i. _____

## Planning

### Goals and Outcomes

15. List an example of a goal and four associated outcomes appropriate for a patient with a sensory alteration.

    a. _____

    b. _____

    c. _____

    d. _____

    e. _____

## Implementation

### Health Promotion

16. List the three recommended vision screening interventions.

    a. _____

    b. _____

    c. _____

17. The most common visual problem is

    _____.

18. Explain how hearing loss can be caused by exposure to excessive noise.

    _____

    _____

    _____

    _____

### Preventive Safety

19. Identify the common injuries due to trauma that result in hearing or vision loss in both adults and children.

    a. Adults:

    _____

    _____

    _____

    b. Children:

    _____

    _____

    _____

### Use of Assistive Devices

20. Explain the measures to take to ensure that assistive devices being used help maintain sensory function at the highest level.

    _____

    _____

    _____

    _____

### Promoting Meaningful Stimulation

21. Briefly explain how the nurse can promote meaningful stimulation for patients with sensory alterations in the following areas:

    a. Vision:

    _____

    _____

    _____

    b. Hearing:

    _____

    _____

    _____

    c. Taste and smell:

    _____

    _____

    _____

    d. Touch:

    _____

    _____

    _____

### Establishing Safe Environments

22. List three methods of establishing a safe environment with regard to the following adaptations.

    a. Visual loss:

    _____

    _____

    _____

b. Reduced hearing:

_____

_____

_____

c. Reduced olfaction:

_____

_____

_____

d. Reduced tactile sensation:

_____

_____

_____

**Promoting Communication**

23. Describe ten communication methods that are appropriate for patients with a hearing impairment.

a. _____

b. _____

c. _____

d. _____

e. _____

f. _____

g. _____

h. _____

i. _____

j. _____

## Acute Care

24. When patients enter acute care settings for therapeutic management of sensory deficits or as a result of traumatic injury, the following approaches are used to maximize sensory function. Briefly explain each.

a. Orientation to the environment:

_____

_____

_____

_____

b. Controlling sensory stimuli:

_____

_____

_____

_____

c. Safety measures:

_____

_____

_____

_____

**Restorative and Continuing Care**

**Maintaining Healthy Lifestyles**

25. After a patient experiences a sensory loss, it becomes important to understand the implications of the loss and to make the adjustments needed to continue a normal lifestyle. Briefly explain each.

a. Understanding sensory loss:

_____

_____

_____

_____

b. Socialization:

_____

_____

_____

_____

c. Promoting self-care:

_____

_____

_____

_____

## Evaluation

**Patient Care**

Only patients themselves will know if their sensory abilities are improved and which interventions or therapies are the most successful.

**Patient Expectations**

26. Patient expectations are one of the evaluative criteria used by the nurse. What questions might you ask to determine if patient expectations have been met?

_____

_____

_____

_____

## Review Questions

Select the appropriate answer, and cite the rationale for choosing that particular answer.

1. All of the following are true of age-related factors that influence sensory function, *except*
   a. Refractive errors are the most common types of visual disorders in children
   b. Visual changes in adulthood include presbyopia
   c. Older adults hear high-pitched sounds best
   d. Neonates are unable to discriminate sensory stimuli

Answer: _____ Rationale:_____
_____
_____

2. Mr. McDonald, a 62-year-old farmer, has been hospitalized for two weeks for thrombophlebitis. He has no visitors, and the nurse notices that he appears bored, restless, and anxious. The type of alteration occurring because of sensory deprivation is:
   a. Affective
   b. Cognitive
   c. Perceptual
   d. Receptual

Answer: _____ Rationale:_____
_____
_____

3. Which of the following would *not* provide meaningful stimuli for a patient?
   a. A clock or calendar with large numbers
   b. A television that is kept on all day at a low volume
   c. Family pictures and personal possessions
   d. Interesting magazines and books

Answer: _____ Rationale:_____
_____
_____

4. Patients with existing sensory loss must be protected from injury. What determines the safety precautions taken?
   a. The existing dangers in the environment
   b. The financial means to make needed safety changes
   c. The nature of the patient's actual or potential sensory loss
   d. The availability of a support system to enable the patient to exist in his or her present environment

Answer: _____ Rationale:_____
_____
_____

5. Mr. Johnson is an 84-year-old postoperative patient with a hearing impairment. Methods to assist communication would include all but one of the following:
   a. Speak quickly and shout.
   b. Face the patient, and stand or sit on the same level.
   c. Rephrase when you are not understood.
   d. Avoid speaking from another room or while walking away.

Answer: _____ Rationale:_____
_____
_____

## Critical Thinking Model for Nursing Care Plan for Disturbed Sensory Perception

Imagine that you are the community health nurse in the Care Plan on pages 1313–1314 of your text. Complete the *planning* phase of the critical thinking model by writing your answers in the appropriate boxes of the model shown. Think about the following:

- In developing Judy's plan of care, what knowledge did you apply?

- In what way might your previous experience assist in developing a plan of care?

- When developing a plan of care, what intellectual and professional standards were applied?

- What critical thinking attitudes might have been applied in Judy's plan of care?

- How will you accomplish the goals?

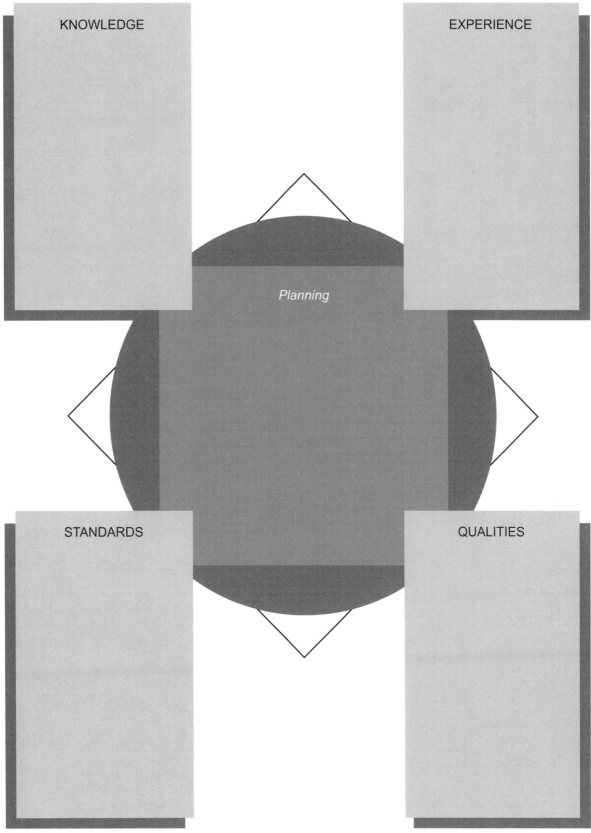

KNOWLEDGE

EXPERIENCE

Planning

STANDARDS

QUALITIES

CHAPTER 47 Critical Thinking Model for Nursing Care Plan for *Disturbed Sensory Perception*
See answers on Evolve site.

# 48

# Care of Surgical Patients

*Preliminary Reading*

Chapter 48, pages 1325–1370

*Comprehensive Understanding*

1. Define *perioperative nursing*.

   _____

   _____

## History of Surgical Nursing

2. Summarize the historical changes that have occurred in surgical nursing.

   _____

   _____

   _____

   _____

   _____

   _____

### Same-Day (Ambulatory) Surgery

3. List the benefits of ambulatory surgery.

   a. _____

   b. _____

   c. _____

   d. _____

## Scientific Knowledge Base

### Classification of Surgery

4. Define the following surgical procedure classifications.

   a. Major:

      _____

      _____

b. Minor:

   _____

   _____

c. Elective:

   _____

   _____

d. Urgent:

   _____

   _____

e. Emergency:

   _____

   _____

f. Diagnostic:

   _____

   _____

g. Ablative:

   _____

   _____

h. Palliative:

   _____

   _____

i. Reconstructive:

   _____

   _____

j. Procurement for transplant:

_____

_____

k. Constructive:

_____

_____

l. Cosmetic

_____

_____

## The Nursing Process in the Preoperative Surgical Phase

### Assessment

An interprofessional team approach is essential. Patients are admitted only hours before the surgical event; thus, you must organize and verify data obtained preoperatively to implement a perioperative care plan.

#### Medical History

5. Identify the data you should collect from the patient's medical history.

_____

_____

_____

_____

#### Risk Factors

6. Briefly explain the following factors that increase the patient's risk in surgery.

a. Age:

_____

_____

_____

_____

b. Nutrition:

_____

_____

_____

_____

c. Obesity:

_____

_____

_____

_____

d. Immunocompetence:

_____

_____

_____

_____

e. Fluid and electrolyte imbalances:

_____

_____

_____

_____

f. Pregnancy:

_____

_____

_____

_____

7. Briefly explain the rationale for assessing the following:

a. Previous surgeries:

_____

_____

_____

_____

b. Perceptions and understanding of surgery:

_____

_____

_____

_____

c. Medication history:

_____

_____

_____

_____

d. Allergies:

_____
_____
_____
_____

e. Smoking habits:

_____
_____
_____
_____

f. Alcohol ingestion and substance use and abuse:

_____
_____
_____
_____

g. Family support:

_____
_____
_____
_____

h. Occupation:

_____
_____
_____
_____

i. Preoperative preparation for pain assessment and management:

_____
_____
_____
_____

**Review of Emotional Health**

8. Briefly explain each of the following factors that must be assessed to understand the impact of surgery on a patient's and family's emotional health:

a. Body image:

_____
_____
_____
_____

b. Coping resources:

_____
_____
_____
_____

**Culture**

9. Cultural differences influence the surgical experience. Give an example.

_____
_____
_____
_____

**Physical Examination**

10. Briefly describe the findings on which you should focus related to the physical examination of the following body systems:

a. General survey:

_____
_____
_____
_____

b. Head and neck:

_____
_____
_____
_____

c. Integument:

_____
_____
_____
_____

d. Thorax and lungs:

_____
_____
_____
_____

e. Heart and vascular system:

_____
_____
_____
_____

f. Abdomen:

_____

_____

_____

_____

g. Neurological status:

_____

_____

_____

_____

## Diagnostic Screening

11. Describe the following routine screening tests for surgical patients.

a. Complete blood count:

_____

_____

b. Serum electrolytes:

_____

_____

c. Coagulation studies:

_____

_____

d. Serum creatinine:

_____

_____

e. Blood urea nitrogen:

_____

_____

f. Glucose:

_____

_____

## Nursing Diagnosis

12. List ten potential or actual nursing diagnoses appropriate for the preoperative patient.

a. _____

b. _____

c. _____

d. _____

e. _____

f. _____

g. _____

h. _____

i. _____

j. _____

## Planning

### Goals and Outcomes

13. Give examples of associated outcomes related to the goal of a preoperative patient being able to verbalize the significance of postoperative exercises.

a. _____

b. _____

c. _____

d. _____

## Implementation

### Informed Consent

14. Surgery cannot be performed until a patient understands the following:

a. _____

b. _____

c. _____

d. _____

e. _____

### Preoperative Teaching

Preparatory information helps patients anticipate the steps of a procedure and thus helps them form realistic images of the surgical experience. When events occur as predicted, patients are better able to cope and attend to the experiences.

15. Describe the criteria that may demonstrate the patient's understanding of the surgical procedure.

a. _____

b. _____

c. _____

d. _____

e. _____

f. _____

g. _____

h. _____

**Acute Care**

**Physical Preparation**

16. Briefly describe the following preoperative preparations:

    a. Maintenance of normal fluid and electrolyte balances:

    _____

    _____

    _____

    _____

    b. Reduction of risk of surgical wound infection:

    _____

    _____

    _____

    _____

    c. Precautions for patient requiring infection-control procedures:

    _____

    _____

    _____

    _____

    d. Prevention of bowel and bladder incontinence:

    _____

    _____

    _____

    _____

    e. Promotion of rest and comfort:

    _____

    _____

    _____

    _____

**Preparation on the Day of Surgery**

17. List nine responsibilities of a nurse caring for a patient on the day of surgery.

    a. _____

    b. _____

    c. _____

d. _____

e. _____

f. _____

g. _____

h. _____

i. _____

**Latex Sensitivity or Allergy**

18. The signs and symptoms of a latex reaction are

_____ .

**Eliminating Wrong Site and Wrong Procedure Surgery**

19. Describe methods to eliminate wrong site and wrong procedure surgery.

    _____

    _____

    _____

    _____

    _____

    _____

## Transport to the Operating Room

20. After the patient leaves the nursing division, the nurse prepares the bed and room for the patient's return if the patient is returning to the same nursing division. List ten pieces of equipment that should be present in the postoperative bedside unit.

    a. _____

    b. _____

    c. _____

    d. _____

    e. _____

    f. _____

    g. _____

    h. _____

    i. _____

    j. _____

## Intraoperative Surgical Phase

21. The nurse functions in one of two roles in the OR: _____ or _____ .

### Preoperative (Holding) Area

22. In the holding area, two nursing responsibilities are _____.

## The Nursing Process in the Intraoperative Surgical Phase

## Assessment

23. The preoperative assessment in the OR is important for the patient's safety because _____.

## Planning

Patient-centred outcomes of preoperative care extend into the intraoperative phase.

## Implementation

### Introduction of Anaesthesia

### General Anaesthesia

24. *General anaesthesia* involves

_____.

### Regional Anaesthesia

25. *Regional anaesthesia* results in

_____.

### Local Anaesthesia

26. *Local anaesthesia* involves

_____.

### *Conscious Sedation*

27. Describe *conscious sedation*, and identify its advantages.

_____
_____
_____
_____
_____
_____

### Positioning the Patient for Surgery

28. Identify factors to consider when positioning the patient for surgery.

_____
_____
_____
_____
_____
_____

### Documentation of Intraoperative Care

During the intraoperative phase, the nursing staff continues the preoperative plan.

Documentation of intraoperative care provides useful data for the nurse who cares for the patient postoperatively.

## Postoperative Surgical Phase

### Immediate Postoperative Recovery

29. Describe the assessment data that you should obtain in the postanaesthesia care unit (PACU).

_____
_____
_____
_____
_____
_____

### Discharge From the Postanaesthesia Care Unit

30. Identify the criteria for discharge from the PACU.

a. _____
b. _____
c. _____
d. _____
e. _____
f. _____
g. _____
h. _____

**Recovery in Ambulatory Surgery**

31. Describe the two phases of postanaesthesia recovery.

    a. Phase I:

    _____

    _____

    _____

    b. Phase II:

    _____

    _____

    _____

32. Describe what the *Postanesthesia Recovery Score* tool is and what minimum score is required for discharge.

    _____

    _____

    _____

    _____

# The Nursing Process in Postoperative Care

## Assessment

33. Explain the frequency of assessments needed during the postoperative period.

    _____

    _____

    _____

    _____

    _____

    _____

    _____

**Respiration**

34. List four major causes of airway obstruction in the postoperative patient.

    a. _____

    b. _____

    c. _____

    d. _____

**Circulation**

35. List four areas to assess to determine a postoperative patient's circulatory status.

    a. _____

    b. _____

    c. _____

    d. _____

36. Describe the characteristic findings associated with postoperative hemorrhage.

    a. Blood pressure:

    _____

    _____

    b. Heart rate and character of pulse:

    _____

    _____

    c. Respiratory rate:

    _____

    _____

    d. Skin:

    _____

    _____

    e. Level of consciousness:

    _____

    _____

**Temperature Control**

37. Explain why patients awakening from surgery often complain of feeling cold.

    _____

    _____

    _____

    _____

38. Define *malignant hyperthermia*.

    _____

    _____

    _____

    _____

**Fluid and Electrolyte Balance**

39. List three areas you should assess to determine fluid and electrolyte alterations.

    a. _____

    b. _____

    c. _____

**Neurological Functions**

40. List the areas of assessment that help to determine a postoperative patient's neurological status.

    a. _____

    b. _____

    c. _____

    d. _____

**Skin Integrity and Condition of the Wound**

41. The nurse assesses the condition of the skin, noting _____, _____, _____, and _____.

42. Describe how the nurse would assess the amount of drainage from a wound.

    _____

    _____

    _____

    _____

**Genitourinary Function**

Depending on the surgery, a patient may not regain voluntary control over urinary function for six to eight hours after anaesthesia.

**Gastrointestinal Function**

43. Distension may occur in the patient who develops a _____.

44. Normally during the immediate recovery phase, faint or absent bowel sounds are auscultated in all four quadrants. Routinely, you auscultate the abdomen to detect return of normal bowel sounds; _____ loud gurgles per minute over each quadrant indicate that peristalsis has returned.

**Pain and Comfort**

45. Pain can be perceived before full consciousness is regained. Acute incisional pain causes patients to become _____ and may be responsible for temporary changes in _____.

Assessment of the patient's discomfort and evaluation of pain relief therapies are essential nursing functions.

# Nursing Diagnosis

46. Identify two actual or potential nursing diagnoses that are appropriate for a postoperative patient.

    a. _____

    b. _____

# Planning

47. List the typical postoperative plans prescribed by surgeons and seen, for example, on clinical pathways.

    a. _____

    b. _____

    c. _____

    d. _____

    e. _____

    f. _____

    g. _____

    h. _____

    i. _____

    j. _____

    k. _____

**Goals and Outcomes**

48. Give five goals of care and associated outcomes for a postoperative patient.

    a. _____

    b. _____

    c. _____

    d. _____

    e. _____

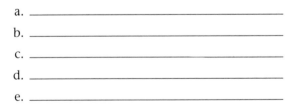

## Implementation

### Health Promotion

49. To prevent respiratory complications, begin pulmonary interventions early. Describe measures that will promote the following.

  a. Airway patency:

  _____
  _____
  _____

  b. Expansion of the lungs:

  _____
  _____
  _____

  c. Removal of pulmonary secretions:

  _____
  _____
  _____

### Preventing Circulatory Complications

50. Briefly describe measures to promote normal venous return and circulatory blood flow.

  a. _____
  b. _____
  c. _____
  d. _____
  e. _____
  f. _____

### Achieving Rest and Comfort

51. List three nonpharmacological pain-relief measures.

  a. _____
  b. _____
  c. _____

### Acute Care

52. Identify two postoperative nursing interventions for the following:

  a. Regulation of temperature:

  _____
  _____

  b. Maintenance of neurological status:

  _____
  _____

  c. Maintenance of fluid and electrolyte balances:

  _____
  _____

### Promoting Wound Healing

You protect the wound and promote healing. A critical time for wound healing is 24 to 72 hours after surgery, after which time a seal is established.

### Maintaining and Enhancing Self-Concept

53. Identify four nursing interventions to help maintain the patient's self-concept.

  _____
  _____
  _____
  _____

## Evaluation

### Patient Care

The nurse evaluates the effectiveness of care provided to the surgical patient on the basis of expected outcomes following nursing interventions.

54. Describe how you should evaluate the ambulatory surgical patient.

  _____
  _____
  _____
  _____
  _____

## Review Questions

Select the appropriate answer, and cite the rationale for choosing that particular answer.

1. Mrs. Yong-Hing, a 45-year-old patient with diabetes, is having a hysterectomy in the morning. Because of her history, the nurse would expect
  a. An increased risk of hemorrhaging
  b. Fluid imbalances
  c. Altered elimination of anaesthetic agents
  d. Impaired wound healing

  Answer: _____ Rationale: _____
  _____
  _____

2. The purposes of the health history for the patient who is to have surgery include all of the following, *except*
   a. Identifying the patient's perception about surgery
   b. Obtaining information about the patient's past experience with surgery
   c. Deciding whether surgery is indicated
   d. Understanding the impact surgery has on the patient's and family's emotional health

Answer: _____ Rationale: _____
_____
_____

3. All of the following patients are at risk for developing serious fluid and electrolyte imbalances during and after surgery, *except*
   a. Patient E, who is 81 years old and is having emergency surgery for a bowel obstruction following four days of vomiting and diarrhea
   b. Patient F, who is 1 year old and is having a cleft palate repair
   c. Patient G, who is 55 years old and has a history of chronic respiratory disease
   d. Patient H, who is 79 years old and has a history of congestive heart failure

Answer: _____ Rationale: _____
_____
_____

4. The primary purpose of postoperative leg exercises is to
   a. Promote venous return
   b. Promote lymphatic drainage
   c. Assess range of motion
   d. Exercise fatigued muscles

Answer: _____ Rationale: _____
_____
_____

5. The PACU nurse notices that the patient is shivering. This is most commonly caused by
   a. The use of a reflective blanket on the OR table
   b. Side effects of certain anaesthetic agents
   c. IV narcotics used for pain management
   d. Malignant hypothermia

Answer: _____ Rationale: _____
_____
_____

## Critical Thinking Model for Nursing Care Plan for Deficient Knowledge Regarding Preoperative and Postoperative Care Requirements

Imagine that you are Joe, the nurse in the Care Plan on pages 1339–1340 of your text. Complete the *evaluation* phase of the critical thinking model by writing your answers in the appropriate boxes of the model shown. Think about the following:

- During evaluation, what knowledge and professional standards were applied to Mrs. Campana's care?

- In what way might Joe's previous experience influence his evaluation of Mrs. Campana's care?

- In what way do critical thinking attitudes play a role in how you approach the evaluation of Mrs. Campana's care plan?

- How might Joe adjust Mrs. Campana's care?

- What knowledge did Joe apply in evaluating Mrs. Campana's care?

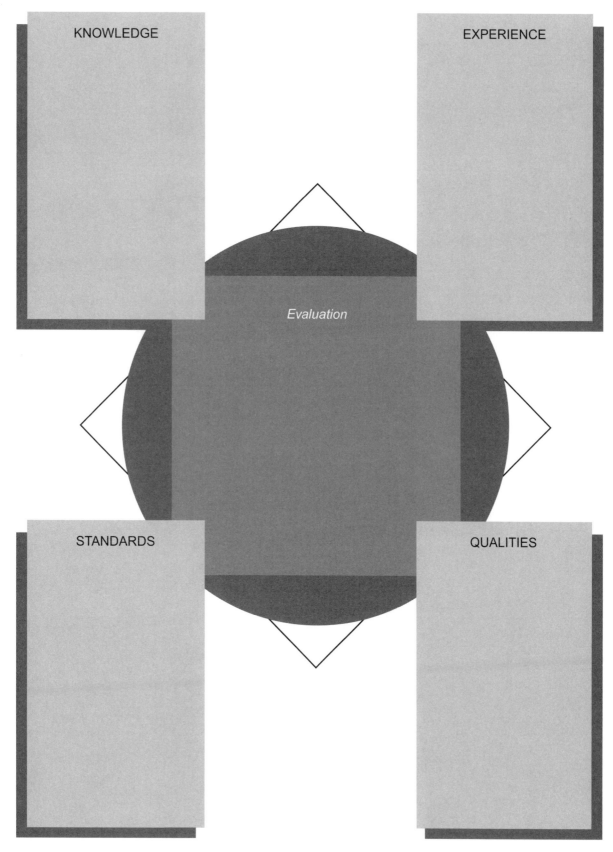

KNOWLEDGE

EXPERIENCE

*Evaluation*

STANDARDS

QUALITIES

CHAPTER 48    Critical Thinking Model for Nursing Care Plan for *Deficient Knowledge Regarding Preoperative and Postoperative Care Requirements*
See answers on Evolve site.

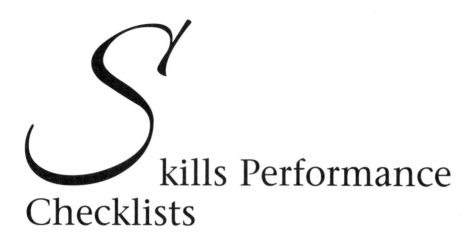

# Skills Performance Checklists

353

STUDENT: _____   DATE: _____

INSTRUCTOR: _____   DATE: _____

## Skill Performance Checklist
## Skill 30-1 Measuring Body Temperature

| | S | U | NP | Comments |
|---|---|---|---|---|
| 1. Assess for temperature alterations and factors that influence body temperature. | ___ | ___ | ___ | _____ |
| 2. Determine any activity that may interfere with accuracy of temperature measurement. | ___ | ___ | ___ | _____ |
| 3. Determine appropriate site and measurement device to be used. | ___ | ___ | ___ | _____ |
| 4. Explain to patient how temperature will be taken and importance of maintaining proper position. | ___ | ___ | ___ | _____ |
| 5. Perform hand hygiene. | ___ | ___ | ___ | _____ |
| 6. Obtain temperature reading: | | | | |
| A. Oral temperature measurement with electronic thermometer | | | | |
| (1) Apply disposable gloves (optional). | ___ | ___ | ___ | _____ |
| (2) Remove thermometer pack from charging unit. Attach oral probe (blue tip) to thermometer unit. Grasp top of probe stem, being careful not to apply pressure on the ejection button. | ___ | ___ | ___ | _____ |
| (3) Slide disposable plastic probe cover over thermometer probe until it locks in place. | ___ | ___ | ___ | _____ |
| (4) Have patient sit or lie in bed. Ask patient to open mouth, then place thermometer probe under tongue in posterior sublingual pocket lateral to centre of lower jaw. | ___ | ___ | ___ | _____ |
| (5) Ask patient to hold thermometer probe with lips closed. | ___ | ___ | ___ | _____ |
| (6) Leave thermometer probe in place until audible signal occurs and temperature appears on digital display. Remove thermometer probe from under the patient's tongue. | ___ | ___ | ___ | _____ |
| (7) Push ejection button on thermometer stem to discard plastic probe cover into appropriate receptacle. | ___ | ___ | ___ | _____ |
| (8) Return thermometer stem to storage well of recording unit. | ___ | ___ | ___ | _____ |
| (9) If gloves were worn, remove and dispose of them in appropriate receptacle. Perform hand hygiene. | ___ | ___ | ___ | _____ |
| (10) Return thermometer to charger. | ___ | ___ | ___ | _____ |
| B. Rectal temperature measurement with electronic thermometer | | | | |
| (1) Prepare for the procedure. Draw curtain around patient's bed or close room door, or do both. | ___ | ___ | ___ | _____ |
| (2) Assist patient to Sims position. | ___ | ___ | ___ | _____ |
| (3) Move aside bed linen to expose only anal area. Drape patient. Remind patient to remain in position until procedure is complete. | ___ | ___ | ___ | _____ |
| (4) Apply disposable gloves. | ___ | ___ | ___ | _____ |
| (5) Remove thermometer pack from charging unit. Attach rectal probe (red tip) to thermometer unit. Grasp top of probe stem. | ___ | ___ | ___ | _____ |
| (6) Slide disposable plastic probe cover over thermometer probe until it locks in place. | ___ | ___ | ___ | _____ |
| (7) Lubricate 2.5 to 3.5 cm of probe for an adult or 1.2 to 2.5 cm for an infant or child. | ___ | ___ | ___ | _____ |
| (8) With nondominant hand, separate buttocks to expose anus. Ask patient to breathe slowly and relax. | ___ | ___ | ___ | _____ |
| (9) Gently insert thermometer in the direction of the umbilicus, 3.5 cm for an adult. | ___ | ___ | ___ | _____ |
| (10) If resistance is felt, withdraw thermometer immediately. Never force thermometer. | ___ | ___ | ___ | _____ |
| (11) Leave thermometer probe in place until audible signal occurs and temperature appears on digital display. Remove thermometer probe from patient's anus. | ___ | ___ | ___ | _____ |
| (12) Push ejection button on thermometer stem to discard plastic probe cover. Wipe probe with alcohol swab. | ___ | ___ | ___ | _____ |

*Continued*

|  | S | U | NP | Comments |
|---|---|---|---|---|

(13) Return thermometer stem to storage well of recording unit. ⎯ ⎯ ⎯ ⎯⎯⎯⎯

(14) Wipe patient's anal area with soft tissue, and discard tissue. Assist patient to a comfortable position, and cover sufficiently with linens. ⎯ ⎯ ⎯ ⎯⎯⎯⎯

(15) Remove and dispose of gloves. Perform hand hygiene. ⎯ ⎯ ⎯ ⎯⎯⎯⎯

(16) Return thermometer to charger. ⎯ ⎯ ⎯ ⎯⎯⎯⎯

C. Axillary temperature measurement with electronic thermometer

(1) Prepare patient for procedure. Draw curtain around patient's bed or close room door, or do both. ⎯ ⎯ ⎯ ⎯⎯⎯⎯

(2) Assist patient to supine or sitting position. ⎯ ⎯ ⎯ ⎯⎯⎯⎯

(3) Move clothing or gown away from patient's shoulder and arm. ⎯ ⎯ ⎯ ⎯⎯⎯⎯

(4) Remove thermometer pack from charging unit. Be sure oral probe (blue tip) is attached to thermometer unit. Grasp top of probe stem. ⎯ ⎯ ⎯ ⎯⎯⎯⎯

(5) Slide disposable plastic probe cover over thermometer probe until it locks in place. ⎯ ⎯ ⎯ ⎯⎯⎯⎯

(6) Raise patient's arm away from torso, and inspect for skin lesions and excessive perspiration. Insert probe into centre of patient's axilla, lower arm over probe, and place arm across chest. ⎯ ⎯ ⎯ ⎯⎯⎯⎯

(7) Hold probe in place until audible signal occurs and temperature appears on digital display. ⎯ ⎯ ⎯ ⎯⎯⎯⎯

(8) Remove probe from axilla. ⎯ ⎯ ⎯ ⎯⎯⎯⎯

(9) Push ejection button on probe to discard plastic probe cover. ⎯ ⎯ ⎯ ⎯⎯⎯⎯

(10) Return probe to storage well of recording unit. ⎯ ⎯ ⎯ ⎯⎯⎯⎯

(11) Assist patient to a comfortable position. ⎯ ⎯ ⎯ ⎯⎯⎯⎯

(12) Perform hand hygiene. ⎯ ⎯ ⎯ ⎯⎯⎯⎯

(13) Return thermometer to charger. ⎯ ⎯ ⎯ ⎯⎯⎯⎯

D. Tympanic membrane temperature with electronic thermometer

(1) Assist patient to a comfortable position with head turned toward the side, away from you. ⎯ ⎯ ⎯ ⎯⎯⎯⎯

(2) Check for the presence of obvious cerumen in the ear canal. ⎯ ⎯ ⎯ ⎯⎯⎯⎯

(3) Remove hand-held thermometer unit from charging base, being careful not to apply pressure on the ejection button. ⎯ ⎯ ⎯ ⎯⎯⎯⎯

(4) Slide disposable speculum cover over tip until it locks into place. ⎯ ⎯ ⎯ ⎯⎯⎯⎯

(5) Insert speculum into ear canal following manufacturer's instructions for tympanic probe positioning: ⎯ ⎯ ⎯ ⎯⎯⎯⎯

a. Pull ear pinna backward, up, and out for adult. For children younger than 2 years, pull pinna backward and point covered speculum tip toward midpoint between eyebrow and sideburn. ⎯ ⎯ ⎯ ⎯⎯⎯⎯

b. Fit probe gently in ear canal, and do not move it. ⎯ ⎯ ⎯ ⎯⎯⎯⎯

c. Point probe toward patient's nose. ⎯ ⎯ ⎯ ⎯⎯⎯⎯

(6) Press scan button on hand-held unit. Leave thermometer probe in place until audible signal occurs and patient's temperature appears on digital display. ⎯ ⎯ ⎯ ⎯⎯⎯⎯

(7) Carefully remove speculum from patient's auditory canal. ⎯ ⎯ ⎯ ⎯⎯⎯⎯

(8) Push ejection button on hand-held unit to discard plastic probe cover. ⎯ ⎯ ⎯ ⎯⎯⎯⎯

(9) If second reading is required, replace probe cover and wait two to three minutes. ⎯ ⎯ ⎯ ⎯⎯⎯⎯

(10) Return hand-held unit to charging base. ⎯ ⎯ ⎯ ⎯⎯⎯⎯

(11) Assist patient to a comfortable position. ⎯ ⎯ ⎯ ⎯⎯⎯⎯

7. Perform hand hygiene. ⎯ ⎯ ⎯ ⎯⎯⎯⎯

8. Discuss findings with patient as needed. ⎯ ⎯ ⎯ ⎯⎯⎯⎯

9. If temperature is being assessed for the first time, establish temperature as baseline if within normal range; document temperature as baseline. ⎯ ⎯ ⎯ ⎯⎯⎯⎯

10. Compare temperature reading with previous baseline and normal temperature range for patient's age group. ⎯ ⎯ ⎯ ⎯⎯⎯⎯

11. Record temperature, and report abnormal findings. ⎯ ⎯ ⎯ ⎯⎯⎯⎯

STUDENT: _____ DATE: _____

INSTRUCTOR: _____ DATE: _____

## Skill Performance Checklist
## Skill 30-2 Assessing the Radial and Apical Pulses

| | S | U | NP | Comments |
|---|---|---|---|---|
| 1. Determine the need to assess radial or apical pulse. | ___ | ___ | ___ | _____ |
| 2. Note risk factors for alterations in apical pulse. | ___ | ___ | ___ | _____ |
| 3. Assess for signs and symptoms of altered stroke volume and cardiac output. | ___ | ___ | ___ | _____ |
| 4. Assess for factors that normally influence pulse rate and rhythm. | ___ | ___ | ___ | _____ |
| 5. Determine previous baseline apical rate (if available) from patient's record. | ___ | ___ | ___ | _____ |
| 6. Explain that pulse or heart rate is to be assessed. Encourage patient to relax and not speak. | ___ | ___ | ___ | _____ |
| 7. Perform hand hygiene. | ___ | ___ | ___ | _____ |
| 8. If necessary, draw curtain around patient's bed or close room door, or do both. | ___ | ___ | ___ | _____ |
| 9. Obtain pulse measurement. | ___ | ___ | ___ | _____ |
|   A. Radial pulse | | | | |
|     (1) Assist patient to supine or sitting position. | ___ | ___ | ___ | _____ |
|     (2) If patient is supine, place patient's forearm straight alongside the body or across lower chest or upper abdomen with wrist extended straight. If patient is sitting, bend patient's elbow 90 degrees and support his or her lower arm on a chair or on your arm. Slightly flex patient's wrist, with palm down. | ___ | ___ | | _____ |
|     (3) Place tips of first two fingers of hand over groove along radial or thumb side of patient's inner wrist. | ___ | ___ | ___ | _____ |
|     (4) Lightly compress your fingertips against patient's radius, obliterate pulse initially, then relax pressure. | ___ | ___ | ___ | _____ |
|     (5) Determine strength of pulse. | ___ | ___ | ___ | _____ |
|     (6) After pulse can be felt regularly, look at watch's second hand and begin to count rate. | ___ | ___ | ___ | _____ |
|     (7) If pulse is regular, count rate for 30 seconds and multiply total by 2. | ___ | ___ | ___ | _____ |
|     (8) If pulse is irregular, count rate for 60 seconds. Assess frequency and pattern of irregularity. Compare bilateral radial pulses. | ___ | ___ | ___ | _____ |
|   B. Apical pulse | | | | |
|     (1) Perform hand hygiene; clean earpieces and diaphragm of stethoscope with alcohol swab. | ___ | ___ | ___ | _____ |
|     (2) Draw curtain around patient's bed or close room door, or do both. | ___ | ___ | ___ | _____ |
|     (3) Assist patient to supine or sitting position. Expose patient's sternum and left side of chest. | ___ | ___ | ___ | _____ |
|     (4) Locate anatomical landmarks to identify the point of maximal impulse. | ___ | ___ | ___ | _____ |
|     (5) Place diaphragm of stethoscope in palm of your hand for five to ten seconds. | ___ | ___ | ___ | _____ |
|     (6) Place diaphragm of stethoscope over point of maximal impulse at the fifth intercostal space at the left midclavicular line, and auscultate for normal $S_1$ and $S_2$ heart sounds. | ___ | ___ | ___ | _____ |
|     (7) When $S_1$ and $S_2$ are heard with regularity, look at watch's second hand and begin to count rate. | ___ | ___ | ___ | _____ |
|     (8) If apical rate is regular, count for 30 seconds, and multiply by 2. | ___ | ___ | ___ | _____ |
|     (9) If rate is irregular or patient is receiving cardiovascular medication, count for 60 seconds. | ___ | ___ | ___ | _____ |
|     (10) Describe pattern of irregularity. | ___ | ___ | ___ | _____ |
|     (11) Replace patient's gown and bed linen; assist patient to a comfortable position. | ___ | ___ | ___ | _____ |
|     (12) Clean earpieces and diaphragm of stethoscope with alcohol swab as necessary. | ___ | ___ | ___ | _____ |
| 10. Perform hand hygiene. | ___ | ___ | ___ | _____ |
| 11. Discuss findings with patient as needed. | ___ | ___ | ___ | _____ |

*Continued*

358

| | S | U | NP | Comments |
|---|---|---|---|---|
| 12. Compare readings with patient's previous baseline or acceptable range of heart rate for patient's age group (or both). | ___ | ___ | ___ | _____ |
| 13. Compare peripheral pulse rate with apical rate, and note discrepancy. | ___ | ___ | ___ | _____ |
| 14. Compare radial pulse equality, and note discrepancy. | ___ | ___ | ___ | _____ |
| 15. Correlate pulse rate with data obtained from blood pressure (BP) and related signs and symptoms. | ___ | ___ | ___ | _____ |
| 16. Record pulse rate with assessment site. | ___ | ___ | ___ | _____ |
| 17. Report abnormal findings to nurse in charge or prescribing health care provider. | ___ | ___ | ___ | _____ |

STUDENT: _____   DATE: _____

INSTRUCTOR: _____   DATE: _____

## Skill Performance Checklist
## Skill 30-3 Assessing Respirations

| | S | U | NP | Comments |
|---|---|---|---|---|
| 1. Determine the need to assess patient's respirations. | ___ | ___ | ___ | _____ |
| 2. Assess pertinent laboratory values. | ___ | ___ | ___ | _____ |
| 3. Determine previous baseline respiratory rate (if available) from patient's record. | ___ | ___ | ___ | _____ |
| 4. Perform hand hygiene. Provide privacy. | ___ | ___ | ___ | _____ |
| 5. Assist patient to a comfortable position, preferably sitting or lying with the head of the bed elevated 45 to 60 degrees. Be sure patient's chest is visible. If necessary, move patient's bed linen or gown. | ___ | ___ | ___ | _____ |
| 6. Place patient's arm in relaxed position across the abdomen or lower chest, or place your hand directly over patient's upper abdomen. | ___ | ___ | ___ | _____ |
| 7. Observe complete respiratory cycle (one inspiration and one expiration). | ___ | ___ | ___ | _____ |
| 8. After cycle is observed, look at watch's second hand and begin to count rate. | ___ | ___ | ___ | _____ |
| 9. If rhythm is regular, count number of respirations in 30 seconds, and multiply by 2. If rhythm is irregular or rate is less than 12 or greater than 20 (or both), count respirations for 60 seconds. | ___ | ___ | ___ | _____ |
| 10. Note depth of respirations. | ___ | ___ | ___ | _____ |
| 11. Note rhythm of ventilatory cycle. | ___ | ___ | ___ | _____ |
| 12. Replace patient's bed linen and gown. | ___ | ___ | ___ | _____ |
| 13. Perform hand hygiene. | ___ | ___ | ___ | _____ |
| 14. Discuss findings with patient as needed. | ___ | ___ | ___ | _____ |
| 15. If respirations are being assessed for the first time, establish rate, rhythm, and depth as baseline if within normal range. | ___ | ___ | ___ | _____ |
| 16. Compare respirations with patient's previous baseline and normal rate, rhythm, and depth. | ___ | ___ | ___ | _____ |
| 17. Record respiratory rate and character and any use of oxygen, and report abnormal findings. | ___ | ___ | ___ | _____ |

STUDENT: _____  DATE: _____

INSTRUCTOR: _____  DATE: _____

## Skill Performance Checklist
## Skill 30-4 Measuring Oxygen Saturation (Pulse Oximetry)

| | S | U | NP | Comments |
|---|---|---|---|---|
| 1. Determine need to measure patient's oxygen saturation ($SpO_2$). | | | | |
| 2. Assess for factors that influence measurement of $SpO_2$. | ___ | ___ | ___ | ___ |
| 3. Review patient's record for prescriber's order. | ___ | ___ | ___ | ___ |
| 4. Determine previous baseline $SpO_2$ (if available) from patient's record. | ___ | ___ | ___ | ___ |
| 5. Perform hand hygiene. | ___ | ___ | ___ | ___ |
| 6. Explain purpose and method of procedure to patient. | ___ | ___ | ___ | ___ |
| 7. Assess site for sensor probe placement. | ___ | ___ | ___ | ___ |
| 8. Assist patient to a comfortable position. If patient's finger is chosen as monitoring site, support patient's lower arm. | ___ | ___ | ___ | ___ |
| 9. Instruct patient to breathe normally. | | | | |
| 10. Use acetone to remove any fingernail polish from digit to be assessed. | ___ | ___ | ___ | ___ |
| 11. Attach sensor probe to monitoring site. Tell patient that clip-on probe will feel like a clothespin on the finger and will not hurt. | ___ | ___ | ___ | ___ |
| 12. Turn on oximeter by activating power. Observe pulse waveform-intensity display and audible beep. Correlate oximeter pulse rate with patient's radial pulse. | ___ | ___ | ___ | ___ |
| 13. Leave probe in place until oximeter readout reaches constant value and pulse display reaches full strength during each cardiac cycle. Read $SpO_2$ on digital display. | ___ | ___ | ___ | ___ |
| 14. Verify $SpO_2$ alarm limits and alarm volume for continuous monitoring. Verify that alarms are on. Assess skin integrity under sensor probe, and relocate sensor probe at least every four hours. | ___ | ___ | ___ | ___ |
| 15. Assist patient in returning to a comfortable position. | ___ | ___ | ___ | ___ |
| 16. Perform hand hygiene. | ___ | ___ | ___ | ___ |
| 17. Discuss findings with patient as needed. | ___ | ___ | ___ | ___ |
| 18. Remove probe and turn oximeter power off after intermittent measurements. Store probe in appropriate location. | ___ | ___ | ___ | ___ |
| 19. Compare $SpO_2$ reading with patient baseline and acceptable values. | ___ | ___ | ___ | ___ |
| 20. Correlate $SpO_2$ reading with $SaO_2$ reading obtained from arterial blood gas measurements, if available. | ___ | ___ | ___ | ___ |
| 21. Correlate $SpO_2$ reading with data obtained from respiratory assessment. | ___ | ___ | ___ | ___ |

STUDENT: _____     DATE: _____

INSTRUCTOR: _____     DATE: _____

## Skill Performance Checklist
## Skill 30-5 Measuring Blood Pressure

| | S | U | NP | Comments |
|---|---|---|---|---|
| 1. Determine the need to assess patient's BP. | ___ | ___ | ___ | _____ |
| 2. Determine best site for BP assessment. | ___ | ___ | ___ | _____ |
| 3. Select appropriate cuff size. | ___ | ___ | ___ | _____ |
| 4. Determine previous baseline BP (if available) from patient's record. | ___ | ___ | ___ | _____ |
| 5. Encourage the patient to avoid exercise and smoking for 30 minutes, and ingestion of caffeine for 60 minutes, before assessment of BP. | ___ | ___ | ___ | _____ |
| 6. Perform hand hygiene. Assist patient to sitting or lying position. Make sure room is warm, quiet, and relaxing. | ___ | ___ | ___ | _____ |
| 7. Explain to patient that BP is to be assessed, and have patient rest at least 5 minutes before measurement is taken. Ask patient not to speak while BP is being measured. | ___ | ___ | ___ | _____ |
| 8. With patient sitting or lying, position patient's forearm or thigh and provide support if needed. | ___ | ___ | ___ | _____ |
| 9. Expose extremity by removing constricting clothing. | ___ | ___ | ___ | _____ |
| 10. Palpate brachial artery or popliteal artery. Position cuff 2.5 cm above site of pulsation. | ___ | ___ | ___ | _____ |
| 11. Centre bladder of cuff above artery. With cuff fully deflated, wrap cuff evenly and snugly around extremity. | ___ | ___ | ___ | _____ |
| 12. To determine BP (two-step method), palpate artery distal to cuff with fingertips of one hand while inflating cuff rapidly to pressure reading that is 30 mm Hg above the point at which pulse disappears. Slowly deflate cuff, and note point when pulse reappears. Deflate cuff fully, and wait 30 seconds. | ___ | ___ | ___ | _____ |
| 13. Place stethoscope earpieces in ears. | ___ | ___ | ___ | _____ |
| 14. Relocate brachial or popliteal artery, and place bell or diaphragm chest piece of stethoscope over it. | ___ | ___ | ___ | _____ |
| 15. Close valve of pressure bulb clockwise until tight. Inflate cuff to 30 mm Hg above palpated systolic pressure. | ___ | ___ | ___ | _____ |
| 16. Slowly release valve, and allow mercury to fall at rate of 2 mm Hg per second. | ___ | ___ | ___ | _____ |
| 17. Note point on manometer when first clear sound is heard. | ___ | ___ | ___ | _____ |
| 18. Continue to deflate cuff, noting point at which muffled or dampened sound appears. | ___ | ___ | ___ | _____ |
| 19. Continue to deflate cuff gradually, noting point at which sound disappears in adults. Listen for 10 to 20 mm Hg after the last sound, then allow remaining air to escape quickly. | ___ | ___ | ___ | _____ |
| 20. Remove cuff from patient's extremity unless measurement must be repeated. If this is the first assessment of the patient, repeat procedure on the other extremity. | ___ | ___ | ___ | _____ |
| 21. Assist patient in returning to a comfortable position, and cover upper arm if previously clothed. | ___ | ___ | ___ | _____ |
| 22. Perform hand hygiene. | ___ | ___ | ___ | _____ |
| 23. Discuss findings with patient as needed. | ___ | ___ | ___ | _____ |
| 24. Compare reading with previous baseline or acceptable BP for patient's age group (or both). | ___ | ___ | ___ | _____ |
| 25. Compare BP readings in both of patient's arms or legs. | ___ | ___ | ___ | _____ |
| 26. Correlate BP with data obtained from pulse assessment and related cardiovascular signs and symptoms. | ___ | ___ | ___ | _____ |
| 27. Inform patient of value of and need for periodic reassessment of BP. | ___ | ___ | ___ | _____ |

STUDENT: _____     DATE: _____

INSTRUCTOR: _____     DATE: _____

## Skill Performance Checklist
## Skill 32-1 Handwashing/Hand Hygiene

| | S | U | NP | Comments |
|---|---|---|---|---|
| 1. Inspect surfaces of hands for breaks or cuts in skin or cuticles. Report and cover lesions before providing patient care. | ___ | ___ | ___ | _____ |
| 2. Inspect hands for visible soiling. | ___ | ___ | ___ | _____ |
| 3. Inspect nails for length and presence of artificial acrylics or chipped nail polish. | ___ | ___ | ___ | _____ |
| 4. Assess patient's risk for or extent of infection. | ___ | ___ | ___ | _____ |
| 5. Push wristwatch and long uniform sleeves above wrists. Remove rings during washing. | ___ | ___ | ___ | _____ |
| 6. If hands are visibly dirty or contaminated with protein-containing material, use plain or antimicrobial soap and water. | ___ | ___ | ___ | _____ |
|   A. Stand in front of sink, keeping hands and uniform away from sink surface. | ___ | ___ | ___ | _____ |
|   B. Turn on water. Turn faucet on, push knee pedals laterally, or press foot pedals to regulate water flow and temperature. | ___ | ___ | ___ | _____ |
|   C. Avoid splashing water onto uniform. | ___ | ___ | ___ | _____ |
|   D. Regulate flow of water so that temperature is warm. | ___ | ___ | ___ | _____ |
|   E. Wet hands and wrists thoroughly under running water. Keep hands and forearms lower than elbows during washing. | ___ | ___ | ___ | _____ |
|   F. Apply a small amount of soap, lathering thoroughly. | ___ | ___ | ___ | _____ |
|   G. Wash hands using plenty of lather and friction for at least 15 seconds. Interlace fingers, and rub palms and back of hands with circular motion at least five times each. Keep fingertips down. Rub knuckles of one hand into the palm of the other; repeat with the other hand. | ___ | ___ | ___ | _____ |
|   H. Rub thumb on one hand with the palm of the other hand; repeat with other hand. | ___ | ___ | ___ | _____ |
|   I. Work the fingertips on one hand into the palm of the other. Massage soap into nail spaces. Repeat with other hand. | ___ | ___ | ___ | _____ |
|   J. Clean fingernails of both hands with orangewood stick or fingernails of other hand and additional soap. | ___ | ___ | ___ | _____ |
|   K. Rinse hands and wrists thoroughly, keeping hands down and elbows up. | ___ | ___ | ___ | _____ |
|   L. Optional: Repeat steps A through J, and extend period of washing if hands are heavily soiled. | ___ | ___ | ___ | _____ |
|   M. Dry hands thoroughly from fingers to wrists and forearms with paper towel, single-use cloth, or warm-air dryer. | ___ | ___ | ___ | _____ |
|   N. Discard paper towel, if used, in proper receptacle. | ___ | ___ | ___ | _____ |
|   O. Turn off water with foot or knee pedals. To turn off hand faucet, use clean, dry paper towel. Avoid touching handles with hands. | ___ | ___ | ___ | _____ |
|   P. If hands are dry or chapped, a small amount of lotion or barrier cream can be applied. | ___ | ___ | ___ | _____ |
|   Q. Inspect surfaces of hands for obvious signs of soil or other contaminants. | ___ | ___ | ___ | _____ |
|   R. Inspect hands for dermatitis or cracked skin. | ___ | ___ | ___ | _____ |
| 7. If hands are not visibly soiled, use an alcohol-based waterless antiseptic for routine decontamination in all clinical situations. | ___ | ___ | ___ | _____ |
|   A. Apply an ample amount of product to the palm of one hand. | ___ | ___ | ___ | _____ |
|   B. Rub hands together, covering all surfaces. | ___ | ___ | ___ | _____ |
|   C. Rub hands together until alcohol is dry. Allow hands to dry before applying gloves. | ___ | ___ | ___ | _____ |
|   D. If hands are dry or chapped, a small amount of lotion or barrier cream can be applied. | ___ | ___ | ___ | _____ |
|   E. Report any dermatitis to employee health or infection control per employer policy. | ___ | ___ | ___ | _____ |

STUDENT: _____ DATE: _____

INSTRUCTOR: _____ DATE: _____

## Skill Performance Checklist
## Skill 32-2 Preparation of a Sterile Field

| | S | U | NP | Comments |
|---|---|---|---|---|
| 1. Prepare sterile field just before planned procedure. | ___ | ___ | ___ | _____ |
| 2. Select clean work surface above waist level. | ___ | ___ | ___ | _____ |
| 3. Assemble equipment. | ___ | ___ | ___ | _____ |
| 4. Check dates on supplies. | ___ | ___ | ___ | _____ |
| 5. Perform hand hygiene. | ___ | ___ | ___ | _____ |
| 6. Place pack with sterile drape on work surface, and open pack. | ___ | ___ | ___ | _____ |
| 7. With fingertips of one hand, pick up folded top edge. | ___ | ___ | ___ | _____ |
| 8. Gently lift drape from its outer cover and let it unfold by itself without touching any object. Discard outer cover with the other hand. | ___ | ___ | ___ | _____ |
| 9. With other hand, grasp adjacent corner of drape and hold it straight up and away from your body. | ___ | ___ | ___ | _____ |
| 10. Holding drape, first position and lay bottom half over intended work surface. | ___ | ___ | ___ | _____ |
| 11. Allow top half of drape to be placed over work surface last. | ___ | ___ | ___ | _____ |
| 12. Grasp 2.5-cm border around edge to position as needed. | ___ | ___ | ___ | _____ |

**ADDING STERILE ITEMS**

| | S | U | NP | Comments |
|---|---|---|---|---|
| 13. Open sterile item while holding outside wrapper in nondominant hand. | ___ | ___ | ___ | _____ |
| 14. Carefully peel wrapper onto nondominant hand. Do not shake. | ___ | ___ | ___ | _____ |
| 15. Making sure that wrapper does not fall down onto sterile field, place item onto field at angle. Do not hold arm over field. | ___ | ___ | ___ | _____ |
| 16. Dispose of wrapper. | ___ | ___ | ___ | _____ |
| 17. Perform procedure using sterile technique. | ___ | ___ | ___ | _____ |

STUDENT: _____  DATE: _____

INSTRUCTOR: _____  DATE: _____

## Skill Performance Checklist
## Skill 32-3 Surgical Hand Hygiene/Hand Hygiene

| | S | U | NP | Comments |
|---|---|---|---|---|
| 1. Consult employer policy regarding required length of scrub time and antiseptic to use for hand antisepsis. | ___ | ___ | ___ | _____ |
| 2. Keep fingernails short, clean, and healthy. Remove artificial nails. | ___ | ___ | ___ | _____ |
| 3. Inspect hands for presence of abrasions, cuts, or open lesions. | ___ | ___ | ___ | _____ |
| 4. Apply surgical shoe covers, cap or hood, face mask, and protective eyewear. | ___ | ___ | ___ | _____ |
| 5. Surgical handwashing: | | | | |
| A. Turn on water using knee or foot controls, and adjust water to comfortable temperature. | ___ | ___ | ___ | _____ |
| B. Wet hands and arms under running lukewarm water, and lather with detergent to 5 cm above elbows. Keep hands above elbows. | ___ | ___ | ___ | _____ |
| C. Rinse hands and arms thoroughly under running water, keeping hands above elbows. | ___ | ___ | ___ | _____ |
| D. Under running water, clean under nails of both hands with nail pick. Discard pick after use. | ___ | ___ | ___ | _____ |
| E. Wet clean sponge, and apply antimicrobial detergent. Scrub the nails of one hand with 15 strokes. Holding sponge perpendicular, scrub the palm, each side of the thumb and all fingers, and the posterior side of the hand with 10 strokes each. The arm is mentally divided into thirds. Scrub each section of the arm ten times. Check manufacturer's recommendations for the duration of the scrub, usually two to six minutes. Rinse sponge, and repeat for other arm. | ___ | ___ | ___ | _____ |
| F. Discard sponge, and rinse hands and arms thoroughly. Turn off water with foot or knee controls, and back into room entrance with hands elevated in front of and away from the body. | ___ | ___ | ___ | _____ |
| G. Walk up to sterile tray and lean forward slightly to pick up a sterile towel. Dry one hand thoroughly, moving from fingers to elbow. Dry in a rotating motion from cleanest to least clean area. | ___ | ___ | ___ | _____ |
| H. Repeat drying method for the other hand, using a different area of the towel or a new sterile towel. | ___ | ___ | ___ | _____ |
| I. Discard towel. | ___ | ___ | ___ | _____ |
| J. Proceed with sterile gowning. | ___ | ___ | ___ | _____ |
| 6. Alternative method of surgical hand hygiene using alcohol-based antiseptic: | | | | |
| A. Wash hands with soap and water for 15 seconds. | ___ | ___ | ___ | _____ |
| B. Clean nails of both hands under running water with disposable nail cleaner. Discard after use, and dry hands with a paper towel. | ___ | ___ | ___ | _____ |
| C. Apply enough alcohol-based waterless antiseptic to one palm to cover both hands thoroughly. Spread antiseptic over all hand and nail surfaces. Allow to air-dry. | ___ | ___ | ___ | _____ |
| D. Repeat the process, and allow hands to air-dry before applying sterile gloves. | ___ | ___ | ___ | _____ |
| E. Report any dermatitis to employee health or infection control per your employer's policy. | ___ | ___ | ___ | _____ |

STUDENT: _____ DATE: _____

INSTRUCTOR: _____ DATE: _____

## Skill Performance Checklist
## Skill 32-4 Applying a Sterile Gown and Performing Closed Gloving

| | S | U | NP | Comments |
|---|---|---|---|---|
| 1. Before entering operating room or treatment area, apply cap, face mask, eyewear, and foot covers. | ___ | ___ | ___ | _____ |
| 2. Perform surgical hand hygiene. | ___ | ___ | ___ | _____ |
| 3. Have circulating nurse open pack containing sterile gown. | ___ | ___ | ___ | _____ |
| 4. Have circulating nurse prepare glove package. Inner glove package is then placed on sterile field created by sterile outer wrapper. | ___ | ___ | ___ | _____ |
| 5. Reach down to sterile gown package; lift gown directly upward and step back from table. | ___ | ___ | ___ | _____ |
| 6. Holding folded gown, locate neckband. Grasp inside front of gown just below neckband. | ___ | ___ | ___ | _____ |
| 7. Allow gown to unfold, keeping inside of gown toward body. Do not touch outside of gown with bare hands or allow it to touch the floor. | ___ | ___ | ___ | _____ |
| 8. With hands at shoulder level, insert each hand through armholes simultaneously. Ask circulating nurse to bring gown over shoulders, leaving sleeves covering hands. | ___ | ___ | ___ | _____ |
| 9. Have circulating nurse tie back of gown at neck and waist. | ___ | ___ | ___ | _____ |
| 10. Closed gloving procedure: | | | | |
| A. With hands covered by sleeves, open inner sterile glove package. | ___ | ___ | ___ | _____ |
| B. With dominant hand inside gown cuff, pick up glove for nondominant hand by grasping folded cuff. | ___ | ___ | ___ | _____ |
| C. Extend nondominant forearm with palm up, and place palm of glove against palm of nondominant hand. Glove fingers will point toward elbow. | ___ | ___ | ___ | _____ |
| D. Grasp back of glove cuff with covered dominant hand, and turn glove cuff over end of nondominant hand and gown cuff. | ___ | ___ | ___ | _____ |
| E. Grasp top of glove and underlying gown sleeve with covered dominant hand. Carefully extend fingers into glove, being sure glove's cuff covers gown's cuff. | ___ | ___ | ___ | _____ |
| F. Repeat steps A through E to glove dominant hand. | ___ | ___ | ___ | _____ |
| G. Adjust fingers until fully extended into both gloves. | ___ | ___ | ___ | _____ |
| 11. For wraparound sterile gowns, take gloved hand and release fastener or ties in front of gown. | ___ | ___ | ___ | _____ |
| 12. Give tie to sterile team member. Allowing margin of safety, turn around to the left, covering back with extended gown flap. Take back tie from team member, and secure tie to gown. Allowing margin of safety, turn around to the left, covering back with extended gown flap. Take back tie from team member, and secure tie to gown. | ___ | ___ | ___ | _____ |

STUDENT: _____   DATE: _____

INSTRUCTOR: _____   DATE: _____

## Skill Performance Checklist
## Skill 32-5 Open Gloving

|  | S | U | NP | Comments |
|---|---|---|---|---|
| 1. Perform thorough hand washing/hand hygiene. | ___ | ___ | ___ | _____ |
| 2. Peel apart sides of outer package of glove wrapper. | ___ | ___ | ___ | _____ |
| 3. Lay inner package on clean, dry flat surface just above waist level. Open package, keeping gloves on wrapper's inside surface. | ___ | ___ | ___ | _____ |
| 4. If gloves are not prepowdered, apply powder lightly to hands over sink or wastebasket. | ___ | ___ | ___ | _____ |
| 5. Identify right and left gloves. | ___ | ___ | ___ | _____ |
| 6. Start by applying glove to dominant hand. With thumb and first two fingers of nondominant hand, grasp edge of cuff of glove for dominant hand, touching only inside surface. | ___ | ___ | ___ | _____ |
| 7. Carefully pull glove over dominant hand, ensuring cuff does not roll up wrist. | ___ | ___ | ___ | _____ |
| 8. With gloved dominant hand, slip fingers underneath second glove's cuff. | ___ | ___ | ___ | _____ |
| 9. Carefully pull second glove over nondominant hand, and do not allow gloved hand to touch any part of exposed nondominant hand. | ___ | ___ | ___ | _____ |
| 10. When both gloves are on, interlock fingers of both hands to secure gloves in position, being careful to touch only sterile sides. | ___ | ___ | ___ | _____ |

### GLOVE DISPOSAL

| | | | | |
|---|---|---|---|---|
| 11. Without touching wrist, grasp outside of one cuff with other gloved hand. | ___ | ___ | ___ | _____ |
| 12. Pull glove off, turning it inside out. Discard in receptacle. | ___ | ___ | ___ | _____ |
| 13. Tuck fingers of bare hand inside remaining glove cuff. Peel glove off, inside out. Discard in receptacle. | ___ | ___ | ___ | _____ |
| 14. Perform hand hygiene. | ___ | ___ | ___ | _____ |

STUDENT: _____  DATE: _____

INSTRUCTOR: _____  DATE: _____

## Skill Performance Checklist
## Skill 33-1 Administering Oral Medications

|  | S | U | NP | Comments |
|---|---|---|---|---|
| 1. Check accuracy and completeness of each medication administration record (MAR) or computer printout against the prescriber's original medication order. Check the patient's name and medication name, dosage, and route and time for administration. Copy or rewrite any portion of the MAR that is difficult to read. | ___ | ___ | ___ | _____ |
| 2. Assess patient for any contraindications to receiving oral medication. Is the patient experiencing nausea or vomiting? Has the patient received a diagnosis of bowel inflammation or reduced peristalsis? Has patient undergone recent gastrointestinal (GI) surgery? Does patient have gastric suction? Is the patient restricted to nothing by mouth? Check the patient's reflexes for swallowing, coughing, and gagging. | ___ | ___ | ___ | _____ |
| 3. Assess the patient's medical history, history of allergies, medication history, and diet history. List the patient's food and drug allergies on each page of the MAR, and prominently display the allergies on the patient's medical record. This information may also be added to an identification bracelet. | ___ | ___ | ___ | _____ |
| 4. Gather information from the patient's physical examination and laboratory data that may influence medication administration (e.g., vital signs, blood glucose levels, electrolyte levels, laboratory findings related to blood clotting times and to renal and liver function). | ___ | ___ | ___ | _____ |
| 5. Assess patient's knowledge regarding health and medication usage. | ___ | ___ | ___ | _____ |
| 6. Assess patient's preferences for fluids. Maintain fluid restriction when applicable. | ___ | ___ | ___ | _____ |
| 7. Prepare medications: | | | | |
| A. Perform hand hygiene. | ___ | ___ | ___ | _____ |
| B. If medication cart is used, move it outside patient's room. | ___ | ___ | ___ | _____ |
| C. Unlock medicine drawer or cart, or log onto the automated medication dispensing system. | ___ | ___ | ___ | _____ |
| D. Prepare medication for one patient at a time. If you are using paper copies of the MAR, keep all pages for one patient together. If you are using the patient's MAR on the computer, view only one computer screen at a time. | ___ | ___ | ___ | _____ |
| E. Select correct medication from a stock supply or a unit-dose drawer. Compare the label on the medication with the MAR or the computer screen. Check expiration date on all medication labels. | ___ | ___ | ___ | _____ |
| F. Calculate the medication dose as necessary. Double-check all calculations, and verify your calculations with another nurse. | ___ | ___ | ___ | _____ |
| G. If you are preparing a controlled substance, check the patient's MAR or computer record to determine the last time the medication was administered. Check the record for the previous medication count, and compare the current count with the supply available. | ___ | ___ | ___ | _____ |
| H. To prepare tablets or capsules from a floor stock bottle, pour required number into the bottle cap, and transfer medication to a medication cup. Do not touch the medication with your fingers. Return extra tablets or capsules to the bottle. Break prescored medications. If necessary, use a gloved hand or clean pillating device. Identify prescored tablets by looking for a line that divides the tablet in half. | ___ | ___ | ___ | _____ |
| I. To prepare unit-dose tablets or capsules, place the packaged tablet or capsule directly into a medicine cup. Do not remove the wrapper. | ___ | ___ | ___ | _____ |
| J. Place all tablets or capsules to be given to patient in one medicine cup, with the patient's identification label attached, except for those medications that require preadministration assessments (e.g., pulse rate or blood pressure); keep medications in their wrappers. After medication administration, remove the patient's identification label, and discard the label in the appropriate confidential waste disposal receptacle. | ___ | ___ | ___ | _____ |

*Continued*

|  | S | U | NP | Comments |
|---|---|---|---|---|

K. If the patient has difficulty swallowing, and liquid medications are not an option, use a pill-crushing device, such as a mortar and pestle to grind the pills. Before using a mortar and pestle, clean them. If a pill-crushing device is not available, place the tablet inside a medication cup, place another cup on top of it, and press on the top cup with a blunt instrument until the pill is crushed. Mix the ground tablet in a small amount of soft food (custard or applesauce).

L. To prepare liquids:
   (1) Gently shake the container. If the medication is in a unit-dose container with the correct amount to administer, no further preparation is needed. If medication is in a multidose bottle, remove the bottle cap from container and place the cap so that the inside of cap is not exposed.
   (2) Hold a multidose bottle with the label against the palm of your hand while pouring.
   (3) Hold medication cup at eye level, and fill to the desired level on the scale. The scale should be even with fluid level at its surface or the base of the meniscus, not at its edges. Draw up volumes of less than 10 mL in a syringe without a needle.
   (4) Discard any excess liquid into a sink. Wipe lip and neck of the multidose bottle with a paper towel.

M. Compare the MAR, computer printout, or computer screen with the prepared medication and container.

N. Return stock containers or unused unit-dose medications to the storage shelf or drawer, and read the labels again.

O. Do not leave medications unattended.

8. Administering medications:
  A. Bring medications to the patient at the correct time.
  B. Identify the patient by using at least two patient identifiers. Compare the patient's name and one other identifier (e.g., the hospital identification number) on the MAR, computer printout, or computer screen against information on the patient's identification bracelet. Ask the patient to state his or her name, if possible, for a third identifier.
  C. Compare the labels of the medications with the MAR at the patient's bedside.
  D. Explain to patient the purpose of each medication and its action. Encourage patient to ask any questions about the medications.
  E. Assist the patient to a sitting position (or side-lying position if sitting is contraindicated).
  F. Administer medications:
    (1) *For tablets*: The patient may wish to hold solid medications in the hand or in a cup before placing in the mouth.
    (2) Offer water or juice to help the patient swallow medications. Give cold carbonated water if it is available and not contraindicated.
    (3) *For sublingual-administered medications*: Have the patient place the medication under the tongue and allow it to dissolve completely. Caution the patient against swallowing the tablet.
    (4) *For buccal medications*: Have the patient place the medication in the mouth against the mucous membranes of the cheek until it dissolves. Avoid administering liquids until the buccal medication has dissolved.
    (5) *For powdered medications*: Mix with liquids at bedside, and give to the patient to drink.
    (6) Caution the patient against chewing or swallowing lozenges.
    (7) Give effervescent powders and tablets immediately after they have dissolved.
  G. If the patient is unable to hold medications in the hand or in a cup, place the medication cup to the patient's lips and gently introduce each medication into the mouth, one at a time. Do not rush.
  H. If a tablet or capsule falls to the floor, discard it, and repeat the preparation.
  I. Stay at the bedside until the patient has completely swallowed each medication. If you are uncertain whether the medication was swallowed, ask the patient to open the mouth.

*Continued*

|  | S | U | NP | Comments |
|---|---|---|---|---|
| J. For highly acidic medications (e.g., aspirin), offer the patient a nonfat snack (e.g., crackers) if it is not contraindicated by the patient's condition. | ___ | ___ | ___ | _____ |
| K. Assist the patient in returning to a comfortable position. | ___ | ___ | ___ | _____ |
| L. Dispose of soiled supplies, and perform hand hygiene. | ___ | ___ | ___ | _____ |
| M. Replenish the stock, such as cups and straws. If a medication cart was used, return the cart to the medication room. Clean the work area. | ___ | ___ | ___ | _____ |
| 9. Evaluate the patient's response to medication at times that correlate with the medication's onset, peak, and duration. | ___ | ___ | ___ | _____ |
| 10. Ask the patient or the patient's family member to identify the medication name and explain the purpose, action, dosage schedule, and potential side effects of drug. | ___ | ___ | ___ | _____ |
| 11. Notify prescriber if the patient exhibits adverse effects of the medication: side effects, toxic effect, or allergic reaction. If any of these occur, withhold further doses of the medication, add allergy information to patient's chart, and notify the prescriber and the pharmacy. | ___ | ___ | ___ | _____ |
| 12. Record the reason any medication was withheld, and follow the employer's policy for proper recording. | ___ | ___ | ___ | _____ |
| 13. Record and report your evaluation of the medication's effect to the prescriber if required (e.g., report urine output following administration of a diuretic if ordered by the prescriber). | ___ | ___ | ___ | _____ |

STUDENT: _____ DATE: _____

INSTRUCTOR: _____ DATE: _____

## Skill Performance Checklist
## Skill 33-2 Administering Ophthalmic Medications

| | S | U | NP | Comments |
|---|---|---|---|---|
| 1. Check the accuracy and completeness of each MAR or computer printout against the prescriber's medication order. Check the patient's name, the medication name and dosage (e.g., number of drops, if a liquid), the eye to be treated (e.g., right, left, or both eyes), and the route and time of administration. Copy or rewrite any portion of the MAR that is difficult to read. | ___ | ___ | ___ | _____ |
| 2. Assess the condition of the patient's external eye structures. (This may also be assessed just before medication instillation.) | ___ | ___ | ___ | _____ |
| 3. Determine whether the patient has any known allergies to eye medications. Also ask whether the patient has an allergy to latex. | ___ | ___ | ___ | _____ |
| 4. Determine whether the patient has any symptoms of visual alterations. | ___ | ___ | ___ | _____ |
| 5. Assess the patient's level of consciousness and ability to follow directions. | ___ | ___ | ___ | _____ |
| 6. Assess the patient's knowledge regarding medication therapy and the desire to self-administer medication. | ___ | ___ | ___ | _____ |
| 7. Assess the patient's ability to manipulate and hold an eyedropper. | ___ | ___ | ___ | _____ |
| 8. Prepare medication. Ensure that you check the label of the medication against the MAR at least two times while preparing medication. | ___ | ___ | ___ | _____ |
| 9. Bring the medication to the patient at correct time, and perform hand hygiene. | ___ | ___ | ___ | _____ |
| 10. Identify the patient by using at least two patient identifiers. Compare the patient's name and one other identifier (e.g., the hospital identification number) on the MAR, computer printout, or computer screen against information on the patient's identification bracelet. Ask the patient to state his or her name, if possible, for a third identifier. | ___ | ___ | ___ | _____ |
| 11. Compare the labels of the medications with the MAR or computer printout at the patient's bedside. | ___ | ___ | ___ | _____ |
| 12. Arrange the medication supplies at the bedside, and put on clean gloves. If eye drops are stored in the refrigerator, allow them to reach room temperature before instilling them. | ___ | ___ | ___ | _____ |
| 13. Gently roll the container. | ___ | ___ | ___ | _____ |
| 14. Explain the procedure to the patient, including positioning and sensations to expect, such as burning or stinging. | ___ | ___ | ___ | _____ |
| 15. Ask the patient to lie supine or to sit back in a chair with the head slightly hyperextended. | ___ | ___ | ___ | _____ |
| 16. If crusts or drainage are present along the eyelid margins or the inner canthus, gently wash them away. Soak any crusts that are dried and difficult to remove by applying a damp washcloth or cotton ball over the eye for a few minutes. Always wipe from the inner to the outer canthus. | ___ | ___ | ___ | _____ |
| 17. Hold a cotton ball or clean tissue in your nondominant hand on the patient's cheekbone just below the lower eyelid. | ___ | ___ | ___ | _____ |
| 18. With the tissue or cotton ball resting below the lower lid, gently press downward with thumb or forefinger against the bony orbit. | ___ | ___ | ___ | _____ |
| 19. Ask the patient to look at the ceiling, and explain steps to the patient. | ___ | ___ | ___ | _____ |
|   A. Instill the eye drops: | | | | |
|     (1) With your dominant hand resting on the patient's forehead, hold the filled medication eyedropper or ophthalmic solution approximately 1 to 2 cm above the conjunctival sac. | ___ | ___ | ___ | _____ |
|     (2) Instill the prescribed number of medication drops into the conjunctival sac. | ___ | ___ | ___ | _____ |
|     (3) If the patient blinks or closes the eye, or if the drops land on the outer lid margins, repeat the procedure. | ___ | ___ | ___ | _____ |
|     (4) After instilling drops, ask the patient to close the eye gently. | ___ | ___ | ___ | _____ |
|     (5) When administering medications that cause systemic effects, apply gentle pressure with your finger and a clean tissue on the patient's nasolacrimal duct for 30 to 60 seconds. | ___ | ___ | ___ | _____ |

*Continued*

380

| | S | U | NP | Comments |
|---|---|---|---|---|

B. Instill eye ointment:
  (1) Ask the patient to look at the ceiling. ___ ___ ___ _____
  (2) Holding the ointment applicator above the lower lid margin, apply a thin stream of ointment evenly along the inner edge of the lower eyelid on conjunctiva from inner canthus to outer canthus. ___ ___ ___ _____
  (3) Have the patient close the eye, and use a cotton ball to rub lid gently in a circular motion, if rubbing is not contraindicated. ___ ___ ___ _____

C. Intraocular disc
  (1) Application:
    (a) Open the package containing the disc. Gently press your fingertip against the disc so it adheres to your finger. Position the convex side of the disc on your fingertip. ___ ___ ___ _____
    (b) With the other hand, gently pull the patient's lower eyelid away from the eye. Ask the patient to look up. ___ ___ ___ _____
    (c) Place the disc in the conjunctival sac, so that it floats on the sclera between the iris and the lower eyelid. ___ ___ ___ _____
    (d) Pull the patient's lower eyelid out and over the disc. ___ ___ ___ _____
  (2) Removal:
    (a) Perform hand hygiene, and put on gloves. ___ ___ ___ _____
    (b) Explain procedure to patient. ___ ___ ___ _____
    (c) Gently pull on the patient's lower eyelid to expose the intraocular disc. ___ ___ ___ _____
    (d) Using your forefinger and thumb of the opposite hand, pinch the disc and lift it out of the patient's eye. ___ ___ ___ _____

20. If excess medication is on eyelid, gently wipe it from inner canthus to outer canthus. ___ ___ ___ _____
21. If patient wears an eye patch, apply a clean patch by placing it over the affected eye so entire eye is covered. Tape securely without applying pressure to eye. ___ ___ ___ _____
22. If patient receives eye medication to both eyes at the same time, use a different tissue or cotton ball for each eye. ___ ___ ___ _____
23. Remove gloves, dispose of soiled supplies in proper receptacle, and perform hand hygiene. ___ ___ ___ _____
24. Note the patient's response to instillation; ask whether the patient felt any discomfort. ___ ___ ___ _____
25. Observe patient's response to medication by assessing any visual changes and noting any side effects. ___ ___ ___ _____
26. Ask the patient to discuss the medication's purpose, action, side effects, and the technique of administration. ___ ___ ___ _____
27. Have patient demonstrate self-administration of next dose. ___ ___ ___ _____
28. Document on the MAR or the computer record the medication, concentration, number of drops, time of administration, and the eye (left, right, or both) that received medication. ___ ___ ___ _____
29. Record the appearance of the eye in the nurses' notes. ___ ___ ___ _____

STUDENT: _____  DATE: _____

INSTRUCTOR: _____  DATE: _____

## Skill Performance Checklist
## Skill 33-3 Using Metered-Dose or Dry Powder Inhalers

|  | S | U | NP | Comments |
|---|---|---|---|---|
| 1. Check the accuracy and completeness of each MAR or computer printout against the prescriber's original medication order. Check the patient's name and medication name, dosage, and route and time of administration. Copy or rewrite any portion of the MAR that is difficult to read. | ___ | ___ | ___ | _____ |
| 2. Assess patient's respiratory pattern, and auscultate the patient's breath sounds. | ___ | ___ | ___ | _____ |
| 3. Assess the patient's ability to hold, manipulate, and depress canister and inhaler. Assess the patient's strength of inhalation. | ___ | ___ | ___ | _____ |
| 4. Assess the patient's readiness to learn: for example, whether the patient asks questions about the medication, disease, or complications; requests education in use of inhaler; is mentally alert; participates in self-care. | ___ | ___ | ___ | _____ |
| 5. Assess patient's ability to learn: The patient should not be fatigued, in pain, or in respiratory distress; assess the patient's level of understanding of technical terms. | ___ | ___ | ___ | _____ |
| 6. Assess the patient's knowledge and understanding of the disease and the purpose and action of the prescribed medications. | ___ | ___ | ___ | _____ |
| 7. Determine the medication schedule and the number of inhalations prescribed for each dose. | ___ | ___ | ___ | _____ |
| 8. Prepare the medication. Ensure that you compare the medication label with the MAR two times during medication preparation. | ___ | ___ | ___ | _____ |
| 9. Identify the patient by using at least two patient identifiers. Compare the patient's name and one other identifier (e.g., the hospital identification number) on the MAR, computer printout, or computer screen against information on the patient's identification bracelet. Ask the patient to state his or her name, if possible, for a third identifier. | ___ | ___ | ___ | _____ |
| 10. Compare the label of medications with the MAR one more time at the patient's bedside. | ___ | ___ | ___ | _____ |
| 11. Instruct the patient in a comfortable environment by sitting in a chair in the hospital room or by sitting at a kitchen table in the patient's home. | ___ | ___ | ___ | _____ |
| 12. Provide adequate time for the teaching session. | ___ | ___ | ___ | _____ |
| 13. Perform hand hygiene, and arrange the equipment needed. | ___ | ___ | ___ | _____ |
| 14. Allow the patient an opportunity to manipulate the inhaler, the canister, and the spacer device. Explain and demonstrate how the canister fits into the inhaler. | ___ | ___ | ___ | _____ |
| A. If the patient is using a metered-dose inhaler (MDI) with or without a spacer, and the inhaler is new or has not been used for several days, push a "test spray" into the air. A test spray is not needed for a dry powder inhaler. | ___ | ___ | ___ | _____ |
| 15. Explain what a metered dose is, and warn the patient about overuse of the inhaler, including medication side effects. | ___ | ___ | ___ | _____ |
| 16. Explain the steps for administering squeeze-and-breathe inhaled dose of medication of MDI (demonstrate steps when possible). | ___ | ___ | ___ | _____ |
| A. Insert the MDI canister into the holder. | ___ | ___ | ___ | _____ |
| B. Remove the mouthpiece cover from the inhaler. | ___ | ___ | ___ | _____ |
| C. Shake the inhaler vigorously five or six times. | ___ | ___ | ___ | _____ |
| D. Have the patient take a deep breath and exhale. | ___ | ___ | ___ | _____ |
| E. Instruct the patient to position the inhaler in one of two ways: | | | | |
| (1) Close the mouth around the MDI, with the opening toward the back of the throat. | ___ | ___ | ___ | _____ |
| (2) Position the device 2 to 4 cm in front of the mouth. | ___ | ___ | ___ | _____ |
| F. With the inhaler properly positioned, have the patient hold it with thumb at the mouthpiece and middle finger at the top. This arrangement is called a three-point or lateral hand position. | ___ | ___ | ___ | _____ |

*Continued*

382

| | S | U | NP | Comments |
|---|---|---|---|---|

G. Instruct patient to tilt the head back slightly, then inhale slowly and deeply through the mouth for three to five seconds while depressing the canister fully. ___ ___ ___ _____

H. Instruct the patient to hold the breath for approximately ten seconds. ___ ___ ___ _____

I. Have the patient remove the MDI from the mouth and to exhale through pursed lips. ___ ___ ___ _____

17. Explain steps to administer MDI by using a spacer, such as an AeroChamber (demonstrate when possible):

A. Remove the mouthpiece cover from the MDI and the mouthpiece of spacer. Inspect the spacer for foreign objects. If the spacer has a valve, ensure the valve is intact. ___ ___ ___ _____

B. Insert the MDI into the end of the spacer. ___ ___ ___ _____

C. Shake the inhaler vigorously five or six times. ___ ___ ___ _____

D. Have the patient exhale completely before closing the mouth around the mouthpiece of the spacer. Avoid covering small exhalation slots with the lips. ___ ___ ___ _____

E. Have the patient depress the medication canister, spraying one puff into the spacer. ___ ___ ___ _____

F. Instruct the patient to inhale deeply and slowly through the mouth for three to five seconds. ___ ___ ___ _____

G. Instruct the patient to hold the breath for ten seconds. ___ ___ ___ _____

H. Instruct the patient to remove the MDI and spacer before exhaling. ___ ___ ___ _____

18. Explain the steps to administer dry powder inhaler or breath-activated MDI (demonstrate when possible):

A. Remove the cover from the mouthpiece. Do not shake the inhaler. ___ ___ ___ _____

B. Prepare medication as directed by the manufacturer (e.g., hold inhaler upright, and turn the wheel to the right and then to the left until a click is heard; load the medication pellet). ___ ___ ___ _____

C. Instruct the patient to exhale away from inhaler before inhalation. ___ ___ ___ _____

D. Position mouthpiece between the patient's lips. ___ ___ ___ _____

E. Instruct the patient to inhale deeply and forcefully through the mouth. ___ ___ ___ _____

F. Instruct the patient to hold breath for five to ten seconds. ___ ___ ___ _____

19. Instruct patient to wait at least 20 to 30 seconds between inhalations. If two medications are to be administered, give the bronchodilator first. ___ ___ ___ _____

20. Instruct the patient against repeating inhalations before the next scheduled dose. ___ ___ ___ _____

21. Instruct patient in cleaning the inhaler:

A. Once a day, the inhaler and its cap should be rinsed in warm running water. The inhaler must be completely dry before use. ___ ___ ___ _____

B. Twice a week, the L-shaped plastic mouthpiece should be washed with mild dishwashing soap and warm water. Rinse and dry well before placing the canister back inside the mouthpiece. ___ ___ ___ _____

22. Ask whether the patient has any questions. ___ ___ ___ _____

23. Have the patient explain and demonstrate the steps in the use of an inhaler. ___ ___ ___ _____

24. Ask the patient to explain the medication schedule, side effects, and when to call health care providers. ___ ___ ___ _____

25. Ask the patient to calculate how many days the inhaler will last. ___ ___ ___ _____

26. After the medication has been taken, assess the patient's respiratory status, including the ease of respirations; auscultate the lungs, and use pulse oximetry to assess the patient's oxygenation status. ___ ___ ___ _____

27. Document the skills that you taught the patient and the patient's ability to perform these skills. ___ ___ ___ _____

28. Document on the MAR or computer record the medication, time of administration, and number of puffs. ___ ___ ___ _____

29. Report any undesirable effects from the medication. ___ ___ ___ _____

STUDENT: _____  DATE: _____

INSTRUCTOR: _____  DATE: _____

## Skill Performance Checklist
## Skill 33-4 Preparing Injections

|  | S | U | NP | Comments |
|---|---|---|---|---|
| 1. Check the accuracy and completeness of each MAR or computer printout against the prescriber's original medication order. Check the patient's name and the medication name, dosage, and route and time of administration. Copy or rewrite any portion of the MAR that is difficult to read. | ___ | ___ | ___ | _____ |
| 2. Review pertinent information related to medication, including its action, purpose, side effects, and nursing implications. | ___ | ___ | ___ | _____ |
| 3. Assess the patient's body build, muscle size, and weight. | ___ | ___ | ___ | _____ |
| 4. Perform hand hygiene, and assemble the medication supplies. | ___ | ___ | ___ | _____ |
| 5. Check the date of expiration on the medication vial or ampule. | ___ | ___ | ___ | _____ |
| 6. Prepare medication: Ensure that you compare the label of the medication with the MAR at least two times while preparing the medication. | ___ | ___ | ___ | _____ |
| A. Ampule preparation | | | | |
| (1) Tap top of ampule lightly and quickly with your finger until the fluid moves from the neck of ampule. | ___ | ___ | ___ | _____ |
| (2) Place a small gauze pad or an unopened alcohol swab around the neck of the ampule. | ___ | ___ | ___ | _____ |
| (3) Snap the neck of the ampule quickly and firmly away from the hands. | ___ | ___ | ___ | _____ |
| (4) Draw up medication quickly, using a filter needle long enough to reach the bottom of the ampule. | ___ | ___ | ___ | _____ |
| (5) Hold the ampule upside down, or set it on a flat surface. Insert the filter needle into centre of the ampule opening. Do not allow the needle tip or shaft to touch the rim of the ampule. | ___ | ___ | ___ | _____ |
| (6) Aspirate the medication into the syringe by gently pulling back on the plunger. | ___ | ___ | ___ | _____ |
| (7) Keep the needle tip under the surface of the liquid. Tip the ampule to bring all fluid within reach of the needle. | ___ | ___ | ___ | _____ |
| (8) If air bubbles are aspirated, do not expel the air into the ampule. | ___ | ___ | ___ | _____ |
| (9) To expel excess air bubbles, remove the needle from the ampule. Hold the syringe with the needle pointing up. Tap the side of the syringe to cause the bubbles to rise toward the needle. Draw back slightly on the plunger, then push the plunger upward to eject the air. Do not eject any fluid. | ___ | ___ | ___ | _____ |
| (10) If the syringe contains excess fluid, dispose of it in a sink. Hold the syringe vertically with the needle tip up and slanted slightly toward the sink. Slowly eject the excess fluid into the sink. Recheck the fluid level in the syringe by holding it vertically. | ___ | ___ | ___ | _____ |
| (11) Cover the needle with its safety sheath or cap. Replace the filter needle with a needle or a needleless access device for injection. | ___ | ___ | ___ | _____ |
| B. Vial containing a solution | | | | |
| (1) Remove the cap covering the top of the unused vial to expose the sterile rubber seal. If a multidose vial has been previously used, the cap has already been removed. Firmly and briskly wipe the surface of the rubber seal with an alcohol swab, and allow it to dry. | ___ | ___ | ___ | _____ |
| (2) Pick up the syringe, and remove the needle cap or the cap covering the needleless vial access device. Pull back on the plunger to draw an amount of air into the syringe equivalent to the volume of medication to be aspirated from the vial. | ___ | ___ | ___ | _____ |
| (3) With the vial on a flat surface, insert the tip of the needle. Ensure the bevelled tip enters first, through the centre of the rubber seal. Apply pressure to the tip of the needle during insertion. | ___ | ___ | ___ | _____ |
| (4) Inject air into the vial's airspace, holding onto the plunger. Hold the plunger with firm pressure; the plunger may be forced backward by air pressure within the vial. | ___ | ___ | ___ | _____ |

*Continued*

384

| | S | U | NP | Comments |
|---|---|---|---|---|

(5) Invert the vial while keeping a firm hold on the syringe and plunger. Hold the vial between the thumb and middle fingers of your nondominant hand. Grasp the end of the syringe barrel and plunger with the thumb and forefinger of your dominant hand to counteract pressure in the vial.

(6) Keep the tip of the needle below the fluid level.

(7) Allow air pressure from the vial to fill the syringe gradually with medication. If necessary, pull back slightly on the plunger to obtain the correct amount of solution.

(8) When the desired volume is obtained, position the needle into the vial's airspace. Tap the side of the syringe barrel carefully to dislodge any air bubbles. Eject any air remaining at the top of the syringe into the vial.

(9) Remove the needle from the vial by pulling back on the barrel of the syringe.

(10) Hold the syringe at eye level, at a 90-degree angle, to ensure the correct volume has been obtained and no air bubbles are present. Remove any remaining air by tapping the barrel to dislodge the air bubbles. Draw back slightly on the plunger; then push the plunger upward to eject the air. Do not eject the fluid. Recheck the volume of medication.

(11) If medication is to be injected into a patient's tissue, change needle to one of the appropriate gauge and length according to the route of medication and the patient's size and weight.

(12) For a multidose vial, make a label that includes the date of mixing, the concentration of the medication per millilitre, and your initials.

C. Vial containing a powder (reconstituting medications)

(1) Remove the cap covering the vial of powdered medication and the cap covering the vial of proper diluent. Firmly wipe both seals with an alcohol swab, and allow to dry.

(2) Draw up diluent into the syringe by following steps 6B (2) through 6B (10).

(3) Insert the tip of the needle through the centre of the rubber seal on the vial of powdered medication. Inject the diluent into the vial. Remove the needle.

(4) Mix the medication thoroughly. Roll the vial in your palms. Do not shake the vial.

(5) Reconstituted medication in the vial is ready to be drawn into a new syringe. Read the label carefully to determine the dose after reconstitution.

(6) Prepare medication in syringe, following steps 6B (2) through 6B (12).

7. Dispose of all soiled supplies. Place broken ampule vials, used vials, and used needles in a puncture-proof and leakproof container. Clean medication work area, and perform hand hygiene.

STUDENT: _____     DATE: _____

INSTRUCTOR: _____     DATE: _____

## Skill Performance Checklist
## Skill 33-5 Administering Injections

| | S | U | NP | Comments |
|---|---|---|---|---|

1. Check accuracy and completeness of each MAR or computer printout against the prescriber's original medication order. Check the patient's name and the medication name, dosage, and route and time of administration. Copy or rewrite any portion of the MAR that is difficult to read.
2. Assess the patient's medical history, medication history, and history of allergies. Determine whether the patient is allergic to any substances and the usual allergic reaction experienced.
3. Check the date of expiration for the medication.
4. Observe patient's verbal and nonverbal responses to receiving an injection.
5. Assess the patient for contraindications.
   A. For subcutaneous injections: Assess the patient for factors such as circulatory shock and reduced local tissue perfusion. Assess the adequacy of the patient's adipose tissue.
   B. For intramuscular injections: Assess the patient for muscle atrophy, reduced blood flow, and circulatory shock.
6. Perform hand hygiene. Aseptically prepare the correct medication dose from an ampule or vial. Ensure all air is expelled from the syringe. Check the label of medication against the MAR two times while preparing the medication. Create a removable label that shows the patient's name, the name of the drug, and the dosage. Apply the label to the removable needle cap.
7. Bring the medication to the patient at the right time, and perform hand hygiene.
8. Close the room curtain or door.
9. Identify the patient by using at least two patient identifiers. Compare the patient's name and one other identifier (e.g., the hospital identification number) on the MAR, computer printout, or computer screen against information on the patient's identification bracelet. Ask the patient to state his or her name, if possible, for a third identifier.
10. Compare the label of the medication with the MAR one more time at the patient's bedside.
11. Describe the steps of the procedure, and inform the patient that the injection will cause a slight burning or stinging sensation.
12. Perform hand hygiene; put on disposable gloves.
13. Keep a sheet or gown draped over the patient's body parts that do not need to be exposed.
14. Select appropriate injection site. Inspect the skin surface over the injection site for bruises, inflammation, and edema.
    A. *Subcutaneous injection:* Palpate the injection site for masses or tenderness. Avoid these areas. For patients who require daily insulin, rotate the injection site daily. Ensure the needle is the correct size by grasping a skin fold at the injection site with your thumb and forefinger. Measure the fold from top to bottom. The needle should be half the length of the skin fold.
    B. *Intramuscular injection:* Note the integrity and size of muscle, and palpate for tenderness or hardness. Avoid these areas. If injections are given frequently, rotate the injection sites. Use the ventrogluteal site if possible.
    C. *Intradermal injection:* Note any lesions or discoloration of patient's forearm. Select an injection site three to four fingerwidths below the antecubital space and a handwidth above the wrist. If the forearm cannot be used, inspect the patient's upper back. If necessary, sites for subcutaneous injections may be used.

*Continued*

|  | S | U | NP | Comments |
|---|---|---|---|---|

15. Assist patient to a comfortable position.    ___ ___ ___ _____
   A. *Subcutaneous injection*: Have the patient relax the arm, leg, or abdomen, depending on the site chosen for injection.    ___ ___ ___ _____
   B. *Intramuscular injection*: Position the patient depending on the site chosen (e.g., have the patient sit, lie flat, lie on one side, or lie prone).    ___ ___ ___ _____
   C. *Intradermal injection*: Have the patient extend the elbow and support the elbow and forearm on a flat surface.    ___ ___ ___ _____
   D. Speak with the patient about a subject of interest. Ask open-ended questions.    ___ ___ ___ _____
16. Relocate the injection site by using anatomical landmarks.    ___ ___ ___ _____
17. Clean the injection site with an antiseptic swab. Touch the swab to the centre of the site, and rotate it outward in a circular direction for about 5 cm.    ___ ___ ___ _____
18. Hold the swab or gauze between the third and fourth fingers of your nondominant hand.    ___ ___ ___ _____
19. Remove the needle cap or sheath from the needle by pulling it straight off.    ___ ___ ___ _____
20. Hold the syringe between the thumb and forefinger of your dominant hand.    ___ ___ ___ _____
   A. *Subcutaneous injection*: Hold the syringe as if you were holding a dart, palm down; or hold the syringe across tops of your fingertips.    ___ ___ ___ _____
   B. *Intramuscular injection*: Hold the syringe as if you were holding a dart, palm down.    ___ ___ ___ _____
   C. *Intradermal injection*: Hold the bevel of the needle pointing up.    ___ ___ ___ _____
21. Administer injection.    ___ ___ ___ _____
   A. Subcutaneous injection
      (1) For an average-size patient, spread the skin tightly across the injection site or pinch the skin with your nondominant hand.    ___ ___ ___ _____
      (2) Inject the needle quickly and firmly at a 45- to 90-degree angle. Then release the skin, if pinched.    ___ ___ ___ _____
      (3) For an obese patient, pinch the skin at the injection site and inject the needle at a 90-degree angle below the tissue fold.    ___ ___ ___ _____
      (4) Inject medication slowly.    ___ ___ ___ _____
   B. Intramuscular injection
      (1) Position your nondominant hand at the proper anatomical landmarks, and pull the skin down approximately 2.5 to 3.5 cm or laterally with the ulnar side of your hand to administer the injection in a Z-track. Hold this position until the medication is injected. Use your dominant hand to insert the needle quickly at a 90-degree angle into the muscle.    ___ ___ ___ _____
      (2) If the patient's muscle mass is small, grasp a body of muscle between your thumb and fingers.    ___ ___ ___ _____
      (3) After needle pierces the skin, grasp the lower end of the syringe barrel with your nondominant hand to stabilize the syringe. Continue to hold the skin tightly with your nondominant hand. Move your dominant hand to the end of the plunger. Do not move the syringe.    ___ ___ ___ _____
      (4) Pull back on the plunger. If no blood appears, inject the medicine slowly, at a rate of 1 mL per 10 seconds.    ___ ___ ___ _____
      (5) Wait ten seconds, and then smoothly and steadily withdraw the needle and release the skin. Apply gentle pressure with dry gauze if desired.    ___ ___ ___ _____
   C. Intradermal injection
      (1) With your nondominant hand, stretch the skin over the injection site with your forefinger or thumb.    ___ ___ ___ _____
      (2) With the needle almost against the patient's skin, insert it slowly at a 5- to 15-degree angle until resistance is felt. Advance the needle through the epidermis to approximately 3 mm below skin surface. The needle tip can be seen through the skin.    ___ ___ ___ _____
      (3) Inject the medication slowly. Normally, resistance is felt. If resistance is not felt, the needle is in too deep; remove and begin again. Your nondominant hand can stabilize the needle during the injection.    ___ ___ ___ _____
      (4) While injecting medication, notice that a small bleb approximately 6 mm in diameter (resembling a mosquito bite) appears on the skin's surface. Instruct the patient that this bleb is a normal finding.    ___ ___ ___ _____

*Continued*

|  | S | U | NP | Comments |
|---|---|---|---|---|

22. Withdraw the needle while applying an alcohol swab or gauze gently over the injection site. ____ ____ ____ _____

23. Apply gentle pressure. Do not massage the injection site. Put on a bandage if needed. ____ ____ ____ _____

24. Assist the patient to a comfortable position. ____ ____ ____ _____

25. Discard the uncapped needle or the needle enclosed in safety shield and attached syringe into a puncture-proof and leakproof receptacle. Do *not* recap the needle. ____ ____ ____ _____

26. Remove disposable gloves, and perform hand hygiene. ____ ____ ____ _____

27. Stay with the patient for three to five minutes to observe for any allergic reactions. ____ ____ ____ _____

28. Periodically return to the patient's room to ask whether the patient feels any acute pain, burning, numbness, or tingling at the injection site. ____ ____ ____ _____

29. Inspect the injection site, noting any bruising or induration. ____ ____ ____ _____

30. Observe the patient's response to medication at times that correlate with the medication's onset, peak, and duration. ____ ____ ____ _____

31. Ask the patient to explain the purpose and effects of the medication. ____ ____ ____ _____

32. For intradermal injections, use a skin pencil and draw a circle around the perimeter of the injection site. Read the site within an appropriate amount of time, which is determined by the type of medication or skin test administered. ____ ____ ____ _____

33. Chart the medication dose, route of administration, site, time, and date of injection on the MAR immediately after giving medication, as per employer policy. ____ ____ ____ _____

34. Document if the scheduled medication is withheld, and record the reason as per employer policy. ____ ____ ____ _____

35. Report any undesirable effects from the medication to the prescriber. ____ ____ ____ _____

36. Record the patient's response to medications in the nurses' notes, and report to prescriber if required. ____ ____ ____ _____

STUDENT: _____ DATE: _____

INSTRUCTOR: _____ DATE: _____

## Skill Performance Checklist
## Skill 33-6 Adding Medications to Intravenous Fluid Containers

|  | S | U | NP | Comments |
|---|---|---|---|---|
| 1. Check the accuracy and completeness of each MAR or computer printout against the prescriber's original medication order. Check the patient's name and the medication name, dosage, and route and time of administration. Copy or rewrite any portion of the MAR that is difficult to read. | ___ | ___ | ___ | _____ |
| 2. Assess the patient's medical history. | ___ | ___ | ___ | _____ |
| 3. Collect information necessary to administer the medication safely, including the medication's action, purpose, side effects, normal dose, time of peak onset, and nursing implications. | ___ | ___ | ___ | _____ |
| 4. When more than one medication is to be added to the intravenous (IV) solution, assess for compatibility of the medications. | ___ | ___ | ___ | _____ |
| 5. Assess patient's systemic fluid balance, as reflected by skin hydration and turgor, body weight, pulse, blood pressure, and ratio of fluid intake to urinary output. | ___ | ___ | ___ | _____ |
| 6. Assess patient's history of medication allergies. | ___ | ___ | ___ | _____ |
| 7. Perform hand hygiene. | ___ | ___ | ___ | _____ |
| 8. Assess the IV insertion site for signs of infiltration or phlebitis. | ___ | ___ | ___ | _____ |
| 9. Assess the patient's understanding of the purpose of the medication therapy. | ___ | ___ | ___ | _____ |
| 10. Prepare prescribed medication; use aseptic techniques. Ensure that you compare the label of the medication with the MAR two times while preparing the medication. | ___ | ___ | ___ | _____ |
| 11. Perform hand hygiene. | ___ | ___ | ___ | _____ |
| 12. Compare the labels of the medication and the IV fluid bag with the MAR or computer printout. | ___ | ___ | ___ | _____ |
| 13. Add the medication to a new container (usually in the medication room or at medication cart): | | | | |
| A. *Solution in a bag*: Locate the medication injection port on the plastic IV solution bag. The port has a small rubber stopper at the end. Do not select the port for the IV tubing insertion or the air vent. | ___ | ___ | ___ | _____ |
| B. *Solution in a bottle*: Locate the injection site on the IV solution bottle, which is often covered by a metal or plastic cap. | ___ | ___ | ___ | _____ |
| C. Wipe the port or injection site with alcohol or an antiseptic swab. | ___ | ___ | ___ | _____ |
| D. Remove the needle cap or sheath from the syringe, and insert the needle of the syringe or the needleless device through the centre of the injection port or site. Inject the medication. | ___ | ___ | ___ | _____ |
| E. Withdraw the syringe from the bag or bottle. | ___ | ___ | ___ | _____ |
| F. Mix the medication and the IV solution by holding the bag or bottle and turning it gently end to end. | ___ | ___ | ___ | _____ |
| G. Complete the medication label by printing the patient's name and dose of medication, date and time of administration, and your initials. Apply the label to the bottle or bag; do not cover essential information on the bottle or bag. Spike the bag or bottle with the IV tubing. | ___ | ___ | ___ | _____ |
| 14. Take the assembled items to patient's bedside at the right time, and perform hand hygiene. | ___ | ___ | ___ | _____ |
| 15. Identify the patient by using at least two patient identifiers. Compare the patient's name and one other identifier (e.g., the hospital identification number) on the MAR, computer printout, or computer screen against information on the patient's identification bracelet. Ask the patient to state his or her name, if possible, for a third identifier. | ___ | ___ | ___ | _____ |
| 16. Prepare the patient by explaining that the medication is to be given through the existing IV line or a new line that will be started. Explain that no discomfort should be felt during the medication infusion. Encourage patient to report symptoms of discomfort. | ___ | ___ | ___ | _____ |
| 17. Connect infusion tubing or spike container to the existing tubing. Regulate infusion at ordered rate. | ___ | ___ | ___ | _____ |

*Continued*

390

|  | S | U | NP | Comments |
|---|---|---|---|---|

18. Add the medication to the existing container.
    A. Prepare a vented IV bottle or plastic bag.
       (1) Check the volume of the solution remaining in the bottle or bag.
       (2) Close off IV infusion clamp.
       (3) Wipe the medication port with an alcohol or antiseptic swab.
       (4) Remove the needle cap or sheath from the syringe; insert the syringe needle or needleless device through the injection port, and inject the medication.
       (5) Withdraw the syringe from the bag or bottle.
       (6) Lower the bag or bottle from the IV pole, and gently mix the medication and IV solution by holding the bag or bottle and turning it gently from end to end. Rehang the bag or bottle.
    B. Complete the medication label, and apply it to the unprinted side of the IV solution bag or bottle. Do not cover the imprinted label of the solution.
    C. Regulate the infusion to the desired rate. Use an IV pump if indicated.
19. Properly dispose of equipment and supplies. Do not recap the needle or syringe. Discard sheathed needles as a unit with the needle covered.
20. Perform hand hygiene.
21. Observe the patient for signs or symptoms of medication reaction.
22. Observe the patient for signs and symptoms of fluid volume excess.
23. Periodically return to the patient's room to assess the IV insertion site and the rate of infusion.
24. Observe the patient for signs or symptoms of IV infiltration.
25. Ensure that a label is applied to the IV tubing; the label must state the date and time that the IV tubing was opened and must be attached to the IV infusion system. Consult employer policy regarding frequency of changing IV tubing.
26. Assess the IV tubing frequently for integrity and occlusions.
27. Ask the patient to explain the purpose and effects of the medication therapy.
28. Record the solution and medication added to parenteral fluid on the appropriate form.
29. Report any adverse effects to the patient's health care provider, and document adverse effects according to institutional policy.

STUDENT: _____ DATE: _____

INSTRUCTOR: _____ DATE: _____

## Skill Performance Checklist
## Skill 33-7 Administering Medications by Intravenous Bolus

|  | S | U | NP | Comments |
|---|---|---|---|---|
| 1. Check the accuracy and completeness of each MAR or computer printout against the prescriber's original medication order. Check the patient's name and the medication name, route, dosage, and time of administration. Copy or rewrite any portion of the MAR that is difficult to read. | ___ | ___ | ___ | _____ |
| 2. Collect the information necessary to administer the medication safely, including action, purpose, side effects, normal dose, time of peak onset, the pace at which to give the medication, and nursing implications, such as the need to dilute the medication or to administer it through a filter. | ___ | ___ | ___ | _____ |
| 3. If pushing medication into an IV line, determine the compatibility of the medication with both the IV fluids ordered and any additives in the IV solution. | ___ | ___ | ___ | _____ |
| 4. Perform hand hygiene. Assess the IV or saline (heparin) lock insertion site for signs of infiltration or phlebitis. | ___ | ___ | ___ | _____ |
| 5. Check the patient's medical history and allergies. | ___ | ___ | ___ | _____ |
| 6. Check the date of expiration for the medication vial or ampule. | ___ | ___ | ___ | _____ |
| 7. Assess the patient's understanding of the purpose of medication therapy. | ___ | ___ | ___ | _____ |
| 8. Prepare the ordered medication from the vial or ampule by using aseptic technique. Check the label of the medication carefully with the MAR two times. Apply a removable label indicating the patient's name and the medication name and dosage to the removable needle cap. | ___ | ___ | ___ | _____ |
| 9. Bring the medication to the patient at the correct time. | ___ | ___ | ___ | _____ |
| 10. Identify the patient by using at least two patient identifiers. Compare the patient's name and one other identifier (e.g., the hospital identification number) on the MAR, computer printout, or computer screen against information on the patient's identification bracelet. Ask the patient to state his or her name, if possible, for a third identifier. | ___ | ___ | ___ | _____ |
| 11. Compare the label of the medications with the MAR at the patient's bedside. | ___ | ___ | ___ | _____ |
| 12. Explain the procedure to the patient. Encourage the patient to report symptoms of discomfort at the IV site. | ___ | ___ | ___ | _____ |
| 13. Perform hand hygiene. Put on gloves. | ___ | ___ | ___ | _____ |
| 14. Administer the medication by IV push (through the existing IV line): |  |  |  |  |
| A. Select the injection port of the IV tubing closest to the patient. Whenever possible, the injection port should accept a needleless syringe. Use the IV filter if required by a medication reference manual or employer policy. | ___ | ___ | ___ | _____ |
| B. Wipe the injection port with an antiseptic swab. Allow to dry. | ___ | ___ | ___ | _____ |
| C. Connect the syringe to the IV line. Insert the needleless tip or a small-gauge needle of a syringe containing the prepared drug through the centre of the injection port. | ___ | ___ | ___ | _____ |
| D. Occlude the IV line by pinching the tubing just above the injection port. | ___ | ___ | ___ | _____ |
| E. Release the tubing, and inject the medication within the amount of time recommended by institutional policy, the pharmacist, or a medication reference manual. Use your watch to time the administration. The IV line can be pinched while medication is being pushed, and released when medication is not being pushed. Allow IV fluids to infuse when the medication is not being pushed. | ___ | ___ | ___ | _____ |
| F. After injecting the medication, release the tubing, withdraw the syringe, and recheck the fluid infusion rate. | ___ | ___ | ___ | _____ |

*Continued*

392

|  | S | U | NP | Comments |
|---|---|---|---|---|

15. Administer medication by IV push (IV lock or needleless system).
   A. Prepare flush solutions according to employer policy. Ensure that a syringe with the correct barrel width is used. Consult employer policy regarding syringes used for delivering IV bolus medications.
      (1) *Saline flush method (preferred)*:
         (a) Prepare two appropriate-sized syringes with 2 to 3 mL of normal saline (0.9%).
      (2) *Heparin flush method (traditional method)*:
         (a) Prepare one appropriate-sized syringe with the ordered amount of heparin flush solution.
         (b) Prepare two syringes with 2 to 3 mL of normal saline (0.9%).
   B. Administer medication:
      (1) Wipe the lock's injection port with an antiseptic swab.
      (2) Insert a syringe containing normal saline into the injection port of the IV lock.
      (3) Pull back gently on the syringe plunger, and look for blood return.
      (4) Flush the IV lock with normal saline by pushing slowly on plunger.
      (5) Remove the saline-filled syringe.
      (6) Clean the lock's injection port with an antiseptic swab.
      (7) Insert the syringe containing the prepared medication into the injection port of the IV lock.
      (8) Inject the medication within the amount of time recommended by institutional policy, the pharmacist, or a medication reference manual. Use a watch to time the administration.
      (9) After administering the bolus, withdraw the syringe.
      (10) Clean the lock's injection port with an antiseptic swab.
      (11) Attach the syringe with normal saline, and inject the normal saline flush at the same rate that the medication was delivered.
      (12) *Heparin flush option*: Insert the needle of the syringe containing the heparin through the diaphragm.
16. Dispose of uncapped needles and syringes in a puncture-proof and leakproof container.
17. Remove and dispose of gloves. Perform hand hygiene.
18. Observe the patient closely for adverse reactions while the medication is administered and for several minutes thereafter.
19. Observe the IV site during injection for sudden swelling.
20. Observe the patient's status after the medication is administered, to evaluate effectiveness of medication.
21. Consult employer policy with regard to the frequency of saline flushes.
22. Ask the patient to explain the medication's purposes and side effects.
23. Record the medication, dose, time, and route on the appropriate form (MAR) or in computer record.
24. Report any adverse reactions immediately to the health care provider because the reactions could be life-threatening. The patient's response may indicate the need for additional medical therapy.
25. Record the patient's response to medication in the nurses' notes.

STUDENT: _____   DATE: _____

INSTRUCTOR: _____   DATE: _____

## Skill Performance Checklist
## Skill 33-8 Administering Intravenous Medications by Piggyback, Intermittent Intravenous Infusion Sets, and Mini-Infusion Pumps

|  | S | U | NP | Comments |
|---|---|---|---|---|
| 1. Check the accuracy and completeness of each MAR or computer printout against the prescriber's original medication order. Check the patient's name and the medication name, dosage, and route and time of administration. Copy or rewrite any portion of the MAR that is difficult to read. | ___ | ___ | ___ | _____ |
| 2. Determine the patient's medical history. | ___ | ___ | ___ | _____ |
| 3. Collect the information necessary to administer the medication safely, including the action, purpose, side effects, normal dose, time of peak onset, and nursing implications, such as the need to dilute the medication or administer it through a filter. | ___ | ___ | ___ | _____ |
| 4. Assess the compatibility of the drug with the existing IV solution. | ___ | ___ | ___ | _____ |
| 5. Assess patency of the patient's existing IV infusion line by the noting infusion rate of the main IV line. | ___ | ___ | ___ | _____ |
| 6. Perform hand hygiene. Assess IV insertion site for signs of infiltration or phlebitis: redness, pallor, swelling, tenderness on palpation. | ___ | ___ | ___ | _____ |
| 7. Assess the patient's history of medication allergies. | ___ | ___ | ___ | _____ |
| 8. Assess the patient's understanding of the purpose of medication therapy. | ___ | ___ | ___ | _____ |
| 9. Prepare the medication. Ensure that you compare the label of the medication with the MAR two times while preparing the medication. | ___ | ___ | ___ | _____ |
| 10. Assemble supplies at the patient's bedside. Prepare the patient by explaining that the medication will be given through the IV equipment. | ___ | ___ | ___ | _____ |
| 11. Perform hand hygiene. | ___ | ___ | ___ | _____ |
| 12. Identify the patient by using at least two patient identifiers. Compare the patient's name and one other identifier (e.g., the hospital identification number) on the MAR, computer printout, or computer screen against information on the patient's identification bracelet. Ask the patient to state his or her name, if possible, for a third identifier. | ___ | ___ | ___ | _____ |
| 13. Compare medication label with MAR at the patient's bedside. | ___ | ___ | ___ | _____ |
| 14. Explain to the patient the purpose of the medication and its side effects. Encourage the patient to report symptoms of discomfort at the injection site. | ___ | ___ | ___ | _____ |
| 15. Administer the infusion. | | | | |
| A. Piggyback or tandem infusion | | | | |
| (1) Connect the infusion tubing to the medication bag. Allow the solution to fill the tubing by opening the regulator flow clamp. Once the tubing is full, close the clamp and cap the end of the tubing. | ___ | ___ | ___ | _____ |
| (2) Hang the piggyback medication bag above the level of the primary fluid bag. (A hook can be used to lower the main bag.) Hang the tandem infusion bag at the same level as the primary fluid bag. | ___ | ___ | ___ | _____ |
| (3) Connect the tubing of the piggyback or tandem infusion to the appropriate connector on the primary infusion line: | | | | |
| (a) *Stopcock*: Wipe the stopcock port with an alcohol swab, and connect the tubing. Turn the stopcock to the open position. | ___ | ___ | ___ | _____ |
| (b) *Needleless system*: Wipe the needleless port, and insert the tip of the piggyback or tandem infusion tubing. | ___ | ___ | ___ | _____ |
| (c) *Tubing port*: Connect the sterile needle to the end of the piggyback or tandem infusion tubing, remove the cap, clean the injection port on the main IV line, and insert the needle or needleless access device through the centre of the port. Secure by taping the connection. | ___ | ___ | ___ | _____ |
| (4) Regulate the flow rate of the medication solution by adjusting the regulator clamp. (Infusion times vary. Refer to a medication reference manual or institutional policy for the safe flow rate.) | ___ | ___ | ___ | _____ |

*Continued*

394

(5) After medication has infused, check the flow regulator on the primary infusion. The primary infusion should automatically begin to flow after the piggyback or tandem solution is empty.

(6) Regulate the main infusion line to the desired rate, if necessary.

(7) Leave the IV piggyback bag and tubing in place for future medication administration, or discard in appropriate containers.

B. Volume-control administration set (e.g., Volutrol)

(1) Assemble the supplies in the medication room.

(2) Prepare medication from a vial or ampule.

(3) Fill the Volutrol with the desired amount of fluid (50–100 mL) by opening the clamp between the Volutrol and the main IV bag.

(4) Close the clamp, and ensure the clamp on the air vent of the Volutrol chamber is open.

(5) Clean the injection port on the top of the Volutrol with an antiseptic swab.

(6) Remove the needle cap or sheath, and insert the syringe needle through the port, then inject medication. Gently rotate the Volutrol between your hands.

(7) Regulate the IV infusion rate to allow the medication to infuse in time recommended by institutional policy, a pharmacist, or a medication reference manual.

(8) Label the Volutrol with the name of the medication, the dosage, the total volume (including the diluent), and the time of administration.

(9) Dispose of the uncapped needle or the needle enclosed in the safety shield and syringe in a proper container. Perform hand hygiene.

C. Mini-infusion administration

(1) Connect prefilled syringe to the mini-infusion tubing.

(2) Carefully apply pressure to the syringe plunger, allowing the tubing to fill with medication.

(3) Place the syringe into mini-infusion pump (follow product directions). Ensure the syringe is secure.

(4) Connect the mini-infusion tubing to the main IV line.

(a) *Stopcock*: Wipe the stopcock port with an alcohol swab, and connect the tubing. Turn the stopcock to the open position.

(b) *Needleless system*: Wipe the needleless port, and insert the tip of the mini-infusion tubing.

(c) *Tubing port*: Connect the sterile needle to the mini-infusion tubing, remove the cap, clean the injection port on the main IV line, and insert the needle through the centre of port. Consider placing tape where the IV tubing enters the port to secure the connection.

(5) Explain the purpose of the medication and the side effects to the patient, and explain that the medication is to be given through the existing IV line. Ask the patient to report any symptoms of discomfort at the injection site.

(6) Hang the infusion pump with the syringe on the IV pole alongside the main IV bag. Set the pump to deliver medication within the time recommended by institutional policy, the pharmacist, or a medication reference manual. Press the button on the pump to begin infusion. Optional: Set the alarm.

(7) After medication has infused, check the flow regulator on the primary infusion. The infusion should automatically begin to flow once the pump stops. Regulate the main infusion line to the desired rate as needed. (Note: If the stopcock is used, turn off the mini-infusion line.)

16. Observe the patient for signs of adverse reactions.

17. During infusion, periodically check the infusion rate and the condition of the IV site.

18. Ask the patient to explain the purpose and side effects of the medication.

STUDENT: _____ DATE: _____

INSTRUCTOR: _____ DATE: _____

## Skill Performance Checklist
## Skill 36-1 Applying Physical Restraints

| | S | U | NP | Comments |
|---|---|---|---|---|
| 1. Assess whether the patient needs a restraint. Does the patient continually try to interrupt needed therapy? Is the patient at risk for injuring self or others? | ___ | ___ | ___ | _____ |
| 2. Assess the patient's behaviour, such as confusion, disorientation, agitation, restlessness, combativeness, or inability to follow directions. Consult with a gerontological nurse specialist if available. | ___ | ___ | ___ | _____ |
| 3. Review your employer's policies regarding restraints. Consider the purpose, type, location, and duration of restraint. Determine whether signed consent for the use of restraint is needed. | ___ | ___ | ___ | _____ |
| 4. Review restraint manufacturer's instructions before entering the patient's room. Determine the most appropriate size of restraint. | ___ | ___ | ___ | _____ |
| 5. Perform hand hygiene, and gather equipment. | ___ | ___ | ___ | _____ |
| 6. Introduce yourself to the patient and family. Assess their feelings about restraint use. Explain that restraint is temporary and is designed to protect the patient from injury. | ___ | ___ | ___ | _____ |
| 7. Inspect the area of the patient's body where the restraint is to be placed. Assess the condition of skin underlying where the restraint is to be applied. | ___ | ___ | ___ | _____ |
| 8. Approach patient in a calm, confident manner. Check the patient's identification by using two identifiers. Explain what you plan to do. | ___ | ___ | ___ | _____ |
| 9. Adjust the bed to proper height, and lower the side rail on the side of patient contact. | ___ | ___ | ___ | _____ |
| 10. Provide privacy. Make sure the patient is comfortable and in proper body alignment. Drape the patient as needed. | ___ | ___ | ___ | _____ |
| 11. Pad the skin and bony prominences (if necessary) before applying restraints. | ___ | ___ | ___ | _____ |
| 12. Apply the appropriate-sized restraint, making sure it does not cover an IV line or other device (e.g., dialysis shunt) and that it does not cover the patient's identification or allergy bracelet. | | | | |
|   A. *Belt restraint*: This device secures the patient to a bed or stretcher. Apply it over the patient's clothes or gown. Remove wrinkles from the front and back of the restraint while placing it around the patient's waist. Bring ties through slots in the belt. Avoid placing the belt across the chest or too tightly across the abdomen. | ___ | ___ | ___ | _____ |
|   B. *Extremity (ankle or wrist) restraint*: This restraint is designed to immobilize one or all extremities. Commercially available limb restraints are composed of sheepskin or foam padding. Wrap the limb restraint around the wrist or ankle with the soft part toward the skin and secure it snugly in place with Velcro straps. | ___ | ___ | ___ | _____ |
|   C. *Mitten restraint*: This thumbless mitten device is used to restrain the patient's hands. Place a hand in the mitten, being sure the mitten end is brought all the way over the wrist. | ___ | ___ | ___ | _____ |
|   D. *Elbow restraint*: This piece of fabric with slots has tongue blades placed so that elbow joint remains rigid. | ___ | ___ | ___ | _____ |
|   E. *Mummy restraint*: The mummy restraint consists of a blanket or sheet. It is opened on the bed or crib with one corner folded toward the centre. Place the child on the blanket with shoulders at the fold and feet toward the opposite corner. With child's right arm straight down against the body, pull the right side of the blanket firmly across the right shoulder and chest, and secure it beneath the left side of the body. Place the left arm straight against the body, and bring the left side of the blanket across the shoulder and chest and beneath the child's body on right side. Fold lower corner, bring it over the child's body, and tuck or fasten it securely with safety pins. | ___ | ___ | ___ | _____ |

*Continued*

|  | S | U | NP | Comments |
|---|---|---|---|---|
| 13. Attach restraints to the bed frame, which moves when the head of the bed is raised or lowered. Do not attach them to side rails. | ___ | ___ | ___ | _____ |
| 14. Secure restraints with a quick-release tie. Do not tie in a knot. | ___ | ___ | ___ | _____ |
| 15. Make sure two fingers will fit under secured restraint. | ___ | ___ | ___ | _____ |
| 16. The proper placement of the restraint, skin integrity, pulses, temperature, colour, and sensation of the restrained body part should be assessed at least every hour or per your employer's policy. | ___ | ___ | ___ | _____ |
| 17. Restraints should be removed at regular intervals (see employer policy). If the patient is violent and noncompliant, remove one restraint at a time or have staff assist while removing restraints. The patient should not be left unattended at this time. | ___ | ___ | ___ | _____ |
| 18. Secure a call light or intercom system within the patient's reach. | ___ | ___ | ___ | _____ |
| 19. Leave the patient's bed or chair with wheels locked. The bed should be in its lowest position. | ___ | ___ | ___ | _____ |
| 20. Perform hand hygiene. | ___ | ___ | ___ | _____ |
| 21. Reassess the patient's status and needs: | | | | |
| A. Inspect the patient for any injuries, including all hazards of immobility, while restraints are in use. | ___ | ___ | ___ | _____ |
| B. Observe IV catheters, urinary catheters, and drainage tubes to ensure that they are positioned correctly and that therapy remains uninterrupted. | ___ | ___ | ___ | _____ |
| C. Regularly reassess the patient's need for continued use of the restraint (for medical or surgical reason) with the intent of discontinuing the restraint at the earliest possible time. | ___ | ___ | ___ | _____ |
| D. Provide sensory stimulation and reorient patient as needed. | ___ | ___ | ___ | _____ |
| 22. Record behaviours that place patient at risk for injury. | ___ | ___ | ___ | _____ |
| A. Describe restraint alternatives attempted and patient's response. | ___ | ___ | ___ | _____ |
| B. Record patient's and family's understanding of and consent to restraint application. | ___ | ___ | ___ | _____ |
| C. Record type and location of the restraint and time applied. | ___ | ___ | ___ | _____ |
| D. Record time of assessments and releases. | ___ | ___ | ___ | _____ |
| E. Document the patient's behaviour after the application of the restraint. | ___ | ___ | ___ | _____ |
| F. Document specific assessments related to orientation, oxygenation, skin integrity, circulation, and positioning. | ___ | ___ | ___ | _____ |
| G. Describe the patient's response when restraints were removed. | ___ | ___ | ___ | _____ |

STUDENT: _____ DATE: _____

INSTRUCTOR: _____ DATE: _____

## Skill Performance Checklist
## Skill 36-2 Seizure Precautions

|  | S | U | NP | Comments |
|---|---|---|---|---|
| 1. Assess seizure history, noting the frequency of seizures, presence of aura, and sequence of events, if known. Assess for medical and surgical conditions that may lead to seizures or exacerbate existing seizure condition. Assess medication history. | — | — | — | _____ |
| 2. Inspect the patient's environment for potential safety hazards if risk for seizure exists, such as a bedside stand or table, an IV pole, or other medical equipment. | — | — | — | _____ |
| 3. Perform hand hygiene, and prepare bed with padded side rails and headboard. Set the bed in the low position, and place the patient in side-lying position when possible. | — | — | — | _____ |
| 4. For patients with a history of seizures, ensure that items such as an airway, suction apparatus, disposable gloves, and pillows are visible in the hospital setting for immediate use. | — | — | — | _____ |
| 5. When a seizure begins, position the patient safely. If the patient is standing or sitting, guide the patient to the floor, and protect his or her head by cradling it in your lap or placing a pillow under the head. Clear the surrounding area of furniture. If the patient is in bed, raise the side rails, add padding, and put the bed in low position. | — | — | — | _____ |
| 6. Provide privacy. | | | | |
| 7. If possible, turn the patient on the side, with the head flexed slightly forward. | — | — | — | _____ |
| 8. Do not restrain the patient. Loosen the patient's clothing. | — | — | — | _____ |
| 9. Do not put anything into the patient's mouth, such as fingers, tongue depressor, or medicine. | — | — | — | _____ |
| 10. Stay with the patient. Observe the sequence and timing of seizure activity. | — | — | — | _____ |
| 11. After the seizure is over, explain what happened and answer the patient's questions. Foster an atmosphere of acceptance and respect. | — | — | — | _____ |
| 12. After the seizure, assist the patient to a position of comfort in bed with padded side rails up and the bed in low position. Place a call light within reach, and provide a quiet, nonstimulating environment. Perform hand hygiene before leaving the room. | — | — | — | _____ |

**STATUS EPILEPTICUS:**

*For a patient experiencing status epilepticus, the following actions are required:*

|  | S | U | NP | Comments |
|---|---|---|---|---|
| 13. Put on disposable gloves, and insert an oral airway when the jaw is relaxed between seizure activities. Hold the airway with curved side up; insert downward until airway reaches the back of the throat, and then rotate and follow the natural curve of the tongue. Do not place fingers near or in the patient's mouth. | — | — | — | _____ |
| 14. Access oxygen and suction equipment. Prepare for IV insertion. | | | | |
| 15. Use pillows or pads to protect the patient from injuring self. | — | — | — | _____ |
| 16. Record the timing of seizure activity and the sequence of events. Record the presence of aura (if any), level of consciousness, posture, colour, movements of extremities, incontinence, and patient's status following the seizure. | — | — | — | _____ |
| 17. Document patient's response and expected or unexpected outcomes. | — | — | — | _____ |
| 18. Report to the physician immediately as seizure begins. Status epilepticus is an emergency situation requiring immediate medical management. | — | — | — | _____ |

STUDENT: _____ DATE: _____

INSTRUCTOR: _____ DATE: _____

## Skill Performance Checklist
## Skill 37-1 Bathing a Patient

| | S | U | NP | Comments |
|---|---|---|---|---|
| 1. Review orders for specific safety measures concerning the patient's movement, positioning, or isolation precautions. | ___ | ___ | ___ | _____ |
| 2. Explain the procedure to the patient, and ask the patient for suggestions on how to prepare supplies. Encourage and promote independence by asking the patient how much of the bath he or she wishes to complete. | ___ | ___ | ___ | _____ |
| 3. Assess the patient's ability to perform self-care, and allow the patient to perform as much of the bath as he or she can. | ___ | ___ | ___ | _____ |
| 4. Assess the patient's tolerance for activity, comfort level, cognitive ability, and musculoskeletal function. | ___ | ___ | ___ | _____ |
| 5. Assess the patient's bathing preferences: frequency, type of hygiene products, and other factors. | ___ | ___ | ___ | _____ |
| 6. Ask whether patient has noticed any skin problems or unusual marks on the skin. Observe the skin throughout the procedure, paying particular attention to areas that were previously soiled, were reddened, or showed early signs of breakdown. | ___ | ___ | ___ | _____ |
| 7. Begin complete or partial bed bath, tub bath, whirlpool bath, or shower. | ___ | ___ | ___ | _____ |
| A. *Complete or partial bed bath*: | | | | |
| (1) Close room doors, and draw room divider curtain. | ___ | ___ | ___ | _____ |
| (2) Prepare equipment and supplies. | ___ | ___ | ___ | _____ |
| (3) For nonambulatory patients, offer a bedpan or urinal. Provide a towel and washcloth for perineal care afterward. | ___ | ___ | ___ | _____ |
| (4) Perform hand hygiene. If the patient's skin is soiled with drainage or body secretions, put on disposable gloves. Ensure the patient is not allergic to latex. | ___ | ___ | ___ | _____ |
| (5) Place hospital bed at appropriate level, and lower side rail closest to you. Assist the patient in assuming a comfortable position that maintains body alignment, preferably supine. Bring the patient, or have the patient move, toward the side of the bed closest to you. | ___ | ___ | ___ | _____ |
| (6) Loosen the top covers. Place the bath blanket over the top sheet. Remove the top sheet from under the blanket. If possible, have the patient hold the bath blanket while you withdraw the sheet. Optional: Use the top sheet when a bath blanket is not available. | ___ | ___ | ___ | _____ |
| (7) If the top sheet is to be reused, fold it for replacement later. If not, place it in linen bag, taking care not to allow linen to contact uniform. | ___ | ___ | ___ | _____ |
| (8) Assist the patient with oral hygiene. See Skill 37-3. | ___ | ___ | ___ | _____ |
| (9) Remove the patient's gown or pyjamas. If the patient has an IV infusing and the gown has snaps, simply unsnap and remove the gown without disconnecting the IV tubing. If the gown does not have snaps, remove gown from the arm without the IV first; then lower the IV container or remove from the pump and slide the gown covering the affected arm over the tubing and container. Rehang the IV container, and check flow rate or reset pump rate. Do not disconnect the tubing. If an extremity is injured or has reduced mobility, begin removal from the unaffected side. | ___ | ___ | ___ | _____ |
| (10) Raise the side rail. Fill a wash basin two-thirds full with warm water. Have the patient place fingers in the water to test temperature. Change the water as necessary throughout the bath. | ___ | ___ | ___ | _____ |
| (11) Remove the pillow, if allowed, and raise the head of the bed 30 to 45 degrees. Place the bath towel under the patient's head. Place a second bath towel over the patient's chest. | ___ | ___ | ___ | _____ |

*Continued*

|  | S | U | NP | Comments |
|---|---|---|---|---|

(12) Immerse the washcloth in warm water, and wring it thoroughly. If desired, fold the washcloth around the fingers of your hand to form a mitt.

(13) Inquire whether the patient is wearing contact lenses. Wash the patient's eyes with plain warm water. Use a different section of the mitt for each eye. Move the mitt from inner to outer canthus. Soak any crusts on eyelid for two to three minutes with the damp cloth before attempting removal. Dry eye thoroughly but gently.

(14) Ask whether the patient prefers to use soap on his or her face. Wash, rinse, and thoroughly dry all areas of the face, neck, and ears. Men may wish to shave at this point or after the bath.

(15) Expose the patient's arm that is farthest from you, and place the bath towel lengthwise under that arm.

(16) Bathe the patient's arm with soap and water, using long, firm strokes from distal to proximal areas. Raise and support the arm as needed while washing the axilla.

(17) Rinse and dry the arm and axilla thoroughly. If the patient uses deodorant or talcum powder, apply it.

(18) Fold the bath towel in half, and lay it on the bed beside the patient. Place a basin on the towel. Immerse the patient's hand in water. Allow the hand to soak for three to five minutes before washing hand and fingernails. Remove the basin, and dry the hand well.

(19) Cover the arm with a bath blanket or towel. Repeat steps 15 through 18 for other arm.

(20) Cover the patient's chest with a bath towel, and fold the bath blanket down to the umbilicus. With one hand, lift the edge of the towel away from the patient's chest. With washcloth or mitted hand, bathe the patient's chest, using long, firm strokes. Take special care to wash skinfolds under a female patient's breasts. Keep the patient's chest covered between wash and rinse periods. Dry well.

(21) Place bath towel lengthwise over the patient's chest and abdomen. (Two towels may be needed.) Fold blanket down to just above the patient's pubic region.

(22) With one hand, lift the bath towel. With the mitted hand, bathe the patient's abdomen, giving special attention to bathing the umbilicus and abdominal folds. Keep the patient's abdomen covered between washing and rinsing. Dry well.

(23) Cover the patient's chest and abdomen with the top of the bath blanket. Expose the patient's far leg by folding the blanket toward the midline. Be sure the other leg and perineum are covered.

(24) Place the bath towel lengthwise under the far leg, and, using firm strokes (unless contraindicated), wash, rinse, and dry thoroughly. Support the leg with one hand if the patient is unable to support it.

(25) Cleanse the foot, making sure to bathe between toes. Clean and clip nails as per physician orders. Dry well. If the skin is dry, apply lotion. Do not massage any reddened area on the patient's skin.

(26) Repeat steps 23 through 25 for the patient's other leg and foot.

(27) Assist the patient in assuming a prone or side-lying position (as applicable). Place towel lengthwise along the patient's side. Put on disposable gloves if you have not done so already.

*Continued*

|  | S | U | NP | Comments |
|---|---|---|---|---|

(28) Wash, rinse, and dry the patient's back from neck to buttocks, using long, firm strokes. Pay special attention to folds of the buttocks and the anus for redness or skin breakdown. Give a back massage. Change bath water if necessary, and put on disposable gloves.

  (a) *Female perineal care*:

    (a1) Assist patient in assuming a dorsal recumbent position, if not contraindicated. Cover the chest and upper extremities with a towel and the lower extremities with a bath blanket. Expose only the genitalia. (If the patient can wash, covering entire body with a bath blanket may be preferable.) Clean the perineal area. Pay special attention to skin folds. If fecal material is present, enclose in a fold of underpad and remove with disposable wipes.

    (a2) Wash labia majora. Wipe from the perineum to the rectum. Repeat on the opposite side, using a different section of the washcloth.

    (a3) Separate the labia with your nondominant hand, exposing the urethral meatus and vaginal orifice. Wash downward from the pubic area toward the rectum in one smooth stroke. Use a separate section of cloth for each stroke. Cleanse thoroughly around the labia minora, clitoris, and vaginal orifice. Dry thoroughly.

    (a4) Assist the patient to a comfortable position.

    (a5) Remove disposable gloves, and perform hand hygiene.

  (b) *Male perineal care*:

    (b1) Lower the side rails, and assist the patient to a supine position. Note restriction in mobility.

    (b2) Gently raise the penis, and place a bath towel underneath. Gently grasp the shaft of the penis. If the patient is uncircumcised, retract the foreskin. If the patient has an erection, defer perineal care until later.

    (b3) Wash the tip of the penis at the urethral meatus first, using a circular motion. Cleanse from the meatus outward. Rinse and dry gently.

    (b4) Return the foreskin to its natural position.

    (b5) Wash the shaft of the penis with gentle but firm downward strokes. Pay special attention to the underlying surface of the penis. Rinse and dry thoroughly.

    (b6) Gently cleanse the scrotum, making sure to wash underlying skin folds. Rinse and dry thoroughly.

    (b7) Inspect the surface of the external genitalia after cleansing.

    (b8) If the patient has bowel or urinary incontinence, apply a thin layer of skin barrier cream to the buttock, anus, and perineal area.

    (b9) Assist the patient to a comfortable position, and cover with the bath blanket.

(29) Assist the patient in dressing. Comb the patient's hair. Women may want to apply makeup, and men may wish to shave at this point. Assist the patient to a chair or wheelchair.

(30) Make the patient's bed.

(31) Remove soiled linen, and place it in a linen bag. Clean and replace the bathing equipment. Replace the call light and the patient's personal possessions. Leave the room as clean and comfortable as possible.

(32) Remove disposable gloves, and perform hand hygiene.

*Continued*

402

|  | S | U | NP | Comments |
|---|---|---|---|---|

B. *Tub or whirlpool bath or shower (verify with employer policy whether a physician's order is needed):*

(1) Check the tub or shower for cleanliness. Use cleaning techniques outlined in employer policy. Place a rubber mat on the tub or shower bottom. Place a disposable bath mat or towel on the floor in front of the tub or shower.

(2) Collect all hygienic aids, toiletry items, and linens requested by the patient. Place within easy reach of the tub or shower.

(3) Assist the patient to the bathroom if necessary. Have the patient wear a robe and slippers to the bathroom.

(4) Demonstrate how to use the call signal for assistance.

(5) Place an "occupied" sign on the bathroom door.

(6) Provide a shower seat or tub chair if needed. Fill the bathtub halfway with warm water. If the patient's sensation is normal, ask the patient to test the water, and adjust the temperature if needed. Explain which faucet controls hot water. If the patient is taking a shower, turn it on and adjust the water temperature before the patient enters the shower stall.

(7) Instruct the patient to use safety bars when getting in and out of the tub or shower. Caution the patient against the use of bath oil in tub water.

(8) Instruct the patient not to remain in tub for more than 20 minutes. Debilitated patients should not be left alone while in the tub. Observe patient's range of motion during the bath.

(9) Return to the bathroom when the patient signals, and knock before entering.

(10) For the patient who is unsteady, drain the tub of water before the patient attempts to get out of it. Place a bath towel over the patient's shoulders. Assist the patient in getting out of the tub as needed, and assist with drying. If the patient is weak or unstable, have another person assist.

(11) Observe the patient's skin, paying particular attention to areas that were previously soiled, reddened, or showed early signs of breakdown.

(12) Assist the patient as needed in donning a clean gown or pyjamas, slippers, and robe. (In a home setting, the patient may don regular clothing.)

(13) Assist the patient to his or her room and a comfortable position in a bed or chair.

(14) Clean the tub or shower according to employer policy. Whirlpool baths may require special cleaning. Remove soiled linen and place it in a linen bag. Discard disposable equipment in the proper receptacle. Place an "unoccupied" sign on the bathroom door. Return supplies to the storage area.

(15) Perform hand hygiene.

8. Record the condition of skin and any significant findings (e.g., reddened areas, bruises, nevi, or joint or muscle pain).

9. Report any evidence of alterations in skin integrity or increased wound secretions to the person in charge or the physician.

10. Record the presence of any abnormal findings (e.g., the character and amount of discharge or condition of the genitalia), and record any related procedure you perform.

11. Record the appearance of a suture line, if present.

12. Report any break in a suture line or the presence of abnormalities to the person in charge or the physician.

13. Record all procedures performed, the amount of assistance provided, and the extent of the patient's participation.

STUDENT: _____ DATE: _____

INSTRUCTOR: _____ DATE: _____

## Skill Performance Checklist
## Skill 37-2 Performing Nail and Foot Care

|  | S | U | NP | Comments |
|---|---|---|---|---|
| 1. Identify patients at risk for foot or nail problems: |  |  |  |  |
| A. Older adult | ___ | ___ | ___ | _____ |
| B. Diabetes mellitus | ___ | ___ | ___ | _____ |
| C. Heart failure or renal disease | ___ | ___ | ___ | _____ |
| D. Cerebrovascular accident (stroke) | ___ | ___ | ___ | _____ |
| 2. Assess the patient's knowledge of foot and nail care practices. | ___ | ___ | ___ | _____ |
| 3. Ask female patients whether they use nail polish and polish remover frequently. | ___ | ___ | ___ | _____ |
| 4. Assess the patient's ability to care for nails or feet. Consider visual alterations, fatigue, and musculoskeletal weakness. | ___ | ___ | ___ | _____ |
| 5. Assess the types of home remedies (e.g., aloe vera, herbal preparations) that the patient uses: |  |  |  |  |
| A. Over-the-counter liquid preparations to remove corns | ___ | ___ | ___ | _____ |
| B. Cutting or shaving corns or calluses with razor blade or scissors | ___ | ___ | ___ | _____ |
| C. Use of oval corn pads | ___ | ___ | ___ | _____ |
| D. Application of adhesive tape | ___ | ___ | ___ | _____ |
| 6. Assess the type of footwear worn by the patient: Are socks worn? Are shoes tight or ill fitting? Are garters or knee-high nylons worn? Is footwear clean? | ___ | ___ | ___ | _____ |
| 7. Observe patient's walking gait. Have the patient walk down a hall or in a straight line (if able). | ___ | ___ | ___ | _____ |
| 8. Assist an ambulatory patient to sit in a bedside chair. Help a bedbound patient to a supine position with the head of the bed elevated. Place a disposable bath mat on the floor under the patient's feet, or place a towel on the mattress. | ___ | ___ | ___ | _____ |
| 9. Obtain a physician's order for cutting patient's nails if your employer policy requires it. | ___ | ___ | ___ | _____ |
| 10. Explain the procedure to the patient, including the fact that proper soaking requires several minutes. | ___ | ___ | ___ | _____ |
| 11. Perform hand hygiene. Arrange equipment on an overbed table. | ___ | ___ | ___ | _____ |
| 12. Fill wash basin with warm water. Test water temperature. | ___ | ___ | ___ | _____ |
| 13. Place the basin on the bath mat or towel. | ___ | ___ | ___ | _____ |
| 14. Fill an emesis basin with warm water, and place the basin on paper towels on the overbed table. | ___ | ___ | ___ | _____ |
| 15. Pull the curtain around the bed, or close the room door (if desired). | ___ | ___ | ___ | _____ |
| 16. Inspect all surfaces of the fingers, toes, feet, and nails. Pay particular attention to areas of dryness, inflammation, or cracking. Also inspect areas between toes, heels, and soles of the feet. | ___ | ___ | ___ | _____ |
| 17. Assess the colour and temperature of toes, feet, and fingers. Assess capillary refill. Palpate radial and ulnar pulses of each hand and dorsalis pedis pulses of feet. | ___ | ___ | ___ | _____ |
| 18. Instruct the patient to place his or her fingers in the emesis basin and to place arms in a comfortable position. Assist the patient in placing feet in the wash basin. | ___ | ___ | ___ | _____ |
| 19. Allow the patient's feet and fingernails to soak for 10 to 20 minutes (unless the patient has diabetes). Rewarm the water after 10 minutes. | ___ | ___ | ___ | _____ |
| 20. Clean gently under the fingernails with an orange stick or the wooden end of a cotton-tipped swab while the patient's fingers are immersed. Remove fingers from emesis basin, and dry fingers thoroughly. | ___ | ___ | ___ | _____ |
| 21. Using nail clippers, clip fingernails straight across and even with tops of the fingers. Using a file, shape the nails straight across. If the patient has circulatory problems, do not cut the nail; only file the nail. | ___ | ___ | ___ | _____ |
| 22. Push the patient's cuticles back gently with the orange stick. Thoroughly dry the patient's hands. | ___ | ___ | ___ | _____ |

*Continued*

|   | S | U | NP | Comments |
|---|---|---|---|---|
| 23. Move the overbed table away from the patient. | ___ | ___ | ___ | _____ |
| 24. Put on disposable gloves, and scrub callused areas of the feet with a washcloth, unless contraindicated. | ___ | ___ | ___ | _____ |
| 25. Clean gently under the toenails with the orange stick. Remove the patient's feet from the basin and dry thoroughly, especially between the toes. | ___ | ___ | ___ | _____ |
| 26. Clean and trim toenails, using the procedures described in steps 21 and 22. Do not file the corners of toenails. | ___ | ___ | ___ | _____ |
| 27. Apply lotion to feet (not between the toes) and hands, and assist the patient back to bed and into a comfortable position. | ___ | ___ | ___ | _____ |
| 28. Remove disposable gloves and place in a receptacle. Clean and return equipment and supplies to the proper place. Dispose of soiled linen in a hamper. Perform hand hygiene. | ___ | ___ | ___ | _____ |
| 29. Inspect the patient's nails and surrounding skin surfaces after soaking and nail trimming. | ___ | ___ | ___ | _____ |
| 30. Ask the patient to explain or demonstrate nail care. | ___ | ___ | ___ | _____ |
| 31. Observe patient's walk or gait after toenail care. | ___ | ___ | ___ | _____ |
| 32. Document the procedure and any observations (e.g., breaks in the skin, inflammation, ulcerations) on the patient's record sheets using the forms provided by your employer or facility. | ___ | ___ | ___ | _____ |
| 33. Report any breaks in the skin or ulcerations to the person in charge or the physician. These breaks are serious in patients with diabetes, peripheral vascular disease, and illnesses that impair circulation. Special foot care treatments may be needed. | ___ | ___ | ___ | _____ |

STUDENT: _____  DATE: _____

INSTRUCTOR: _____  DATE: _____

## Skill Performance Checklist
## Skill 37-3 Providing Oral Hygiene

|  | S | U | NP | Comments |
|---|---|---|---|---|
| 1. Determine the patient's oral hygiene practices: |  |  |  |  |
| A. Frequency of tooth brushing and flossing | — | — | — | _____ |
| B. Type of toothpaste or dentifrice used | — | — | — | _____ |
| C. Last dental visit | — | — | — | _____ |
| D. Frequency of dental visits | — | — | — | _____ |
| E. Type of mouthwash or moistening preparation such as over-the-counter saliva substitutes or sugar-free gum with xylitol | — | — | — | _____ |
| 2. Assess the risk for oral hygiene problems. | — | — | — | _____ |
| 3. Assess the patient's risk for aspiration: impaired swallowing, reduced gag reflex. | — | — | — | _____ |
| 4. Assess the patient's ability to grasp and manipulate a toothbrush. (For older adults, try a 30-second tooth brushing assessment.) | — | — | — | _____ |
| 5. Prepare equipment at the bedside. | — | — | — | _____ |
| 6. Perform hand hygiene, and put on disposable gloves. | — | — | — | _____ |
| 7. Inspect integrity of the lips, teeth, buccal mucosa, gums, palate, and tongue. | — | — | — | _____ |
| 8. Identify the presence of common oral problems: |  |  |  |  |
| A. Dental caries—chalky white discoloration of a tooth or the presence of brown or black discoloration | — | — | — | _____ |
| B. Gingivitis—inflammation of gums | — | — | — | _____ |
| C. Periodontitis—receding gum lines, inflammation, gaps between teeth | — | — | — | _____ |
| D. Halitosis—bad breath | — | — | — | _____ |
| E. Cheilosis—cracking of the lips | — | — | — | _____ |
| F. Stomatitis—inflammation of the mouth | — | — | — | _____ |
| G. Dry, cracked, coated tongue | — | — | — | _____ |
| 9. Explain the procedure to the patient, and discuss preferences regarding the use of hygienic aids. | — | — | — | _____ |
| 10. Raise the bed to a comfortable working position. Raise the head of the bed (if allowed) and lower the side rail. Move the patient, or help the patient move closer. A side-lying position can be used. | — | — | — | _____ |
| 11. Place paper towels on overbed table, and arrange other necessary equipment within easy reach. | — | — | — | _____ |
| 12. Place a towel over the patient's chest. | — | — | — | _____ |
| 13. Apply toothpaste to the toothbrush while holding the brush over the emesis basin. Pour a small amount of water over toothpaste. | — | — | — | _____ |
| 14. Patient may assist by brushing. Hold (or have patient hold if able to) the toothbrush bristles at a 45-degree angle to the gum line. Be sure tips of bristles rest against and penetrate under gum line. Brush inner and outer surfaces of upper and lower teeth by brushing from gum to crown of each tooth. Clean the biting surfaces of teeth by holding the top of the bristles parallel with teeth and brushing gently back and forth. Brush sides of the teeth by moving bristles back and forth. | — | — | — | _____ |
| 15. Have the patient hold the brush at a 45-degree angle and lightly brush over the surface and sides of the tongue. Avoid initiating gag reflex. | — | — | — | _____ |
| 16. Allow the patient to rinse the mouth thoroughly by taking several sips of water, swishing water across all tooth surfaces, and spitting into the emesis basin. | — | — | — | _____ |
| 17. Allow the patient to gargle and rinse the mouth with mouthwash as desired. | — | — | — | _____ |
| 18. Assist in wiping the patient's mouth. | — | — | — | _____ |
| 19. Allow the patient to floss, or assist patient with flossing. | — | — | — | _____ |
| 20. Allow the patient to rinse the mouth thoroughly with cool water and spit into the emesis basin. Assist in wiping patient's mouth. | — | — | — | _____ |
| 21. Ask the patient whether any area of the oral cavity feels uncomfortable or irritated. Inspect the oral cavity. | — | — | — | _____ |

*Continued*

406

|  | S | U | NP | Comments |
|---|---|---|---|---|

22. Assist the patient to a comfortable position, remove the emesis basin and bedside table, raise the side rail (if used), and lower the bed to the original position. ____ ____ ____ _____

23. Wipe off overbed table. Discard soiled linens and paper towels in appropriate containers. Remove and dispose of soiled gloves. Return equipment to the proper place. ____ ____ ____ _____

24. Remove gloves, and perform hand hygiene. ____ ____ ____ _____

25. Ask the patient to describe proper hygiene techniques. ____ ____ ____ _____

26. Record all procedures on a flow sheet provided by your employer or facility. Note the condition of the oral cavity in the patient care notes. ____ ____ ____ _____

27. Report any bleeding or the presence of lesions to the person in charge or the physician. ____ ____ ____ _____

STUDENT: _____ DATE: _____

INSTRUCTOR: _____ DATE: _____

## Skill Performance Checklist
## Skill 37-4 Performing Mouth Care for an Unconscious or Debilitated Patient

| | S | U | NP | Comments |
|---|---|---|---|---|
| 1. Assess the patient's risk for oral hygiene problems. | ___ | ___ | ___ | _____ |
| 2. Explain the procedure to the patient. | ___ | ___ | ___ | _____ |
| 3. Test for the presence of a gag reflex by placing a tongue blade on the back half of the patient's tongue. | ___ | ___ | ___ | _____ |
| 4. Raise the bed to the appropriate working height; lower the head of bed (if patient's condition permits) and then lower the side rail. | ___ | ___ | ___ | _____ |
| 5. Pull the curtain around the bed, or close the room door. | ___ | ___ | ___ | _____ |
| 6. Perform hand hygiene, and put on disposable gloves. | ___ | ___ | ___ | _____ |
| 7. Place paper towels on an overbed table and arrange equipment. If needed, turn on a suction machine and connect tubing to the suction catheter. | ___ | ___ | ___ | _____ |
| 8. Position the patient on the side (Sims' position), close to the side of the bed. Turn the patient's head toward the dependent side. Move patient close to side of the bed. Raise the side rail. | ___ | ___ | ___ | _____ |
| 9. Place a towel under the patient's head, and place an emesis basin under the chin. | ___ | ___ | ___ | _____ |
| 10. Carefully separate upper and lower teeth with padded tongue blade by inserting the blade, quickly but gently, between the back molars. Do not use your fingers. Insert blade when patient is relaxed, if possible. Do not use force. | ___ | ___ | ___ | _____ |
| 11. Inspect the condition of the oral cavity. | ___ | ___ | ___ | _____ |
| 12. Clean the mouth, using a toothbrush or sponge Toothette swabs moistened with a chlorhexidine solution (if patient can tolerate it); otherwise, moisten with water. Clean chewing and inner and outer tooth surfaces. Swab the roof of the mouth, gums, insides of cheeks, and tongue, but avoid stimulating the gag reflex (if present). Moisten a clean swab or a Toothette swab with water to rinse. (A bulb syringe can also be used to rinse.) Repeat rinse several times. | ___ | ___ | ___ | _____ |
| 13. Suction secretions as they accumulate, if necessary. | | | | |
| 14. Apply a thin layer of water-soluble jelly to the lips. | ___ | ___ | ___ | _____ |
| 15. Inform the patient that the procedure is completed. | ___ | ___ | ___ | _____ |
| 16. Put on clean gloves, and inspect the oral cavity. | ___ | ___ | ___ | _____ |
| 17. Ask the debilitated patient whether his or her mouth feels clean. | ___ | ___ | ___ | _____ |
| 18. Reposition patient comfortably, raise the side rail as appropriate or as ordered, and return the bed to the original position. | ___ | ___ | ___ | _____ |
| 19. Clean equipment, and return it to the proper place. Place soiled linen in the proper receptacle. | ___ | ___ | ___ | _____ |
| 20. Remove and discard gloves. Perform hand hygiene. | ___ | ___ | ___ | _____ |
| 21. Assess the patient's respirations on an ongoing basis. | ___ | ___ | ___ | _____ |
| 22. Record the procedure, including pertinent observations (e.g., the presence of bleeding gums, dry mucosa, ulcerations, or crusts on the tongue). | ___ | ___ | ___ | _____ |
| 23. Report any unusual findings to the person in charge or the physician. | ___ | ___ | ___ | _____ |

STUDENT: _____  DATE: _____

INSTRUCTOR: _____  DATE: _____

## Skill Performance Checklist
## Skill 37-5 Making an Occupied Bed

| | S | U | NP | Comments |
|---|---|---|---|---|
| 1. Assess the potential for patient incontinence or for excess drainage on bed linen. | ___ | ___ | ___ | _____ |
| 2. Check the chart for orders or specific precautions concerning movement and positioning. | ___ | ___ | ___ | _____ |
| 3. Explain the procedure to the patient, noting that he or she will be asked to turn on the side and to roll over linen. | ___ | ___ | ___ | _____ |
| 4. Perform hand hygiene, and put on gloves. (Gloves are worn only if linen is soiled or if contact with body secretions is possible.) | ___ | ___ | ___ | _____ |
| 5. Assemble equipment, and arrange it on a bedside chair or table. Remove unnecessary equipment such as a dietary tray or items used for hygiene. | ___ | ___ | ___ | _____ |
| 6. Draw the room curtain around the bed, or close the room door. | ___ | ___ | ___ | _____ |
| 7. Adjust the bed height to a comfortable working position. Lower any raised side rail on one side of the bed. Remove the call light. | ___ | ___ | ___ | _____ |
| 8. Loosen top linen at the foot of the bed. | ___ | ___ | ___ | _____ |
| 9. Remove bedspread and blanket separately. If they are soiled, place them in a soiled linen bag. Do not allow soiled linen to contact uniform. Do not fan or shake linen. | ___ | ___ | ___ | _____ |
| 10. If the blanket and bedspread are to be reused, fold them by bringing the top and bottom edges together. Fold the farthest side over onto the nearer bottom edge. Bring top and bottom edges together again. Place folded linen over the back of a chair. | ___ | ___ | ___ | _____ |
| 11. Cover the patient with a bath blanket in the following manner: Unfold the bath blanket over the top sheet. Ask the patient to hold the top edge of the bath blanket. If the patient is unable to help, tuck the top of the bath blanket under the patient's shoulder. Grasp the top sheet under the bath blanket at the patient's shoulders, and bring the sheet down to the foot of the bed. Remove the sheet, and discard it in a linen bag. | ___ | ___ | ___ | _____ |
| 12. With assistance from another person, slide the mattress toward the head of the bed. | ___ | ___ | ___ | _____ |
| 13. Position the patient on the far side of the bed, turned onto his or her side and facing away from you. Be sure the side rail in front of the patient is up. Adjust the pillow under the patient's head. | ___ | ___ | ___ | _____ |
| 14. Loosen bottom bed linens, moving from head to foot of the bed. With seam side down (facing the mattress), fan-fold bottom sheet and drawsheet toward patient—first drawsheet, then bottom sheet. Tuck edges of linen just under buttocks, back, and shoulders. Do not fan-fold the mattress pad if it is to be reused. | ___ | ___ | ___ | _____ |
| 15. Wipe off any moisture on the exposed mattress with a towel and appropriate disinfectant. | ___ | ___ | ___ | _____ |
| 16. Put clean linen on the exposed half of the bed: | | | | |
| A. Place a clean mattress pad on the bed by folding it lengthwise with centre crease in the middle of the bed. Fan-fold the top layer over the mattress. (If pad part is reused, simply smooth out any wrinkles.) | ___ | ___ | ___ | _____ |
| B. Unfold bottom sheet lengthwise so that centre crease is situated lengthwise along the centre of the bed. Fan-fold the sheet's top layer toward the centre of the bed alongside the patient. Smooth the bottom layer of the sheet over the closest side of the mattress. Pull the fitted sheet smoothly over mattress ends. Allow the edge of the flat unfitted sheet to hang about 25 cm over the mattress edge. The lower hem of the bottom flat sheet should lie seam down and even with the bottom edge of the mattress. | ___ | ___ | ___ | _____ |

*Continued*

|  | S | U | NP | Comments |
|---|---|---|---|---|

17. Mitre the bottom flat sheet at the head of the bed:
    A. Face the head of the bed diagonally. Place your hand away from the head of the bed under the top corner of the mattress, near the mattress edge, and lift. ___ ___ ___ _____
    B. With your other hand, tuck the top edge of the bottom sheet smoothly under the mattress so that side edges of the sheet above and below the mattress would meet if brought together. ___ ___ ___ _____
    C. Face the side of the bed, and pick up the top edge of the sheet approximately 45 cm from top of mattress. ___ ___ ___ _____
    D. Lift the sheet, and lay it on top of the mattress to form a neat triangular fold, with the lower base of the triangle even with the mattress side edge. ___ ___ ___ _____
    E. Tuck the lower edge of the sheet, which is hanging free below the mattress, under the mattress. Tuck with your palms down, without pulling triangular fold. ___ ___ ___ _____
    F. Hold the portion of the sheet covering the side of mattress in place with one hand. With the other hand, pick up the top of triangular linen fold and bring it down over the side of the mattress. Tuck this portion under the mattress. ___ ___ ___ _____
18. Tuck the remaining portion of the sheet under the mattress, moving toward the foot of the bed. Keep the linen smooth. ___ ___ ___ _____
19. *(Optional)* Open drawsheet so that it unfolds in half. Lay centre fold along the middle of the bed lengthwise, and position the sheet so that it will be under the patient's buttocks and torso. Fan-fold the top layer toward the patient, with the edge along the patient's back. Smooth the bottom layer out over the mattress, and tuck the excess edge under the mattress (keep your palms down). ___ ___ ___ _____
20. Place waterproof pad over drawsheet, with centre fold against the patient's side. Fan-fold the top layer toward the patient. ___ ___ ___ _____
21. Have the patient roll slowly toward you, over the layers of linen. Raise the side rail on the working side of the bed, and go to the other side of the bed. ___ ___ ___ _____
22. Lower the side rail. Assist the patient in positioning on the other side, over the folds of linen. Loosen the edges of soiled linen from under the mattress. ___ ___ ___ _____
23. Remove soiled linen by folding it into a bundle or square, with soiled side turned in. Discard in a linen bag. If necessary, wipe the mattress with antiseptic solution, and dry the mattress surface before putting on new linen. ___ ___ ___ _____
24. Pull clean, fan-folded linen smoothly over the edge of the mattress from head to foot of the bed. ___ ___ ___ _____
25. Assist the patient in rolling back into the supine position. Reposition pillow. ___ ___ ___ _____
26. Pull the fitted sheet smoothly over the mattress ends. Mitre the top corner of the bottom sheet. When tucking the corner, be sure the sheet is smooth and free of wrinkles. ___ ___ ___ _____
27. Facing the side of the bed, grasp the remaining edge of the bottom flat sheet. Lean back; keeping your back straight, pull while tucking excess linen under the mattress. Proceed from head to foot of the bed. (Avoid lifting the mattress during tucking to ensure fit.) ___ ___ ___ _____
28. Smooth out the fan-folded drawsheet or waterproof pad over the bottom sheet. Grasp the edge of the sheet with your palms down, lean back, and tuck the sheet under the mattress. Tuck from middle to top and then to bottom. ___ ___ ___ _____
29. Place the top sheet over the patient with centre fold lengthwise down the middle of the bed. Open the sheet from head to foot, and unfold it over the patient. ___ ___ ___ _____
30. Ask the patient to hold the clean top sheet, or tuck the sheet around the patient's shoulders. Remove the bath blanket and discard in the linen bag. ___ ___ ___ _____
31. Place a blanket on the bed, unfolding it so that the crease runs lengthwise along the middle of the bed. Unfold the blanket to cover the patient. The top edge should be parallel with the edge of the top sheet and 15 to 20 cm from the top sheet's edge. ___ ___ ___ _____

*Continued*

|  | S | U | NP | Comments |
|---|---|---|---|---|

32. Place the bedspread over the bed according to step 31. Be sure that the top edge of the bedspread extends about 2.5 cm above the blanket's edge. Tuck the top edge of the bedspread over and under the top edge of the blanket.

33. Make a cuff by turning the edge of the top sheet down over the edge of the blanket and bedspread.

34. Standing on one side at the foot of the bed, lift the mattress corner slightly with one hand and tuck top linens under the mattress. Tuck the top sheet and blanket under together. Be sure that linens are loose enough to allow movement of the patient's feet. Making a horizontal toe pleat is an option.

35. Make a modified mitred corner with the top sheet, blanket, and bedspread:
    A. Pick up the side edge of the top sheet, blanket, and bedspread approximately 45 cm from the foot of the mattress. Lift the linen to form a triangular fold, and lay it on the bed.
    B. Pick up the lower edge of the sheet, which is hanging free below the mattress, and tuck it under the mattress. Do not pull the triangular fold.
    C. Pick up the triangular fold, and bring it down over the mattress while holding the linen in place along the side of the mattress. Do not tuck the tip of the triangle.

36. Raise the side rail. Make the other side of the bed; spread out sheet, blanket, and bedspread evenly. Fold the top edge of bedspread over the blanket, and make cuff with top sheet (see step 33). Make a modified mitred corner at foot of bed (see step 35).

37. Change pillowcase, and fit pillow corners evenly in corners of pillowcase.
    A. Have the patient raise his or her head. While supporting the patient's neck with one hand, remove the pillow. Allow the patient to lower the head.
    B. Remove soiled pillowcase by grasping the pillow at the open end with one hand and pulling the case back over the pillow with the other hand. Discard the case in the linen bag.
    C. Grasp the clean pillowcase at the centre of the closed end. Gather the case, turning it inside out of the hand holding it. With the same hand, pick up the middle of one end of the pillow. Pull the pillowcase down over the pillow with the other hand.
    D. Be sure pillow corners fit evenly into the corners of the pillowcase. Place the pillow under the patient's head.

38. Place the call bell within the patient's reach, and return the bed to a comfortable position.

39. Open the room curtains, and rearrange furniture. Place personal items within the patient's easy reach on the overbed table or bedside stand. Return the bed to a comfortable height.

40. Discard dirty linen in a hamper or chute, remove your gloves, and perform hand hygiene.

41. Ask whether the patient feels comfortable.

42. While you are performing this skill, inspect the patient's skin for areas of irritation.

43. Observe the patient for signs of fatigue, dyspnea, pain, or discomfort throughout the skill.

STUDENT: _____   DATE: _____

INSTRUCTOR: _____   DATE: _____

## Skill Performance Checklist
## Skill 38-1 Suctioning

| | S | U | NP | Comments |
|---|---|---|---|---|
| 1. Assess for signs and symptoms of upper and lower airway obstruction necessitating nasotracheal or orotracheal suctioning; abnormal respiratory rate; adventitious sounds; nasal secretions, gurgling, drooling; restlessness; gastric secretions or vomitus in the mouth; and coughing without clearing secretions from the airway. | — | — | — | _____ |
| 2. Assess for signs and symptoms associated with hypoxia and hypercapnia: decreased $SpO_2$, increased pulse and blood pressure, increased respiratory rate, apprehension, anxiety, decreased ability to concentrate, lethargy, decreased level of consciousness (especially acute), increased fatigue, dizziness, behavioural changes (especially irritability), dysrhythmias, pallor, and cyanosis. | — | — | — | _____ |
| 3. Determine factors that normally influence upper or lower airway functioning: fluid status; lack of humidity; pulmonary disease, chronic obstructive pulmonary disorder, and pulmonary infection; anatomy; changes in level of consciousness; and decreased cough or gag reflex, allergies, sinus drainage. | — | — | — | _____ |
| 4. Identify contraindications to nasotracheal suctioning: occluded nasal passages; nasal bleeding, epiglottitis, or croup; acute head, facial, or neck injury or surgery, coagulopathy, or bleeding disorder; irritable airway or laryngospasm or bronchospasm; gastric surgery with high anastomosis; or myocardial infarction. | — | — | — | _____ |
| 5. Examine sputum microbiology data. | — | — | — | _____ |
| 6. Assess the patient's understanding of the procedure. | — | — | — | _____ |
| 7. Obtain a physician's order if indicated by employer policy. | — | — | — | _____ |
| 8. Explain to the patient how the procedure will help clear the airway and relieve breathing problems and that temporary coughing, sneezing, gagging, or shortness of breath is normal. Encourage the patient to cough out secretions. Have the patient practise coughing, if able. Splint surgical incisions, if necessary. | — | — | — | _____ |
| 9. Explain the importance of coughing, and encourage coughing during the procedure. | — | — | — | _____ |
| 10. Help the patient to assume a position comfortable for you and the patient (usually semi-Fowler's or sitting upright with head hyperextended, unless contraindicated). | — | — | — | _____ |
| 11. Place a pulse oximeter on the patient's finger. Take a reading, and leave the pulse oximeter in place. | — | — | — | _____ |
| 12. Place a towel across the patient's chest. | — | — | — | _____ |
| 13. Perform hand hygiene. Apply mask, goggles, or face shield if splashing is likely. | — | — | — | _____ |
| 14. Connect one end of the connecting tubing to the suction machine, and place the other end in a convenient location near the patient. Turn on the suction device, and set the vacuum regulator to appropriate negative pressure (pressure may vary; refer to employer policy). | — | — | — | _____ |
| 15. If indicated, increase supplemental oxygen therapy to 100% or as ordered by the physician. Encourage the patient to breathe deeply. | — | — | — | _____ |
| 16. Preparation for all types of suctioning:<br>A. Open the suction kit or catheter, using aseptic technique. If a sterile drape is available, place it across the patient's chest or on the overbed table. Do not allow the suction catheter to touch any nonsterile surfaces. | — | — | — | _____ |
| B. Unwrap or open a sterile basin, and place it on the bedside table. Fill it with about 100 mL of sterile normal saline (NS) solution or water. | — | — | — | _____ |
| C. Turn on suction device. Set regulator to appropriate negative pressure: 100 to 150 mm Hg for adults. | — | — | — | _____ |

*Continued*

414

| | S | U | NP | Comments |
|---|---|---|---|---|

17. Suction airway.
   A. Oropharyngeal suctioning:
      (1) Put on clean disposable gloves. Put on mask or face shield.     ___ ___ ___ _____
      (2) Attach the suction catheter to connecting tubing. Check that equipment is functioning properly by suctioning a small amount of water or NS from the basin.     ___ ___ ___ _____
      (3) Remove oxygen mask, if present. Keep the oxygen mask near the patient's face. A nasal cannula may remain in place (if present).     ___ ___ ___ _____
      (4) Insert the catheter into the patient's mouth. With suction applied, move the catheter around the mouth, including pharynx and gum line, until secretions are cleared.     ___ ___ ___ _____
      (5) Encourage the patient to cough, and repeat suctioning if needed. Replace oxygen mask, if used.     ___ ___ ___ _____
      (6) Suction water from the basin through the catheter until the catheter is cleared of secretions.     ___ ___ ___ _____
      (7) Place the catheter in a clean, dry area for reuse.     ___ ___ ___ _____
   B. Nasopharyngeal and nasotracheal suctioning:
      (1) Open the lubricant. Squeeze a small amount onto the open sterile catheter package.     ___ ___ ___ _____
      (2) Put a sterile glove on each hand, or put a nonsterile glove on your nondominant hand and a sterile glove on your dominant hand.     ___ ___ ___ _____
      (3) Pick up the suction catheter with your dominant hand without touching nonsterile surfaces. Pick up connecting tubing with your nondominant hand. Secure the catheter to the tubing.     ___ ___ ___ _____
      (4) Check that the equipment is functioning properly by suctioning a small amount of NS solution from the basin.     ___ ___ ___ _____
      (5) Lightly coat the distal 6 to 8 cm of the catheter with water-soluble lubricant.     ___ ___ ___ _____
      (6) Remove the oxygen delivery device, if applicable, with your nondominant hand. Without applying suction and using your dominant thumb and forefinger, gently insert the catheter into the patient's naris during inhalation.     ___ ___ ___ _____
      (7) *Nasopharyngeal*: Follow the natural course of the naris; slightly slant the catheter downward and advance to the back of the pharynx. In adults, insert the catheter about 16 cm; in older children, 8 to 12 cm; in infants and young children, 4 to 8 cm. The rule of thumb is to insert the catheter a distance from the tip of the nose (or mouth) to angle of the mandible.     ___ ___ ___ _____
         (a) Apply intermittent suction for up to 10 to 15 seconds by placing and releasing your nondominant thumb over the catheter vent. Slowly withdraw the catheter while rotating it back and forth between your thumb and forefinger.     ___ ___ ___ _____
      (8) *Nasotracheal*: Follow the natural course of the naris, and advance the catheter slightly slanted and downward to just above the entrance into the trachea. Allow the patient to take a breath. Quickly insert catheter approximately 20 cm (in adult) into the trachea. The patient will begin to cough. *Note*: In older children, advance 16 to 20 cm; in young children and infants, 8 to 14 cm.     ___ ___ ___ _____
         (a) *Positioning option for nasotracheal suctioning*: In some instances, turning the patient's head to the right helps you suction the left mainstem bronchus; turning the head to the left helps you suction the right mainstem bronchus. If resistance is felt after insertion of the catheter for the maximum recommended distance, the catheter has probably hit the carina. Pull the catheter back 1 to 2 cm before applying suction.     ___ ___ ___ _____
         (b) Apply intermittent suction for up to 10 to 15 seconds by placing and releasing your nondominant thumb over the vent of the catheter and slowly withdrawing the catheter while rotating it back and forth between your dominant thumb and forefinger. Encourage the patient to cough. Replace the oxygen device, if applicable.     ___ ___ ___ _____
      (9) Rinse the catheter and connecting tubing with NS or water until cleared.     ___ ___ ___ _____

*Continued*

|  | S | U | NP | Comments |
|---|---|---|---|---|

(10) Assess for need to repeat the suctioning procedure. Allow adequate time (at least one minute) between suction passes for ventilation and oxygenation. Ask the patient to breathe deeply and cough.

C. Artificial-airway suctioning:

    (1) Put on face shield.

    (2) Put one sterile glove on each hand, or put a nonsterile glove on your nondominant hand and a sterile glove on your dominant hand.

    (3) Pick up the suction catheter with your dominant hand without touching nonsterile surfaces. Pick up the connecting tubing with your nondominant hand. Secure the catheter to the tubing.

    (4) Check that equipment is functioning properly by suctioning a small amount of saline from the basin.

    (5) Hyperinflate or hyperoxygenate the patient, or do both, before suctioning, using manual resuscitation bag-valve device connected to the oxygen source on the mechanical ventilator. Some mechanical ventilators have a button that, when pushed, delivers oxygen for a few minutes and then resets to the previous value.

    (6) If the patient is receiving mechanical ventilation, open the swivel adapter or, if necessary, remove the oxygen or humidity delivery device with your nondominant hand.

    (7) Without applying suction, gently but quickly insert the catheter, using your dominant thumb and forefinger, into the artificial airway (it is best to time catheter insertion with inspiration) until resistance is met or the patient coughs; then pull back 1 cm.

    (8) Apply intermittent suction by placing and releasing your nondominant thumb over the vent of the catheter; slowly withdraw the catheter while rotating it back and forth between your dominant thumb and forefinger. Encourage the patient to cough. Watch for respiratory distress.

    (9) If the patient is receiving mechanical ventilation, close the swivel adapter or replace the oxygen delivery device.

    (10) Encourage the patient to breathe deeply, if able. Some patients respond well to several manual breaths from the mechanical ventilator or bag-valve device.

    (11) Rinse the catheter and connecting tubing with NS until clear. Use continuous suction.

    (12) Assess the patient's cardiopulmonary status. Repeat steps 17C (5) through 17C (11) (see illustration in text, page 910) once or twice more to clear secretions. Allow adequate time (at least one full minute) between suction passes for ventilation and reoxygenation. Perform oropharyngeal and nasopharyngeal suctioning (steps 17A and 17B in text illustration, page 910). Do not suction nose again after suctioning mouth.

18. Complete the procedure:

    A. Disconnect the catheter from the connecting tubing. Roll the catheter around the fingers of your dominant hand. Pull the glove off inside out so that the catheter remains in the glove. Pull off the other glove over the first glove in the same way to contain contaminants. Discard gloves into an appropriate receptacle. Turn off the suction device.

    B. Remove the towel or drape, and discard it in an appropriate receptacle.

    C. Reposition the patient as indicated by the condition. Put on clean gloves for the patient's personal care (e.g., oral hygiene).

    D. If indicated, readjust oxygen supply to the original level.

    E. Discard the remainder of NS into an appropriate receptacle. If the basin is disposable, discard into an appropriate receptacle. If the basin is reusable, rinse and place in soiled utility room.

    F. Remove and discard the face shield, and perform hand hygiene.

    G. Place an unopened suction kit on the suction machine table or at the head of bed, according to institution preference.

19. Compare the patient's vital signs and $SpO_2$ saturation before and after suctioning.

20. Ask the patient whether breathing is easier and whether congestion is decreased.

21. Observe airway secretions.

22. Record the amount, consistency, colour, and odour of secretions, and patient's response to procedure; document patient's pre-suctioning and post-suctioning cardiopulmonary status.

STUDENT: _____ DATE: _____

INSTRUCTOR: _____ DATE: _____

## Skill Performance Checklist
## Skill 38-2 Care of an Artificial Airway

| | S | U | NP | Comments |
|---|---|---|---|---|
| 1. Perform cardiopulmonary assessment: | | | | |
| A. Auscultate lung sounds. | — | — | — | _____ |
| B. Assess condition and patency of airway and surrounding tissues. | — | — | — | _____ |
| C. Note type and size of tube, movement of tube, and cuff size. | — | — | — | _____ |
| 2. Explain the procedure to the patient and family. | — | — | — | _____ |
| 3. Position the patient—usually supine or semi-Fowler's. | — | — | — | _____ |
| 4. Place a towel across the patient's chest. | — | — | — | _____ |
| 5. Perform hand hygiene. Apply mask, goggles, or face shield (if indicated). | — | — | — | _____ |
| 6. Perform airway care: | | | | |
| A. Endotracheal (ET) tube care: | | | | |
| (1) Observe for signs and symptoms of the need to perform care of the artificial airway: | | | | |
| (a) Soiled or loose tape | — | — | — | _____ |
| (b) Pressure sores on nares, lip, or corner of mouth | — | — | — | _____ |
| (c) Unstable tube | — | — | — | _____ |
| (d) Excessive secretions | — | — | — | _____ |
| (2) Identify factors that increase risk of complications from ET tubes: | | | | |
| (a) Type and size of tube | — | — | — | _____ |
| (b) Movement of tube up and down trachea | — | — | — | _____ |
| (c) Cuff size | — | — | — | _____ |
| (d) Duration of placement | — | — | — | _____ |
| (3) Determine proper ET tube depth as noted by number of centimetres at lip or gum line. This line is marked on the tube and recorded in the patient's record at time of intubation. | — | — | — | _____ |
| (4) Suction ET tube: | — | — | — | _____ |
| (a) Instruct the patient not to bite or move the ET tube with the tongue or pull on tubing; removal of tape can be uncomfortable. | — | — | — | _____ |
| (b) Leave the Yankauer suction catheter connected to the suction source. | — | — | — | _____ |
| (5) Prepare method to secure the ET tube (check employer policy): | | | | |
| (a) *Tape method*: Cut a piece of tape long enough to go completely around the patient's head, from naris to naris, plus 15 cm (for an adult, about 30 to 60 cm). Lay adhesive side up on the bedside table. Cut and lay 8 to 16 cm of tape, adhesive side down, in the centre of the long strip to prevent the tape from sticking to the patient's hair. | — | — | — | _____ |
| (b) *Commercially available ET tube holder*: Open the package per manufacturer's instructions. Set the device aside with the head guard in place and the Velcro strips open. | — | — | — | _____ |
| (6) Put on clean gloves, and instruct an assistant to apply gloves and hold the ET tube firmly at the patient's lips. Note the number marking on the ET tube at the gum line. | — | — | — | _____ |
| (7) Remove old tape or device: | | | | |
| (a) *Tape*: Carefully remove tape from the ET tube and the patient's face. If the tape is difficult to remove, moisten it with a soapy wet washcloth, water, or adhesive tape remover. Discard tape in an appropriate receptacle if nearby. If not, place soiled tape on the bedside table or on the distant end of the towel. | — | — | — | _____ |
| (b) *Commercially available device*: Remove Velcro strips from the ET tube, and remove the ET tube holder from the patient. | — | — | — | _____ |
| (8) Use adhesive remover swab to remove excess secretions or adhesive left on the patient's face. Wash adhesive remover from face. | — | — | — | _____ |
| (9) Remove oral airway or bite block, if present. | — | — | — | _____ |

*Continued*

|  | S | U | NP | Comments |
|---|---|---|---|---|

(10) Clean the mouth, gums, and teeth opposite the ET tube with non-alcoholic-based mouthwash solution and toothpaste on toothbrush or Toothette. Brush teeth as indicated. If necessary, administer oropharyngeal suctioning with a Yankauer catheter.

(11) Note "cm" ET tube marking at the lips or gums. With the help of the assistant, move the ET tube to the opposite side or centre of the mouth. Do not change tube depth.

(12) Repeat oral cleaning on the opposite side of the mouth.

(13) Clean the face and neck with a soapy washcloth; rinse and dry. Shave a male patient as necessary.

(14) Use a small amount of skin protectant or liquid adhesive on a clean 2 × 2 gauze, and dot on the upper lip (with oral ET tube) or across the nose (with nasal ET tube) and from cheeks to ear. Allow to dry completely.

(15) Secure ET tube.
 (a) Tube method:
  (a1) Slip tape under the patient's head and neck, adhesive side up. Do not twist the tape or catch hair. Do not allow tape to stick to itself. It helps to stick tape gently to the tongue blade, which serves as a guide as the tape is passed behind the patient's head. Centre tape so that double-faced tape extends around the back of the neck from ear to ear.
  (a2) On one side of the patient's face, secure tape from ear to naris (with nasal ET tube) or to the edge of the mouth (with oral ET tube). Tear remaining tape in half lengthwise, forming two pieces that are 1 to 2 cm wide. Secure the bottom half of the tape across the upper lip (with oral ET tube) or across the top of the nose (with nasal ET tube). Wrap the top half of tape around the tube. Tape should encircle tube at least two times for security.
  (a3) Gently pull the other side of tape firmly to pick up slack, and secure to the remaining side of the face. Have the assistant release hold when the tube is secure. You may want the assistant to help reinsert the oral airway.
 (b) Commercially available device:
  (b1) Place the ET tube through the opening designed to secure the ET tube. Ensure that the pilot balloon to the ET tube is accessible.
  (b2) Place the Velcro strips of the ET holder under the patient at the occipital region of the head.
  (b3) Verify that the ET tube is at the established position, using the lip or gum line as a guide.
  (b4) Secure the Velcro strips at the base of the patient's head. Leave 1 cm slack in the strips.
  (b5) Verify that the tube is secure and that it does not move forward from the patient's mouth or backward down into the patient's throat. Ensure that there are no pressure areas on the oral mucosa or occipital region of the head.

(16) Clean the oral airway in warm, soapy water, and rinse well. A solution of half hydrogen peroxide and half NS aids in removal of crusted secretions. A mouthwash rinse will freshen patient's mouth. Shake excess water from oral airway. Be sure to rinse hydrogen peroxide mixture from airway.

(17) For an unconscious patient, reinsert the oral airway without pushing the tongue into the oropharynx.

B. Tracheostomy care:
 (1) Observe for signs and symptoms of the need to perform tracheostomy care:
  (a) Soiled or loose ties or dressing
  (b) Nonstable tube
  (c) Excessive secretions

*Continued*

|  | S | U | NP | Comments |
|---|---|---|---|---|

(2) Suction tracheostomy. Before removing gloves, remove soiled tracheostomy dressing and discard in a glove with the coiled catheter.

(3) Prepare equipment.

   (a) Open sterile tracheostomy kit. Open two 4 × 4 gauze packages, using aseptic technique, and pour NS on one package. Leave the second package dry. Open two packages of cotton-tipped swabs, and pour NS on one package. Do not recap NS.

   (b) Open the sterile tracheostomy package.

   (c) Unwrap the sterile basin, and pour approximately 0.5 to 2 cm of normal saline into it.

   (d) Open the small sterile brush package, and place it aseptically into the sterile basin.

   (e) Prepare a length of twill tape long enough to go around the patient's neck two times, approximately 60 to 75 cm for an adult. Cut ends on the diagonal. Lay aside in a dry area.

   (f) If using a commercially available tracheostomy tube holder, open the package according to the manufacturer's directions.

(4) Apply sterile gloves. Keep your dominant hand sterile throughout the procedure.

(5) Hyperoxygenate the patient if the patient has oxygen saturation levels below 92%. Apply the oxygen source loosely over the tracheostomy if the patient desaturates during the procedure.

(6) If a nondisposable inner cannula is used:

   (a) While touching only the outer aspect of the tube, remove the inner cannula with your nondominant hand. Drop the inner cannula into NS basin.

   (b) Place the tracheostomy collar or T tube and ventilator oxygen source over or near the outer cannula. (*Note:* T tube and ventilator oxygen devices cannot be attached to all outer cannulas when the inner cannula is removed.)

   (c) To prevent oxygen desaturation in affected patients, quickly pick up the inner cannula and use a small brush to remove secretions from inside and outside the cannula.

   (d) Hold the inner cannula over the basin, and rinse with NS, using your nondominant hand to pour.

   (e) Replace the inner cannula, and secure the "locking" mechanism. Reapply the ventilator or oxygen sources.

(7) If a disposable inner cannula is used:

   (a) Remove the cannula from the manufacturer's packaging.

   (b) While touching only the outer aspect of the tube, withdraw the inner cannula and replace with the new cannula. Lock into position.

   (c) Dispose of the contaminated cannula in an appropriate receptacle, and apply oxygen source.

(8) Using NS-saturated cotton-tipped swabs and 4 × 4 gauze, clean the exposed outer cannula surfaces and stoma under the faceplate, extending 5 to 10 cm in all directions from the stoma. Clean in a circular motion from the stoma site outward, using your dominant hand to handle sterile supplies.

(9) Using dry 4 × 4 gauze, pat lightly at skin and exposed outer cannula surfaces.

(10) Secure tracheostomy.

   (a) *Tracheostomy tie method*:

      (a1) Instruct assistant, if available, to hold the tracheostomy tube securely in place while ties are cut.

      (a2) Take the prepared tie, insert one end of the tie through the faceplate eyelet, and pull ends even.

      (a3) Slide both ends of the tie behind the patient's head and around the neck to the other eyelet, and insert one tie through the second eyelet.

      (a4) Pull snugly.

      (a5) Tie ends securely in a double square knot, allowing space for only one loose or two snug fingerwidths in tie.

      (a6) Insert fresh tracheostomy dressing under the clean ties and faceplate.

*Continued*

420

| | S | U | NP | Comments |
|---|---|---|---|---|
| (b) *Tracheostomy tube holder method*: | | | | |
| (b1) While wearing gloves, maintain a secure hold on the tracheostomy tube. This can be done with an assistant or, when an assistant is not available, by leaving the old tracheostomy tube holder in place until the new device is secure. | ___ | ___ | ___ | _____ |
| (b2) Align strap under the patient's neck. Ensure that Velcro attachments are positioned on either side of the tracheostomy tube. | ___ | ___ | ___ | _____ |
| (b3) Place the narrow end of ties under and through the faceplate eyelets. Pull the ends even, and secure with Velcro closures. | ___ | ___ | ___ | _____ |
| (b4) Verify that there is space for only one loose or two snug fingerwidths under the neck strap. | ___ | ___ | ___ | _____ |
| 7. Position the patient comfortably, and assess respiratory status. | ___ | ___ | ___ | _____ |
| 8. Replace any oxygen delivery devices. | ___ | ___ | ___ | _____ |
| 9. Remove and discard gloves. Replace the caps on the hydrogen peroxide and NS. Perform hand hygiene. | ___ | ___ | ___ | _____ |
| 10. Compare respiratory assessments made before and after the procedure. | ___ | ___ | ___ | _____ |
| 11. Observe depth and position of tubes. | ___ | ___ | ___ | _____ |
| 12. Assess the security of the tape or commercial ET or ET tube holder by tugging at the tube. | ___ | ___ | ___ | _____ |
| 13. Assess the skin around the mouth and the oral mucosa (with ET tube) and the tracheostomy stoma for drainage, pressure, and signs of irritation. | ___ | ___ | ___ | _____ |
| 14. Record respiratory assessments before and after care. | ___ | ___ | ___ | _____ |
| 15. Record ET tube care: depth of ET tube, frequency and extent of care, patient tolerance, and any complications related to presence of the tube. | ___ | ___ | ___ | _____ |
| 16. Record tracheostomy care: type and size of tracheostomy tube, frequency and extent of care, patient tolerance, and any complications related to presence of the tube. | ___ | ___ | ___ | _____ |

STUDENT: _____    DATE: _____

INSTRUCTOR: _____    DATE: _____

## Skill Performance Checklist
## Skill 38-3 Care of Patients With Chest Tubes

| | S | U | NP | Comments |
|---|---|---|---|---|
| 1. Perform hand hygiene, and assess patient for respiratory distress and chest pain, breath sounds over affected lung area, and vital signs. | ___ | ___ | ___ | _____ |
| A. Pulmonary status: Assess for respiratory distress, chest pain, breath sounds over affected lung area, and stable vital signs. Signs and symptoms of increased respiratory distress or chest pain include decreased breath sounds over the affected and nonaffected lungs, marked cyanosis, asymmetrical chest movements, presence of subcutaneous emphysema around tube insertion site or neck, hypotension, and tachycardia. | ___ | ___ | ___ | _____ |
| B. Measure vital signs and SpO$_2$. | ___ | ___ | ___ | _____ |
| C. Pain: If possible, ask the patient to rate the level of pain on a scale of 0 to 10. | ___ | ___ | ___ | _____ |
| 2. Observe the following: | | | | |
| A. Chest tube dressing and site surrounding tube insertion | ___ | ___ | ___ | _____ |
| B. Tubing, for kinks, dependent loops, or clots | ___ | ___ | ___ | _____ |
| C. Chest drainage system, which should be upright and below level of tube insertion | ___ | ___ | ___ | _____ |
| 3. Provide two shodded hemostats or approved clamps for each chest tube, and attach them to the top of the patient's bed with adhesive tape. Chest tubes are clamped only under specific circumstances per physician order or nursing policy and procedure: | ___ | ___ | ___ | _____ |
| A. To assess air leak | ___ | ___ | ___ | _____ |
| B. To quickly empty or change disposable systems; performed by a nurse who has received education in the procedure | ___ | ___ | ___ | _____ |
| C. To assess whether the patient is ready to have the chest tube removed (which is done by physician's order); the patient is monitored for recurrent pneumothorax | ___ | ___ | ___ | _____ |
| 4. Position patient in one of the following ways: | | | | |
| A. Semi-Fowler's position to evacuate air (pneumothorax) | ___ | ___ | ___ | _____ |
| B. High-Fowler's position to drain fluid (hemothorax, effusion) | ___ | ___ | ___ | _____ |
| 5. Maintain the tube connection between the chest and drainage tubes; ensure that it is intact and taped. Check patency of air vents in system: | ___ | ___ | ___ | _____ |
| A. The water-sealed vent must be without occlusion. | ___ | ___ | ___ | _____ |
| B. The suction-control chamber vent must be without occlusion when suction is used. | ___ | ___ | ___ | _____ |
| C. Confirm that valves are unobstructed. Waterless systems have relief valves without caps. For dry suction systems, the positive pressure relief valve must remain unobstructed. | ___ | ___ | ___ | _____ |
| 6. Avoid excess tubing; the tubing should be laid horizontally across the patient's bed or chair before dropping vertically into the drainage bottle. If the patient is in a chair and the tubing is coiled, lift the tubing every 15 minutes to promote drainage. | ___ | ___ | ___ | _____ |
| 7. Adjust the tubing to hang in a straight line from the top of the mattress to the drainage chamber. If the chest tube is draining fluid, indicate time (e.g., 0900 hours) that drainage began on the drainage bottle's adhesive tape or on the write-on surface of the disposable commercial system. Check institutional policy before stripping or milking chest tubes. | ___ | ___ | ___ | _____ |
| 8. Perform hand hygiene. | ___ | ___ | ___ | _____ |
| 9. Evaluate: | | | | |
| A. Vital signs and pulse oximetry as ordered or if patient's condition changes. | ___ | ___ | ___ | _____ |
| B. Chest tube dressing. | ___ | ___ | ___ | _____ |
| C. Tubing: It should be free of kinks and dependent loops. | ___ | ___ | ___ | _____ |

*Continued*

|  | S | U | NP | Comments |
|---|---|---|---|---|
| D. Chest drainage system: It should be upright and below the level of tube insertion. Note the presence of clots or debris in tubing. | ___ | ___ | ___ | _____ |
| E. Water seal for fluctuations with the patient's inspiration and expiration: | | | | |
| (1) Waterless system: diagnostic indicator for fluctuations with patient's inspirations and expirations | ___ | ___ | ___ | _____ |
| (2) Water-seal system: bubbling in the water-seal chamber | ___ | ___ | ___ | _____ |
| (3) Water-seal system: bubbling in the suction-control chamber (when suction is used) | ___ | ___ | ___ | _____ |
| F. Waterless system: Bubbling is diagnostic indicator. | ___ | ___ | ___ | _____ |
| G. Waterless system: The suction control (float ball) indicates the amount of suction that the patient's intrapleural space is receiving. | ___ | ___ | ___ | _____ |
| H. Type and amount of fluid drainage: Note colour and amount of drainage, patient's vital signs, and skin colour. The normal amount of drainage is as follows: | ___ | ___ | ___ | _____ |
| (1) In the adult: less than 50 to 200 mL/hour immediately after surgery in a mediastinal chest tube; approximately 500 mL in the first 24 hours. | ___ | ___ | ___ | _____ |
| (2) Between 100 and 300 mL of fluid may drain in a pleural chest tube in an adult during the first 3 hours after insertion. You can expect 500 to 1000 mL in the first 24 hours. Drainage is grossly bloody during the first several hours after surgery and then changes to serous. Remember that a sudden gush of drainage may be retained blood and not active bleeding. This increase in drainage can result from patient's position changes. | ___ | ___ | ___ | _____ |
| I. Observe the patient for decreased respiratory distress and chest pain; auscultate lung sounds over the affected area, and monitor $SpO_2$. | ___ | ___ | ___ | _____ |
| J. Pain: Ask the patient to evaluate pain on a level of 0 to 10. | ___ | ___ | ___ | _____ |
| 10. Record in nurse's notes patency of chest; presence, type, and amount of drainage; presence of fluctuations; patient's vital signs; chest dressing status, amount of suction and water seal; and level of comfort. | ___ | ___ | ___ | _____ |

STUDENT: _____   DATE: _____

INSTRUCTOR: _____   DATE: _____

## Skill Performance Checklist
## Skill 38-4 Applying a Nasal Cannula or Oxygen Mask

| | S | U | NP | Comments |
|---|---|---|---|---|
| 1. Inspect the patient for signs and symptoms associated with hypoxia and the presence of airway secretions. | ___ | ___ | ___ | _____ |
| 2. Obtain the patient's most recent $SpO_2$ or arterial blood gas values. Review patient's medical record for the medical order for oxygen, noting delivery method, flow rate, and duration of oxygen therapy. | ___ | ___ | ___ | _____ |
| 3. Explain to the patient and family what the procedure entails and the purpose of oxygen therapy. | ___ | ___ | ___ | _____ |
| 4. Perform hand hygiene. | ___ | ___ | ___ | _____ |
| 5. Attach the oxygen delivery device to the oxygen tubing, and attach the tubing to the humidified oxygen source, adjusted to the prescribed flow rate. | ___ | ___ | ___ | _____ |
| 6. Place tips of the cannula into the patient's nares. Adjust the elastic headband or plastic slide until the cannula fits snugly and comfortably. | ___ | ___ | ___ | _____ |
| 7. Maintain sufficient slack on the oxygen tubing, and secure tubing to the patient's clothes. | ___ | ___ | ___ | _____ |
| 8. Observe for proper function of oxygen delivery device: | | | | |
| A. Nasal cannula: cannula is positioned properly in the nares. | ___ | ___ | ___ | _____ |
| B. Nonrebreathing mask: apply mask over patient's mouth and nose to form a tight seal. The valves on the mask close, so exhaled air does not enter reservoir bag. | ___ | ___ | ___ | _____ |
| C. Partial rebreathing mask: apply mask over patient's mouth and nose to form a tight seal. Ensure that the bag remains partially inflated. | ___ | ___ | ___ | _____ |
| D. Venturi mask: apply mask over patient's mouth and nose to form a tight seal. Select appropriate flow rate. | ___ | ___ | ___ | _____ |
| 9. Check the cannula every eight hours. Keep the humidification jar filled at all times. | ___ | ___ | ___ | _____ |
| 10. Observe the patient's nares and the superior surface of both ears for skin breakdown. | ___ | ___ | ___ | _____ |
| 11. Perform hand hygiene. | ___ | ___ | ___ | _____ |
| 12. Verify oxygen flow rate, proper setup, and physician's orders. | ___ | ___ | ___ | _____ |
| 13. Inspect the patient for relief of symptoms. | ___ | ___ | ___ | _____ |
| 14. Record oxygen delivery device and litre flow in medical record. Document patient and family education. Report oxygen delivery device, litre flow, and response to changes in therapy to oncoming shift. | ___ | ___ | ___ | _____ |

STUDENT: _____  DATE: _____

INSTRUCTOR: _____  DATE: _____

## Skill Performance Checklist
## Skill 38-5 Using Home Oxygen Equipment

|  | S | U | NP | Comments |
|---|---|---|---|---|
| 1. While the patient is in the hospital, determine the patient's and family's ability to use oxygen equipment correctly. In the home setting, reassess for appropriate use of equipment. | ___ | ___ | ___ | _____ |
| 2. Assess the home environment for adequate electrical service if an oxygen concentrator is used. | ___ | ___ | ___ | _____ |
| 3. Assess patient's and family's ability to observe for signs and symptoms of hypoxia. | ___ | ___ | ___ | _____ |
| 4. Determine appropriate resources in the community for equipment and assistance, including maintenance and repair services and the medical equipment supplier. | ___ | ___ | ___ | _____ |
| 5. In case of power failure, determine appropriate backup system when a compressor is used. Have a spare oxygen tank available. | ___ | ___ | ___ | _____ |
| 6. Perform hand hygiene. | ___ | ___ | ___ | _____ |
| 7. Place the oxygen delivery system in a clutter-free environment that is well ventilated; away from walls, drapes, bedding, and combustible materials; and at least 2.5 m from a heat source. | ___ | ___ | ___ | _____ |
| 8. Demonstrate steps for preparation and completion of oxygen therapy. |  |  |  |  |
| A. Compressed oxygen system: |  |  |  |  |
| (1) Turn the cylinder valve counterclockwise two to three turns with the wrench. Store the wrench with the oxygen tank. | ___ | ___ | ___ | _____ |
| (2) Check cylinders by reading the amount on the pressure gauge. | ___ | ___ | ___ | _____ |
| B. Oxygen concentrator system: |  |  |  |  |
| (1) Plug the concentrator into an appropriate outlet. | ___ | ___ | ___ | _____ |
| (2) Turn on the power switch. | ___ | ___ | ___ | _____ |
| (3) Alarm will sound for a few seconds. | ___ | ___ | ___ | _____ |
| C. Liquid oxygen system: |  |  |  |  |
| (1) Check liquid system by depressing the button at the lower right corner and reading the dial on the stationary oxygen reservoir or ambulatory tank. | ___ | ___ | ___ | _____ |
| (2) Collaborate with the medical equipment provider to supply instruction on refilling the ambulatory tank. | ___ | ___ | ___ | _____ |
| (3) Refilling the oxygen tank: |  |  |  |  |
| (a) Wipe both filling connectors with a clean, dry, lint-free cloth. | ___ | ___ | ___ | _____ |
| (b) Turn off the flow selector of the ambulatory unit. | ___ | ___ | ___ | _____ |
| (c) Attach the ambulatory unit to the stationary reservoir by inserting the adapter of the ambulatory tank into the adapter of the stationary reservoir. | ___ | ___ | ___ | _____ |
| (d) Open the fill valve on the ambulatory tank, and apply firm pressure to the top of the stationary reservoir. Stay with the unit while it is filling. You will hear a loud hissing noise. The tank fills in about two minutes. | ___ | ___ | ___ | _____ |
| (e) Disengage the ambulatory unit from the stationary reservoir when the hissing noise changes and a vapour cloud begins to form from the stationary unit. | ___ | ___ | ___ | _____ |
| (f) Wipe both filling connectors with a clean, dry, lint-free cloth. | ___ | ___ | ___ | _____ |
| 9. Connect the oxygen delivery device to the oxygen system. | ___ | ___ | ___ | _____ |
| 10. Adjust to the prescribed flow rate (litres per minute). | ___ | ___ | ___ | _____ |
| 11. Place the oxygen delivery device on the patient. | ___ | ___ | ___ | _____ |
| 12. Perform hand hygiene. | ___ | ___ | ___ | _____ |
| 13. Instruct the patient and family not to change the oxygen flow rate. | ___ | ___ | ___ | _____ |
| 14. Guide the patient and family as they perform each step. Provide written material for reinforcement and review. | ___ | ___ | ___ | _____ |
| 15. Instruct the patient or family to notify the physician if signs or symptoms of hypoxia or respiratory tract infection occur. | ___ | ___ | ___ | _____ |

*Continued*

426

| | S | U | NP | Comments |
|---|---|---|---|---|
| 16. Discuss emergency plans for power loss, natural disaster, and acute respiratory distress. Instruct the patient or family to call 911 and notify the physician and home care employer. | ___ | ___ | ___ | _____ |
| 17. Instruct the patient in safe home oxygen practices, including not allowing smoking in the home, keeping oxygen tanks away from open flames, and storing tanks upright. | ___ | ___ | ___ | _____ |
| 18. Monitor rate of oxygen delivery. | ___ | ___ | ___ | _____ |
| 19. Record the patient's and family's ability to safely use the home oxygen equipment. Report the type of home oxygen equipment to be used, the patient's and family's understanding of how to use the equipment, knowledge of safety guidelines and unexpected outcomes, and ability to demonstrate proper use of the oxygen delivery device. | ___ | ___ | ___ | _____ |

STUDENT: _____  DATE: _____

INSTRUCTOR: _____  DATE: _____

## Skill Performance Checklist
## Skill 39-1 Initiating a Peripheral Intravenous Infusion

|  | S | U | NP | Comments |
|---|---|---|---|---|
| 1. Review the physician's order for the type and amount of intravenous (IV) fluid, rate of fluid administration, and purpose of infusion. Follow ten rights for administration of medications. | —— | —— | —— | _____ |
| 2. Observe the patient for signs and symptoms indicating fluid or electrolyte imbalances that may be affected by IV fluid administration: |  |  |  |  |
| A. Peripheral edema | —— | —— | —— | _____ |
| B. Greater than 20% change in body weight | —— | —— | —— | _____ |
| C. Dry skin and mucous membranes | —— | —— | —— | _____ |
| D. Distended neck veins | —— | —— | —— | _____ |
| E. Blood pressure changes | —— | —— | —— | _____ |
| F. Irregular pulse rhythm; tachycardia | —— | —— | —— | _____ |
| G. Auscultation of abnormal lung sounds | —— | —— | —— | _____ |
| H. Decreased skin turgor | —— | —— | —— | _____ |
| I. Thirst | —— | —— | —— | _____ |
| J. Anorexia, nausea, and vomiting | —— | —— | —— | _____ |
| K. Decreased urine output | —— | —— | —— | _____ |
| L. Behavioural changes | —— | —— | —— | _____ |
| 3. Assess the patient's prior or perceived experience with IV therapy and arm placement preference. | —— | —— | —— | _____ |
| 4. Determine whether the patient is to undergo any planned surgeries or is to receive blood infusion later. | —— | —— | —— | _____ |
| 5. Assess laboratory data and patient's history of allergies. | —— | —— | —— | _____ |
| 6. Assess for the following risk factors: child or older adult, presence of heart failure or renal failure, or low platelet count. | —— | —— | —— | _____ |
| 7. Prepare the patient and family by explaining the procedure, its purpose, and what is expected of the patient. | —— | —— | —— | _____ |
| 8. Perform hand hygiene. | —— | —— | —— | _____ |
| 9. Assist the patient to a comfortable sitting or supine position. | —— | —— | —— | _____ |
| 10. Organize equipment on a clean, clutter-free bedside stand or overbed table. | —— | —— | —— | _____ |
| 11. Change the patient's gown to a more easily removable gown with snaps at the shoulder, if available. | —— | —— | —— | _____ |
| 12. Check IV solution, using the rights of medication administration. Make sure prescribed additives (e.g., potassium, vitamins) have been added. Check solution for colour, clarity, and expiration date. Check bag for leaks, which is best if done before reaching the bedside. | —— | —— | —— | _____ |
| 13. Open sterile packages, using sterile aseptic technique. | —— | —— | —— | _____ |
| 14. Open the infusion set, maintaining sterility of both ends of tubing. Many sets allow for priming of tubing without removal of end cap. | —— | —— | —— | _____ |
| 15. Place a roller clamp about 2 to 5 cm below the drip chamber, and move the roller clamp to closed position. | —— | —— | —— | _____ |
| 16. Remove the protective sheath over the IV bag tubing port. For bottled IV solution, remove the metal cap and the metal and rubber discs beneath the cap. Use caution to avoid touching the exposed opening. | —— | —— | —— | _____ |
| 17. Insert the infusion set into the fluid bag or bottle by removing the protector cap from the tubing insertion spike (keeping the spike sterile), and inserting the spike into the opening of the IV bag. Cleanse the rubber stopper on the glass-bottled solution with antiseptic, and insert the spike into the black rubber stopper of the IV bottle. Hang the solution container on the IV pole at a minimum height of 90 cm above the planned insertion site. | —— | —— | —— | _____ |
| 18. Compress the drip chamber and release, allowing it to fill one-third to one-half full. Open the clamp and prime the infusion tubing by filling with IV solution, carefully inverting valves and ports in sequence as the solution moves through the tubing. | —— | —— | —— | _____ |

*Continued*

428

|  | S | U | NP | Comments |
|---|---|---|---|---|

19. Remove the tubing protector cap (some tubing can be primed without removal), and slowly release the roller clamp to allow fluid to travel from the drip chamber through the tubing to the needle adapter. Return the roller clamp to the closed position after the tubing is primed (filled with IV fluid). ___ ___ ___ _____

20. Be certain that the tubing is clear of air and air bubbles. To remove small air bubbles, firmly tap the IV tubing where air bubbles are located. Check the entire length of tubing to ensure that all air bubbles are removed. ___ ___ ___ _____

21. Replace the tubing cap protector on the end of the tubing. ___ ___ ___ _____

22. *Optional*: Prepare normal saline lock for infusion. If a loop or short extension tubing is needed, use a sterile technique to connect the IV plug to the loop or short extension tubing. Inject 1 to 3 mL of normal saline through the plug and through the loop or short extension tubing. ___ ___ ___ _____

23. Put on disposable gloves. Eye protection and a mask may be worn if splash or spray of blood is possible. *Note*: Gloves can be left off to locate a vein but must be put on before the site is prepared. ___ ___ ___ _____

24. Identify an accessible vein for IV placement. Place a tourniquet 10 to 15 cm above the proposed insertion site. Position the tourniquet so that the ends are away from the site. Check for the presence of the radial pulse. *Option:* Apply a blood pressure (BP) cuff instead of a tourniquet. Inflate the cuff to a level just below the patient's normal diastolic pressure. Maintain inflation at that pressure until the venipuncture is completed. ___ ___ ___ _____

25. Select the vein. Common IV sites for the adult include cephalic, basilic, and median cubital veins:
    A. Use the most distal site in the patient's nondominant arm, if possible. ___ ___ ___ _____
    B. Avoid areas that are painful to palpation. ___ ___ ___ _____
    C. Select a vein large enough for catheter placement. ___ ___ ___ _____
    D. Choose a site that will not interfere with the patient's activities of daily living or planned procedures. ___ ___ ___ _____
    E. Use the fingertips to palpate the vein by pressing downward and noting the resilient, soft, bouncy feeling as the pressure is released. ___ ___ ___ _____
    F. Promote venous distension by instructing the patient to open and close the fist several times, lowering the patient's arm in a dependent position, applying warmth to the arm for several minutes, and rubbing or stroking the patient's arm from distal to proximal below the proposed site. ___ ___ ___ _____
    G. Avoid sites distal to the previous venipuncture site, sclerosed or hardened cordlike veins, infiltrated site or phlebitic vessels, bruised areas, and areas of venous valves or bifurcation. Avoid veins in the antecubital fossa and ventral surface of the wrist. ___ ___ ___ _____
    H. Avoid fragile dorsal veins in older adults and vessels in an extremity with compromised circulation (e.g., in cases of mastectomy, dialysis graft, or paralysis). ___ ___ ___ _____

26. Release tourniquet temporarily. Clip arm hair with scissors (if necessary). Do not shave the area. ___ ___ ___ _____

27. (If area of insertion appears to need cleansing, use soap and water first.) Cleanse the insertion site, using a firm, circular motion (centre to outward) in concentric circles 5 to 7.5 cm from the insertion site. Use antiseptic preparation as a single agent or in combination, according to employer policy. Two percent chlorhexidine gluconate is the antiseptic cleansing agent of choice. Povidone-iodine is a topical anti-infective agent that reduces skin surface bacteria; 70% alcohol is another antiseptic cleansing agent. Povidone-iodine must dry to be effective in reducing microbial counts. Avoid touching the cleansed site. Allow the site to dry for at least two minutes. If the skin is touched after cleansing, repeat cleansing procedure. ___ ___ ___ _____

28. Reapply tourniquet or BP cuff. ___ ___ ___ _____

*Continued*

| | S | U | NP | Comments |
|---|---|---|---|---|

29. Perform venipuncture. Anchor the vein by placing your thumb over the vein beneath the insertion site and by stretching the skin against the direction of insertion 5 to 7.5 cm distal to the site. Warn the patient of a sharp stick. Puncture skin and vein, holding the catheter at a 10- to 30-degree angle with bevel pointed upward.

    A. *Butterfly needle*: Hold the needle at a 10- to 30-degree angle with bevel up, slightly distal to the actual site of venipuncture.

    B. *Needleless over-the-needle catheter (ONC) safety device:* Insert ONC with bevel up, at a 10- to 30-degree angle, slightly distal to the actual site of venipuncture in the direction of the vein.

30. Look for blood return through the tubing of the butterfly needle or flashback chamber of the ONC, indicating that the needle has entered the vein. Lower the catheter or needle until almost flush with the skin. Advance the butterfly needle, or loosen stylet and advance ONC until hub is near the insertion site. Do not reinsert the stylet once it is loosened. (Advance the safety device by using the push-tab to thread the catheter.)

31. Stabilize the catheter. Apply gentle but firm pressure with the index finger of your nondominant hand 3 cm above the insertion site. Release the tourniquet or BP cuff using your dominant hand, and retract the stylet from ONC. Do not recap the stylet. For a safety device, slide the catheter off the stylet while gliding the protective guard over the stylet. A click indicates that the device is locked over the stylet.

32. Quickly connect the adapter of the primed fluid administration set or saline lock to the hub of the ONC or butterfly tubing. Be sure the connection is secure. Do not touch the point of entry of the adapter.

33. Release the roller clamp slowly to begin infusion at a rate to maintain patency of the IV line.

    A. *Intermittent infusion*: Continue to stabilize the catheter with your nondominant hand, and attach the injection cap of the adapter. Insert prefilled flush solution into the injection cap. Flush slowly. Maintain thumb pressure on the syringe during withdrawal, or close the clamp on the extension tubing of the injection cap while still flushing the last 0.2 to 0.4 mL of flush solution.

34. Tape or secure the catheter.

    A. *If applying transparent dressing*: Secure the catheter with your nondominant hand while preparing to apply dressing. Tape over catheter hub.

    B. *If applying a gauze dressing*:

        (1) Tape the IV catheter. Place a narrow piece (1 cm wide) of sterile tape under the hub of the catheter with adhesive side up, and criss-cross tape over the hub to form a chevron.

        (2) Place tape only on the catheter, never over the insertion site. Secure the site to allow easy visual inspection and early recognition of infiltration and phlebitis. Avoid applying tape around the extremity.

    C. Observe the site for swelling.

35. Apply sterile dressing over the site.

    A. Transparent dressing:

        (1) Carefully remove adherent backing. Apply one edge of dressing, and then gently smooth remaining dressing over the site, leaving the end of the catheter hub uncovered.

        (2) Take a 2.5-cm piece of tape and place over the IV tubing or extension set. Do not apply tape over transparent dressing.

        (3) Apply chevron and place only over the tape, not the transparent dressing.

    B. Sterile gauze dressing:

        (1) Fold $2 \times 3 \times 2$ gauze in half, and cover with a 2.5-cm-wide piece of sterile tape extending about 2.5 cm from each side. Place under tubing–catheter hub junction. Place a $2 \times 2$ gauze pad over venipuncture site and catheter hub. Secure edges with tape.

        (2) Curl a loop of tubing alongside the arm, and place a second piece of tape directly over the $2 \times 2$ gauze, securing tubing in two places.

*Continued*

| | S | U | NP | Comments |
|---|---|---|---|---|

36. Prepare the equipment according to expected frequency of use:
    A. *For IV fluid administration*: Adjust the flow rate to correct drops per minute or connect to electronic infusion device. ___ ___ ___ _____
    B. *For intermittent use*: Saline lock. Flush with 3 mL of sterile normal saline at prescribed frequency or per employer policy. ___ ___ ___ _____
37. Label dressing with date, time, gauge size and length of catheter, placement of IV line and dressing, and your initials. ___ ___ ___ _____
38. Dispose of used needles in an appropriate sharps container. Discard supplies. Remove gloves, and perform hand hygiene. ___ ___ ___ _____
39. Observe the patient every hour to determine whether fluid is infusing correctly: ___ ___ ___ _____
    A. Check whether the correct amount of solution is infused as prescribed by looking at the time tape. ___ ___ ___ _____
    B. Count the flow or check the rate on the infusion pump. ___ ___ ___ _____
    C. Check the patency of the IV catheter or needle. ___ ___ ___ _____
    D. Observe the patient for signs of discomfort. ___ ___ ___ _____
    E. Inspect the insertion site for absence of phlebitis, infiltration, or inflammation. ___ ___ ___ _____
40. Document IV insertion including date, time, device selected (size, type, length, brand), site, number of attempts, name and professional designation. A special parenteral therapy flow sheet may be used. Record patient's response to intravenous fluid, amount infused, and integrity and patency of system every four hours or according to employer policy. ___ ___ ___ _____
41. Observe the patient every hour to determine response to therapy (i.e., measure vital signs, conduct postprocedure assessments). ___ ___ ___ _____

STUDENT: _____     DATE: _____

INSTRUCTOR: _____     DATE: _____

## Skill Performance Checklist
## Skill 39-2 Regulating Intravenous Flow Rates

| | S | U | NP | Comments |
|---|---|---|---|---|
| 1. Check the patient's medical record for the correct solution, additives, and time of infusion. The usual order includes solution for 24 hours, usually divided into 2 or 3 L. On occasion, an intravenous (IV) order contains only 1 L to keep the vein open (KVO). An order also indicates the time over which each litre is to infuse. | ___ | ___ | ___ | _____ |
| 2. Perform hand hygiene. Observe for patency of the IV line and the needle or catheter. | ___ | ___ | ___ | _____ |
|   A. Open the drip regulator and observe for rapid flow of fluid from the solution into the drip chamber, and then close the drip regulator to the prescribed rate. | ___ | ___ | ___ | _____ |
| 3. Check the patient's knowledge of how positioning of the IV site affects flow rate. | ___ | ___ | ___ | _____ |
| 4. Verify with the patient how the venipuncture site feels (e.g., determine whether the patient is experiencing pain or a burning sensation). | ___ | ___ | ___ | _____ |
| 5. Have paper and pencil to calculate the flow rate, or use a calculator. | ___ | ___ | ___ | _____ |
| 6. Check calibration (drop factor) in drops per millilitre (gtt/mL) of the infusion set: | | | | |
|   A. *Microdrip*: 60 gtt/mL | ___ | ___ | ___ | _____ |
|   B. *Macrodrip*: 15 gtt/mL or 10 gtt/mL, depending on manufacturer (will be stated on package) | ___ | ___ | ___ | _____ |
| 7. Calculate flow rate (hourly volume) of the prescribed infusion. Flow rate (mL/hr) = total infusion (volume in millilitres) per hours of infusion (time to be infused). | ___ | ___ | ___ | _____ |
| 8. Read the physician's orders, and follow ten rights for the correct solution and proper additives. | ___ | ___ | ___ | _____ |
| 9. Determine how long each litre of fluid should run. IV fluids are usually ordered by rate, such as 100 mL/hr. On occasion, however, IV fluids are ordered over a period of time, such as 1000 mL 5% dextrose in water with 20 mmol potassium chloride over eight hours. | ___ | ___ | ___ | _____ |
| 10. Place adhesive or fluid indicator tape on the IV bottle or bag next to volume markings. | ___ | ___ | ___ | _____ |
| 11. Select one of the following formulas to calculate minute rate (gtt/min) on the basis of the drop factor of the infusion set: | | | | |
|   A. mL/hr/60 min = mL/min, and drop factor · mL/min = gtt/min | ___ | ___ | ___ | _____ |
|   B. Alternative: mL/hr · drop factor/60 min = gtt/min. Using this formula, calculate minute flow rate for bottle 1:1000 mL with 20 mmol potassium chloride:<br>*Microdrip:*<br>125 mL/hr · 60 gtt/mL = 7500 gtt/hr<br>7500 gtt ÷ 60 minutes = 125 gtt/min<br>*Macrodrip:*<br>125 mL/hr · 15 gtt/mL = 1875 gtt/hr<br>1875 gtt ÷ 60 minutes = 31 gtt/min | ___ | ___ | ___ | _____ |
| 12. Establish flow rate by counting drops in the drip chamber for one minute by watch; then adjust the roller clamp to increase or decrease the rate of infusion. | ___ | ___ | ___ | _____ |

*Continued*

432

| | S | U | NP | Comments |
|---|---|---|---|---|

13. Follow this procedure for the infusion controller or pump:
   A. Place the IV infusion tubing within the ridges of the control box in the direction of flow (i.e., the portion of tubing nearest the IV bag at the top and the portion of tubing nearest the patient at the bottom). Close the control chamber door. Turn on the pump. Select required drops per minute or volume per hour and volume to be infused. Open the rate-control clamp, and press the start button.
   B. Monitor infusion rates and IV site for complications according to employer policy.
   C. Assess patency and integrity of the system when the alarm sounds.
14. Follow this procedure for a volume-control device:
   A. Place the volume-control device between the IV bag and insertion spike of the infusion set, using sterile technique.
   B. Place a two-hour allotment of fluid into the chamber device.
   C. Assess the system at least hourly; add fluid to the volume-control device as needed. Regulate flow rate.
15. Record name of solution, rate of infusion, drops/minute, and mL/hour in nurses' notes or flow sheet every four hours or according to patient's condition and to employer policy. Immediately record in nurses' notes or flow sheet any new intravenous fluid rates. Document use of any electronic infusion device or controlling device, and record number on that device.
16. Evaluate infusion site for signs of infiltration, inflammation, clot in catheter, or kink or knot in infusion tubing.

STUDENT: _____ DATE: _____

INSTRUCTOR: _____ DATE: _____

## Skill Performance Checklist
## Skill 39-3 Maintenance of Intravenous System

| | S | U | NP | Comments |
|---|---|---|---|---|

**CHANGING INTRAVENOUS SOLUTION:**

1. Check physician's orders. ___ ___ ___ _____

2. If the order is written for KVO or to keep open, contact the physician for clarification of the rate of the infusion. Note date and time when solution was last changed. ___ ___ ___ _____

3. Determine the compatibility of all IV fluids and additives by consulting appropriate literature or the pharmacy. ___ ___ ___ _____

4. Determine the patient's understanding of the need for continued IV therapy. ___ ___ ___ _____

5. Assess patency of the current IV access site. ___ ___ ___ _____

6. Have the next solution prepared and accessible at least one hour before needed. Check that the solution is correct and properly labelled. Check the solution expiration date and for the presence of precipitate and discoloration. ___ ___ ___ _____

7. Prepare to change solution when less than 50 mL of fluid remains in the bottle or bag or when a new type of solution is ordered. ___ ___ ___ _____

8. Prepare the patient and family by explaining the procedure, its purpose, and what is expected of the patient. ___ ___ ___ _____

9. Ensure that the drip chamber is at least half full. ___ ___ ___ _____

10. Perform hand hygiene. ___ ___ ___ _____

11. Prepare the new solution for changing. If using a plastic bag, remove the protective cover from the IV tubing port. If using a glass bottle, remove the metal cap and the metal and rubber discs. ___ ___ ___ _____

12. Move the roller clamp to stop the flow rate. ___ ___ ___ _____

13. Remove the old IV fluid container from the IV pole. ___ ___ ___ _____

14. Quickly remove the spike from the old solution bag or bottle, and, without touching the tip, insert the spike into the new bag or bottle. ___ ___ ___ _____

15. Hang the new bag or bottle of solution on the IV pole. ___ ___ ___ _____

16. Check for air in the tubing. If bubbles form, they can be removed by closing the roller clamp, stretching the tubing downward, and tapping the tubing with your finger (the bubbles rise in the fluid to the drip chamber). For larger amounts of air, swab the injection port below the air with alcohol, and allow to dry. Connect a syringe to this port, and aspirate the air into the syringe. Reduce air in tubing by priming slowly instead of allowing a wide-open flow. ___ ___ ___ _____

17. Ensure drip chamber is one-third to half full. If the drip chamber is too full, pinch off tubing below the drip chamber, invert the container, squeeze the drip chamber, hang up the bottle, and release the tubing. ___ ___ ___ _____

18. Regulate flow to the prescribed rate. ___ ___ ___ _____

19. Mark the date and time on label, and tape it on bag. Do not use felt-tipped pens or permanent markers on IV bags. ___ ___ ___ _____

20. Observe the patient for signs of overhydration or dehydration to determine response to IV fluid therapy. ___ ___ ___ _____

21. Observe IV system for patency and development of complications (e.g., infiltration or phlebitis). ___ ___ ___ _____

**CHANGING INTRAVENOUS TUBING:**

22. Determine when a new infusion set is needed:
    A. Employer policy will indicate the frequency of routine change for IV administration sets and saline flush tubing. ___ ___ ___ _____
    B. Puncture of infusion tubing necessitates immediate change. ___ ___ ___ _____
    C. Contamination of tubing necessitates immediate change. ___ ___ ___ _____
    D. Occlusions in existing tubing can occur after infusion of packed red blood cells, whole blood, albumin, or other blood components. ___ ___ ___ _____

23. Prepare the patient and family by explaining the procedure, its purpose, and what is expected of the patient. ___ ___ ___ _____

24. Perform hand hygiene. ___ ___ ___ _____

*Continued*

| | S | U | NP | Comments |
|---|---|---|---|---|

25. Open the new infusion set, keeping protective coverings over the infusion spike and distal adapter. Secure all junctions with Luer-Loks, clasping devices, or threaded devices.
26. Apply nonsterile disposable gloves. ___ ___ ___ _____
27. If the catheter hub is not visible, remove IV dressing while maintaining the stability of the catheter. If transparent dressing must be removed, place a small piece of sterile tape across the hub temporarily to anchor the catheter during disconnection. Do not remove tape securing the needle or catheter to the skin with gauze dressing. ___ ___ ___ _____
28. For IV continuous infusion:
    A. Move the roller clamp on new IV tubing to the closed position. ___ ___ ___ _____
    B. Slow the rate of infusion by regulating the drip rate on the old tubing. Maintain KVO rate. ___ ___ ___ _____
    C. Compress and fill the drip chamber. ___ ___ ___ _____
    D. Remove the IV container from the pole, invert the container, and remove old tubing from the container. Carefully hold the container while hanging or taping the drip chamber on the IV pole 1 m above the IV site. ___ ___ ___ _____
    E. Place the insertion spike of the new tubing into the old solution bag opening, and hang the solution bag on the IV pole. ___ ___ ___ _____
    F. Compress and release the drip chamber on the new tubing. Slowly fill the drip chamber one-third to half full. ___ ___ ___ _____
    G. Slowly open the roller clamp, remove the protective cap from the needle adapter (if necessary), and flush the new tubing with solution. Replace the cap. ___ ___ ___ _____
    H. Turn the roller clamp on the old tubing to the closed position. ___ ___ ___ _____
29. For saline lock:
    A. If a loop or short extension tubing is needed because of an awkward IV site placement, use sterile technique to connect the new injection cap to the loop or tubing. ___ ___ ___ _____
    B. Swab the injection cap with recommended solution for 15 seconds. Insert the syringe with 1 to 3 mL saline, and inject through the injection cap into the loop or short extension tubing. Connect tubing to injection cap. ___ ___ ___ _____
30. Stabilize the hub of the catheter, and apply pressure over the vein just above the catheter tip, at least 3 cm above the insertion site. Gently disconnect old tubing from the catheter hub. Maintain stability of the hub, and quickly insert the adapter of new tubing or saline lock into the hub. ___ ___ ___ _____
31. Open the roller clamp on new tubing. Allow solution to run rapidly for 30 to 60 seconds. ___ ___ ___ _____
32. Regulate the IV drip according to physician's orders, and monitor the rate hourly. ___ ___ ___ _____
33. Apply new dressing, if necessary. ___ ___ ___ _____
34. Discard old tubing in a proper container. ___ ___ ___ _____
35. Remove and dispose of gloves. Perform hand hygiene. ___ ___ ___ _____
36. Evaluate the flow rate and observe the connection site for leakage. ___ ___ ___ _____

**DISCONTINUING PERIPHERAL INTRAVENOUS ACCESS:**

37. Check physician's order for discontinuing IV therapy.
38. Explain the procedure to the patient. Explain that the affected extremity must be held still and how long the procedure will take. ___ ___ ___ _____
39. Perform hand hygiene, and put on disposable gloves. ___ ___ ___ _____
40. Turn the IV tubing roller clamp to the closed position. Remove the tape securing the tubing. ___ ___ ___ _____
41. Remove the IV site dressing and tape while stabilizing the catheter. ___ ___ ___ _____
42. With dry gauze or an alcohol swab held over the site, apply light pressure and withdraw the catheter, using a slow, steady movement, keeping the hub parallel to the skin. ___ ___ ___ _____
43. Apply pressure to the site for two to three minutes, using the dry, sterile gauze pad. Secure with tape. ___ ___ ___ _____
44. Inspect the catheter for intactness, noting tip integrity and length. ___ ___ ___ _____
45. Discard used supplies. ___ ___ ___ _____
46. Remove and discard gloves, and perform hand hygiene. ___ ___ ___ _____
47. Instruct the patient to report any redness, pain, drainage, or swelling that may occur after catheter removal. ___ ___ ___ _____
48. Record changing of tubing and solution on patient's record. A special parenteral therapy flow sheet may be used. ___ ___ ___ _____
49. Place a piece of tape or preprinted label with the date and time of tubing change, and attach tape to tubing below the level of drip chamber. ___ ___ ___ _____

STUDENT: _____  DATE: _____

INSTRUCTOR: _____  DATE: _____

## Skill Performance Checklist
## Skill 39-4 Changing a Peripheral Intravenous Dressing

|  | S | U | NP | Comments |
|---|---|---|---|---|
| 1. Determine when dressing was last changed. Many institutions require that the nurse record the date and time on the dressing when the device is first placed. | ___ | ___ | ___ | _____ |
| 2. Perform hand hygiene. Observe the present dressing for moisture and intactness. | ___ | ___ | ___ | _____ |
| 3. Observe the IV system for proper functioning or complications: kinks in infusion tubing or IV catheter. Palpate the catheter site through the intact dressing for inflammation or subjective complaints of pain or burning sensation. | ___ | ___ | ___ | _____ |
| 4. Inspect the exposed catheter site for swelling or blanching. | ___ | ___ | ___ | _____ |
| 5. Assess patient's understanding of need for continued IV infusion. | ___ | ___ | ___ | _____ |
| 6. Explain procedure and purpose to the patient and family. Explain that the affected extremity must be held still and how long the procedure will take. | ___ | ___ | ___ | _____ |
| 7. Put on disposable gloves. | ___ | ___ | ___ | _____ |
| 8. Remove tape, gauze, or transparent dressing from the old dressing, one layer at a time, leaving tape (if present) that secures the IV catheter in place. Be cautious if catheter tubing becomes tangled or attached to dressing. When removing transparent dressing, hold the catheter hub and tubing with your nondominant hand. | ___ | ___ | ___ | _____ |
| 9. Observe the insertion site for signs and symptoms of infection (redness, swelling, and exudate). If they are present, remove the catheter, and insert a new IV line in another site. | ___ | ___ | ___ | _____ |
| 10. If infiltration, phlebitis, or clot occurs, or if otherwise ordered by physician, stop infusion and discontinue IV therapy. Restart new IV line if continued therapy is necessary. Place a moist, warm compress over an area of phlebitis. | ___ | ___ | ___ | _____ |
| 11. If IV fluid is infusing properly, gently remove tape securing the catheter. Stabilize the needle or catheter with one hand. Use adhesive remover to cleanse skin and remove adhesive residue, if needed. | ___ | ___ | ___ | _____ |
| 12. Stabilize the catheter at all times with one finger over the catheter until tape or dressing is replaced. | ___ | ___ | ___ | _____ |
| 13. Use circular motion, cleanse the peripheral IV insertion site with an antiseptic swab, starting at the insertion site and working outward, creating concentric circles. Allow swab solution to air-dry completely. | ___ | ___ | ___ | _____ |
| 14. Apply new transparent or gauze dressing. | ___ | ___ | ___ | _____ |
| 15. Remove and discard gloves. | ___ | ___ | ___ | _____ |
| 16. Anchor IV tubing with additional pieces of tape. When using transparent polyurethane dressing, minimize the tape placed over dressing. | ___ | ___ | ___ | _____ |
| 17. Write insertion date, date and time of dressing change, size and gauge of catheter, and your initials directly on dressing. Apply arm board, commercial housing device, or both if the site is affected by joint motion. | ___ | ___ | ___ | _____ |
| 18. Discard used equipment, and perform hand hygiene. | ___ | ___ | ___ | _____ |
| 19. Observe functioning and patency of the IV system in response to changing dressing. | ___ | ___ | ___ | _____ |
| 20. Monitor the patient's body temperature. | ___ | ___ | ___ | _____ |
| 21. Record appearance of IV site, type of dressing, and status of IV fluid infusion. | ___ | ___ | ___ | _____ |

STUDENT: _____  DATE: _____

INSTRUCTOR: _____  DATE: _____

## Skill Performance Checklist
## Skill 42-1 Aspiration Precautions

|  | S | U | NP | Comments |
|---|---|---|---|---|
| 1. Give patients who are not alert within the first 24 hours after a stroke nothing by mouth (NPO), and monitor closely. | ___ | ___ | ___ | _____ |
| 2. Assess patients who are at increased risk of aspiration for signs and symptoms of dysphagia (e.g., cough, pharyngeal pooling, change in voice after swallowing). | ___ | ___ | ___ | _____ |
| 3. Observe the patient during mealtime for signs of dysphagia, and allow the patient to attempt to feed himself or herself. Observe as the patient eats foods of various consistencies and drinks liquids. Note at the end of the meal whether the patient becomes tired. | ___ | ___ | ___ | _____ |
| 4. Ask the patient about any difficulties with chewing or swallowing various foods with different textures. | ___ | ___ | ___ | _____ |
| 5. Ensure the clinical bedside screening trial is conducted by a speech language pathologist or appropriately trained specialist. | ___ | ___ | ___ | _____ |
| 6. Elevate the head of the patient's bed so that hips are flexed at a 90-degree angle and the head is flexed slightly forward, or help the patient to the same position in a chair. | ___ | ___ | ___ | _____ |
| 7. The clinical bedside screening trial involves giving 5 to 10 mL of water and if that is well tolerated is followed by a small cup (50 mL) of water. | ___ | ___ | ___ | _____ |
| 8. For a patient who may feed himself or herself, explain that you are initially observing while the patient eats. | ___ | ___ | ___ | _____ |
| A. Observe as patient consumes various consistencies of food and liquids, watching for signs of dysphagia. | ___ | ___ | ___ | _____ |
| B. Note at the end of the meal if patient becomes tired. | ___ | ___ | ___ | _____ |
| C. Report signs and symptoms of dysphagia. | ___ | ___ | ___ | _____ |
| D. Place identification on patient's record indicating that dysphagia is present. | ___ | ___ | ___ | _____ |
| 9. For patients who require supervision or assistance with eating because dysphagia and risk of aspiration have been identified, explain that you will assist them with their meal. | ___ | ___ | ___ | _____ |
| A. Perform hand hygiene. | ___ | ___ | ___ | _____ |
| B. As ordered or recommended by the feeding/swallowing team, add thickener to thin liquids to create the consistency of nectar, honey, or pudding. | ___ | ___ | ___ | _____ |
| C. Place ½ to 1 teaspoon of food on unaffected side of the mouth, allowing utensil to touch the mouth or tongue. | ___ | ___ | ___ | _____ |
| D. Place hand on throat to gently palpate swallowing event as it occurs. Swallowing twice is often necessary to clear the pharynx. | ___ | ___ | ___ | _____ |
| E. Provide verbal coaching and positive reinforcement while feeding patient. | ___ | ___ | ___ | _____ |
| • Feel the food in your mouth. | ___ | ___ | ___ | _____ |
| • Chew and taste the food. | ___ | ___ | ___ | _____ |
| • Raise your tongue to the roof of your mouth. | ___ | ___ | ___ | _____ |
| • Think about swallowing. | ___ | ___ | ___ | _____ |
| • Close your mouth, and swallow. | ___ | ___ | ___ | _____ |
| • Swallow again. | ___ | ___ | ___ | _____ |
| • Cough to clear airway. | ___ | ___ | ___ | _____ |
| F. Observe patient for coughing, choking, gagging, and drooling of food; suction airway as necessary. | ___ | ___ | ___ | _____ |

*Continued*

438

| | S | U | NP | Comments |
|---|---|---|---|---|
| G. Provide rest periods as necessary during meal to avoid rushed or forced feeding. | ___ | ___ | ___ | _____ |
| H. Using a penlight and tongue blade, gently inspect patient's oral cavity during and after the meal to detect pockets of food. | ___ | ___ | ___ | _____ |
| I. Ask patient to remain sitting upright for at least 30 minutes after the meal. | ___ | ___ | ___ | _____ |
| J. Help patient to perform hand hygiene and mouth care. | ___ | ___ | ___ | _____ |
| K. Record intake, and report any observations indicative of feeding and swallowing difficulties. | ___ | ___ | ___ | _____ |
| L. Ensure return of patient's tray to appropriate place, and perform hand hygiene. | ___ | ___ | ___ | _____ |
| 10. Weigh patient weekly at the same time on the same scale. | ___ | ___ | ___ | _____ |
| 11. Document the following in the patient's chart: patient's tolerance of various food textures, amount of assistance required, position during meal, absence or presence of any symptoms of dysphagia, and amount eaten. | ___ | ___ | ___ | _____ |
| 12. Report any coughing, gagging, choking, or swallowing difficulties to the nurse in charge or the health care provider. | ___ | ___ | ___ | _____ |

STUDENT: _____ DATE: _____

INSTRUCTOR: _____ DATE: _____

## Skill Performance Checklist
## Skill 42-2 Blood Glucose Monitoring

| | S | U | NP | Comments |
|---|---|---|---|---|
| 1. Assess understanding of procedure and purpose. Determine whether patient with diabetes mellitus understands how to perform test and realizes importance of glucose monitoring. | ___ | ___ | ___ | _____ |
| 2. Determine whether specific conditions have to be met before or after sample collection (e.g., with fasting, after meals, after certain medications, before insulin doses). | ___ | ___ | ___ | _____ |
| 3. Determine whether risks exist for performing skin puncture (e.g., low platelet count, anticoagulant therapy, bleeding disorders). | ___ | ___ | ___ | _____ |
| 4. Assess area of skin that you will use as puncture site. Inspect the patient's fingers, toes, and heel. Alternative sites are the palm, arm, and thigh. Avoid areas that have bruises and open lesions. | ___ | ___ | ___ | _____ |
| 5. Review health care provider's order for times and frequency of measurement. | ___ | ___ | ___ | _____ |
| 6. If diabetic patient performs test at home, assess patient's ability to handle skin-puncturing device. If patient chooses, he or she may wish to continue self-testing while in hospital. | ___ | ___ | ___ | _____ |
| 7. Expected outcomes after completion of procedure:<br>A. Puncture site shows no evidence of bleeding or tissue damage.<br>B. Blood glucose level is normal.<br>C. Patient demonstrates procedure.<br>D. Patient explains test results. | ___ | ___ | ___ | _____ |
| 8. Explain procedure and purpose to patient or family, or both. Offer patient and family opportunity to practise testing procedures. Provide resources and teaching aids for patient. | ___ | ___ | ___ | _____ |
| 9. Perform hand hygiene. | ___ | ___ | ___ | _____ |
| 10. Instruct patient to perform hand hygiene with soap and warm water, if patient is able. | ___ | ___ | ___ | _____ |
| 11. Position patient comfortably in chair or in semi-Fowler's position in bed. | ___ | ___ | ___ | _____ |
| 12. Remove test strip from container; then tightly seal cap. Check the code on the test strip vial. | ___ | ___ | ___ | _____ |
| 13. Turn on glucose meter, if necessary. Some monitors are activated when the test strip is inserted and therefore do not have a specific on–off switch. | ___ | ___ | ___ | _____ |
| 14. Insert strip into glucose meter (refer to manufacturer's directions), and make necessary adjustments. | ___ | ___ | ___ | _____ |
| 15. Remove unused glucose test strip from meter and place on paper towel or clean, dry surface with test pad facing up (see manufacturer's directions). | ___ | ___ | ___ | _____ |
| 16. Apply disposable gloves. | ___ | ___ | ___ | _____ |
| 17. Choose puncture site. Puncture site should be vascular. In adults, select lateral side of finger; be sure to avoid central tip of finger, which has a denser nerve supply. | ___ | ___ | ___ | _____ |
| 18. Hold the finger that you will puncture in dependent position while gently massaging finger toward puncture site. | ___ | ___ | ___ | _____ |
| 19. Clean site with antiseptic swab, and allow it to dry completely. | ___ | ___ | ___ | _____ |
| 20. Remove cover of lancet or blood-letting device. Hold lancet perpendicular to puncture site, and pierce finger or heel quickly in one continuous motion (do not force lancet). | ___ | ___ | ___ | _____ |
| 21. Place blood-letting device firmly against side of finger and push release button, causing needle to pierce skin. | ___ | ___ | ___ | _____ |
| 22. Wipe away first droplet of blood with cotton ball. (See manufacturer's directions for meter used.) | ___ | ___ | ___ | _____ |
| 23. Lightly squeeze puncture site (without touching) until a second large droplet of blood has formed. Repuncturing is necessary if large enough drop does not form to ensure accurate test results. (See manufacturer's direction regarding how blood is applied.) | ___ | ___ | ___ | _____ |

*Continued*

440

| | S | U | NP | Comments |
|---|---|---|---|---|
| 24. Obtain test results. | ___ | ___ | ___ | _____ |
| A. Be sure meter is still on. Bring test strip in the meter (in this example, an Accu-Check) to the drop of blood. The blood will be absorbed into the test strip (see manufacturer's instructions). | ___ | ___ | ___ | _____ |
| (1) Do not scrape blood onto the test strips or apply blood to wrong side of test strip. This prevents accurate glucose measurement. Ensure enough blood is applied to completely fill the test window. Otherwise a false reading or error message will be displayed. | ___ | ___ | ___ | _____ |
| B. The blood glucose test result will appear on the screen (see step 24B illustration, textbook page xx). Some devices beep when measurement is completed. | ___ | ___ | ___ | _____ |
| 25. Turn meter off. Dispose of test strip, lancet, and gloves in proper receptacle. | ___ | ___ | ___ | _____ |
| 26. Discuss test results with patient. | ___ | ___ | ___ | _____ |
| 27. Re-inspect puncture site for bleeding or tissue injury. | ___ | ___ | ___ | _____ |
| 28. Compare glucose meter reading with normal blood glucose levels and previous test results. | ___ | ___ | ___ | _____ |
| 29. Ask patient to discuss procedure. | ___ | ___ | ___ | _____ |
| 30. Ask patient to explain test and results. | ___ | ___ | ___ | _____ |
| 31. In nurses' notes or special flow sheet, record procedure, glucose level, and action taken for abnormal range. | ___ | ___ | ___ | _____ |
| 32. Describe response, including appearance of puncture site, in nurses' notes. | ___ | ___ | ___ | _____ |
| 33. Record and report abnormal blood glucose levels. | ___ | ___ | ___ | _____ |

STUDENT: _____  DATE: _____

INSTRUCTOR: _____  DATE: _____

## Skill Performance Checklist
## Skill 42-3 Inserting a Small-Bore Nasoenteric or Oral Tube for Enteral Feeding

| | S | U | NP | Comments |
|---|---|---|---|---|
| 1. Assess patient for the need for enteral feeding: NPO or insufficient intake for more than five days, functional gastrointestinal tract, unable to ingest sufficient nutrients. | ___ | ___ | ___ | _____ |
|    A. Review physician's order for insertion of tube and enteral feeding schedule. | | | | |
| 2. Explain procedure to patient. | ___ | ___ | ___ | _____ |
| 3. Assess patency of nares. Have patient close each nostril alternately and breathe. Examine each naris for patency and skin breakdown. | ___ | ___ | ___ | _____ |
| 4. Assess for gag reflex. Place tongue blade in patient's mouth, touching uvula to induce a gag response. | | | | |
| 5. Review patient's medical history for nasal problems (e.g., nosebleeds, oral or facial surgery, facial trauma, past history of aspiration, or anticoagulation therapy). | ___ | ___ | ___ | _____ |
| 6. Perform hand hygiene. | | | | |
| 7. Auscultate abdomen for bowel sounds. | ___ | ___ | ___ | _____ |
| 8. Explain procedure to patient and how to communicate during intubation by raising index finger to indicate gagging or discomfort. | ___ | ___ | ___ | _____ |
| 9. Stand on same side of bed as naris for insertion, and assist patient to high-Fowler's position, unless contraindicated. Place pillow behind head and shoulders. | ___ | ___ | ___ | _____ |
| 10. Place absorbent pad over patient's chest. Keep facial tissues within reach. | ___ | ___ | ___ | _____ |
| 11. Determine length of tube to be inserted, and mark with tape. | ___ | ___ | ___ | _____ |
|    A. Traditional method for placing the tube to the stomach: Measure distance from tip of nose to earlobe and then to xiphoid process of sternum. If placing the tube to small bowel (duodenum), follow employer-specific protocol. | | | | |
| 12. Prepare nasogastric or nasointestinal tube for insertion according to manufacturer recommendation. | | | | |
|    A. Do not ice plastic tubes. | ___ | ___ | ___ | _____ |
|    B. Perform hand hygiene, and put on gloves. | ___ | ___ | ___ | _____ |
|    C. If long-term tube, inject 10 mL of water from 30-mL or larger catheter-tip syringe into the tube, and insert stylet or guide wire. | | | | |
|    D. Make certain that guide wire is securely positioned against weighted tip and that connections are snugly fitted together. | ___ | ___ | ___ | _____ |
| 13. Cut tape 10 cm long, or prepare tube fixation device. Split one end of tape lengthwise for 5 cm. | ___ | ___ | ___ | _____ |
| 14. Dip tube with surface lubricant into glass of water. If tube is not prelubricated, use water-soluble lubricant. | ___ | ___ | ___ | _____ |
| 15. Insert tube through nostril to back of throat (posterior nasopharynx). Aim back and down toward ear. | ___ | ___ | ___ | _____ |
| 16. Have patient flex head toward chest after tube has passed through nasopharynx. | ___ | ___ | ___ | _____ |
| 17. Emphasize need to mouth-breathe and swallow during the procedure (when possible). | ___ | ___ | ___ | _____ |
| 18. When tip of tube reaches the carina (about 25 cm in an adult), stop insertion, hold end of tube near ear, and listen for air exchange from the distal portion of the tube. | ___ | ___ | ___ | _____ |
| 19. Advance tube each time patient swallows until desired length has been passed. | ___ | ___ | ___ | _____ |
| 20. Check for position of tube in back of throat with penlight and tongue blade. | ___ | ___ | ___ | _____ |
| 21. Perform measures to verify placement of tube. Secure tube before X-ray examination, because it may become dislodged during procedure. | ___ | ___ | ___ | _____ |

*Continued*

442

| | S | U | NP | Comments |
|---|---|---|---|---|

22. After gastric aspirates are obtained, anchor tube to nose and avoid pressure on nares. Mark exit site with indelible ink. Select one of the following options:

   A. Apply tape.

     (1) Apply tincture of benzoin or other skin adhesive on tip of patient's nose and tube, and allow it to become "tacky." ___ ___ ___ _____

     (2) Place the intact end of tape over bridge of patient's nose. Wrap each of the 5-cm strips around tube as it exits nose. Change position of tube at naris every eight hours. ___ ___ ___ _____

   B. Apply tube fixation device using shaped adhesive patch.

     (1) Apply wide end of patch to bridge of nose. ___ ___ ___ _____

     (2) Slip connector around tube as it exits nose. ___ ___ ___ _____

23. A second anchoring of tube against cheek with gauze and transparent dressing may be advised. Do not allow tube to rest over bony points. ___ ___ ___ _____

24. For intestinal placement, position patient on right side when possible until radiological confirmation of correct placement has been verified. ___ ___ ___ _____

25. Remove gloves, perform hand hygiene, and assist patient to a comfortable position. ___ ___ ___ _____

26. Obtain X-ray film of abdomen. ___ ___ ___ _____

27. Perform hand hygiene. Apply clean gloves, and administer oral hygiene. Cleanse tubing at nostril. ___ ___ ___ _____

28. Remove gloves, dispose of equipment, and perform hand hygiene. ___ ___ ___ _____

29. Inspect naris and oropharynx for any irritation after insertion. ___ ___ ___ _____

30. Ask if patient feels comfortable. ___ ___ ___ _____

31. Observe patient for any difficulty breathing, coughing, or gagging. ___ ___ ___ _____

32. Auscultate lung sounds. ___ ___ ___ _____

33. Record and report type and size of tube placed, location of distal tip of tube, patient's tolerance of procedure, pH value, and confirmation of tube position by X-ray examination. ___ ___ ___ _____

STUDENT: _____  DATE: _____

INSTRUCTOR: _____  DATE: _____

## Skill Performance Checklist
## Skill 42-4 Administering Enteral Feedings via Nasoenteric Tube

| | S | U | NP | Comments |
|---|---|---|---|---|
| 1. Assess patient's need for enteral tube feedings: impaired swallowing, tracheostomy, decreased level of consciousness, head or neck surgery, facial trauma, surgical procedures involving upper alimentary canal. | ___ | ___ | | _____ |
| 2. Evaluate patient's nutritional status. Obtain baseline weight and laboratory values (e.g., albumin, transferrin, prealbumin). Assess patient for fluid volume excess or deficit, electrolyte abnormalities, and metabolic abnormalities, such as hyperglycemia. | ___ | ___ | ___ | _____ |
| 3. Verify physician's order for formula, rate, route, and frequency and for laboratory data and bedside assessments, such as finger-stick blood glucose measurement. | ___ | ___ | ___ | _____ |
| 4. Explain procedure to patient. | ___ | ___ | ___ | _____ |
| 5. Perform hand hygiene. | ___ | ___ | ___ | _____ |
| 6. Auscultate for bowel sounds before feeding. | ___ | ___ | ___ | _____ |
| 7. Prepare feeding container to administer formula. | | | | |
| A. Check expiration date on formula and integrity of container. | ___ | ___ | ___ | _____ |
| B. Have tube feeding formula at room temperature. | ___ | ___ | ___ | _____ |
| C. Perform hand hygiene, and apply gloves. | ___ | ___ | ___ | _____ |
| D. Shake formula container well, and fill feeding container with formula. Open stopcock on tubing, and fill with formula to remove air. | ___ | ___ | ___ | _____ |
| E. Connect tubing to container as needed, or prepare ready-to-hang container. | ___ | ___ | ___ | _____ |
| 8. For intermittent feeding, have syringe ready, and ensure formula is at room temperature. | ___ | ___ | ___ | _____ |
| 9. Place patient in high-Fowler's position, or elevate head of bed at least 45 degrees. | ___ | ___ | ___ | _____ |
| 10. Verify tube placement. Consider the results from pH testing together with the aspirate's appearance. | ___ | ___ | ___ | _____ |
| 11. Check pH of aspirate; confirm measurement of length of tube from naris to tip of connection port; ensure original mark is in the same position. | ___ | ___ | ___ | _____ |
| 12. Check for gastric residual. | | | | |
| A. Draw 30 mL of air with syringe. Connect to end of feeding tube. Flush tube with air. | ___ | ___ | ___ | _____ |
| B. Pull back evenly to aspirate gastric contents. | ___ | ___ | ___ | _____ |
| (1) If checking for gastric residual when a small-bore tube is in place, consult employer policy. Remember that tube location is important. A tube in the small bowel would have ongoing secretions and much more residual, and therefore checking residuals would not be necessary. | | | | |
| C. Return aspirated contents to stomach if specified by employer policy. | ___ | ___ | ___ | _____ |
| 13. Flush tubing with 30 to 50 mL of tap water at room temperature. | ___ | ___ | ___ | _____ |
| 14. Label feeding tube bag. Complete and post nutrition label on bag to indicate type of formula, rate, time, and date. | ___ | ___ | ___ | _____ |
| 15. Initiate feeding. | | | | |
| A. Syringe or intermittent feeding | | | | |
| (1) Pinch proximal end of the feeding tube. | ___ | ___ | ___ | _____ |
| (2) Remove plunger from syringe, and attach barrel of syringe to end of tube. | ___ | ___ | ___ | _____ |
| (3) Fill syringe with measured amount of formula. Release tube and hold syringe high enough to allow it to empty gradually by gravity and refill; repeat until prescribed amount has been delivered to the patient. | ___ | ___ | ___ | _____ |
| (4) If feeding bag is used, hang feeding bag on an IV pole. Fill bag with prescribed amount of formula, and allow bag to empty gradually over at least 30 minutes, depending on the amount of feeding. | ___ | ___ | ___ | _____ |
| (5) Document tube assessment for placement, formula infusing, and infusion rate; elevate head of bed at least 45 degrees. | ___ | ___ | ___ | _____ |

*Continued*

444

| | S | U | NP | Comments |
|---|---|---|---|---|

B. Continuous-drip method

   (1) Prime and hang feeding bag and tubing.    ____  ____  ____  _____

   (2) Connect distal end of tubing to the proximal end of the feeding tube.    ____  ____  ____  _____

   (3) Connect tubing through infusion pump and set rate.    ____  ____  ____  _____

   (4) Do NOT hang any longer than a four-hour supply, to decrease risk of food spoilage or gastrointestinal infection or upset.    ____  ____  ____  _____

16. Advance the rate of tube feeding gradually.    ____  ____  ____  _____

17. After intermittent infusion or at end of continuous infusion, flush nasoenteral tubing with water. On average, 30 mL of water is used, but the amount can vary from 10 mL to over 30 mL. Repeat every four to six hours. Remove gloves, and perform hand hygiene.    ____  ____  ____  _____

18. When tube feedings are not being administered (e.g., they may be held before tests or procedures such as extubation), cap or clamp the proximal end of the feeding tube.    ____  ____  ____  _____

19. Rinse bag and tubing with water whenever feedings are interrupted or every 8 hours.    ____  ____  ____  _____

20. Change bag and tubing every 24 hours.    ____  ____  ____  _____

21. Measure amount of aspirate (residual) every 8 to 12 hours.    ____  ____  ____  _____

22. Monitor finger-stick blood glucose level every 6 hours until maximum administration rate is reached and maintained for 24 hours.    ____  ____  ____  _____

23. Monitor intake and output every 8 hours, and compute 24-hour totals.    ____  ____  ____  _____

24. Weigh patient daily until maximum administration rate is reached and maintained for 24 hours; then weigh patient three times per week.    ____  ____  ____  _____

25. Observe patient's respiratory status.    ____  ____  ____  _____

26. Observe return of normal laboratory values.    ____  ____  ____  _____

27. Record amount and type of feeding and patient's response to tube feeding, patency of tube, and any side effects.    ____  ____  ____  _____

28. Report patient's tolerance and adverse effects.    ____  ____  ____  _____

STUDENT: _____ DATE: _____

INSTRUCTOR: _____ DATE: _____

## Skill Performance Checklist
## Skill 42-5 Administering Enteral Feedings via Gastrostomy or Jejunostomy Tubes

| | S | U | NP | Comments |
|---|---|---|---|---|
| 1. Assess patient's need for enteral tube feedings: impaired swallowing, decreased level of consciousness, surgical procedures involving upper alimentary tract, need for long-term enteral nutrition. | ___ | ___ | ___ | _____ |
| 2. Obtain baseline weight and laboratory values. | ___ | ___ | ___ | _____ |
| 3. Verify physicians' order for formula, rate, route, and frequency. | ___ | ___ | ___ | _____ |
| 4. Perform hand hygiene. | ___ | ___ | ___ | _____ |
| 5. Explain procedure to patient. | ___ | ___ | ___ | _____ |
| 6. Auscultate for bowel sounds before feeding. Consult physician if bowel sounds are absent. | ___ | ___ | ___ | _____ |
| 7. Assess gastrostomy or jejunostomy site for breakdown, irritation, or drainage. | ___ | ___ | ___ | _____ |
| 8. Perform hand hygiene, and apply gloves. | ___ | ___ | ___ | _____ |
| 9. Prepare feeding container to administer formula. | | | | |
|    A. Have tube feeding at room temperature. | ___ | ___ | ___ | _____ |
|    B. Connect tubing to container as needed, or prepare ready-to-hang container. | ___ | ___ | ___ | _____ |
|    C. Shake formula container well, and fill container with formula. | ___ | ___ | ___ | _____ |
| 10. For intermittent feeding, have syringe ready, and be sure formula is at room temperature. | ___ | ___ | ___ | _____ |
| 11. Elevate head of bed 30 to 45 degrees. | ___ | ___ | ___ | _____ |
| 12. Apply gloves, and verify tube placement. | | | | |
|    A. Gastrostomy tube: Attach syringe and aspirate gastric secretions; observe their appearance, and check pH. Return aspirated contents to stomach unless volume exceeds 100 mL or specified amount based on patient's age. If the volume is greater than 100 mL or the specified amount on two consecutive assessments, hold feeding, and notify the physician. | ___ | ___ | ___ | _____ |
|    B. Jejunostomy tube: Aspirate intestinal secretions, observe their appearance and check pH. | ___ | ___ | ___ | _____ |
| 13. Flush with 30 mL of room-temperature tap water. | ___ | ___ | ___ | _____ |
| 14. Initiate feeding. | | | | |
|    A. Syringe or intermittent feeding | | | | |
|      (1) Pinch proximal end of the gastrostomy or jejunostomy feeding tube. | ___ | ___ | ___ | _____ |
|      (2) Remove plunger from syringe, and attach barrel of syringe to end of tube, then fill syringe with formula. | ___ | ___ | ___ | _____ |
|      (3) Release tube, and hold syringe high enough to allow it to empty gradually by gravity, then refill; repeat until prescribed amount has been delivered to patient. | ___ | ___ | ___ | _____ |
|    B. Continuous-drip method | | | | |
|      (1) Verify that volume in container is sufficient for length of feeding (four to eight hours; check manufacturer's recommendations). | ___ | ___ | ___ | _____ |
|      (2) Hang container on IV pole, and clear tubing of air. | ___ | ___ | ___ | _____ |
|      (3) Thread tubing into pump according to manufacturer's directions. | ___ | ___ | ___ | _____ |
|      (4) Connect tubing to end of gastrostomy or jejunostomy tube. | ___ | ___ | ___ | _____ |
|      (5) Begin infusion at prescribed rate. | ___ | ___ | ___ | _____ |
| 15. Administer water via feeding tube as ordered with or between feedings. | ___ | ___ | ___ | _____ |
| 16. Flush feeding tube with 30 mL of water every four to six hours and before and after administering medications via feeding tube. | ___ | ___ | ___ | _____ |
| 17. When tube feeding is not being administered, cap or clamp the proximal end of the feeding tube. | ___ | ___ | ___ | _____ |
| 18. Rinse container and tubing with warm water after all intermittent feedings. | ___ | ___ | ___ | _____ |

*Continued*

|  | S | U | NP | Comments |
|---|---|---|---|---|

19. Assess skin around tube exit site. Before site has healed, clean with normal saline. The skin around the tube should be cleansed daily with warm water and mild soap once site has healed. Fully healed tubing exit site is left open to air. Before healing, a small precut gauze dressing may be applied to exit site and secured with tape. The dressing is assessed for drainage and changed daily and as needed. If patient received nasogastric feedings before tube insertion and then undergoes a procedure, tube is not used for first four to six hours after procedure. (Patient will be on NPO status the night before the procedure. Postprocedure documentation—as per employer policy—will indicate when to use tube.) Feeding will resume at previous nasogastric rates once it is safe to begin feeding.

20. Dispose of supplies, and perform hand hygiene.

21. Evaluate patient's tolerance to tube feeding. Measure the amount of aspirate every 8 to 12 hours.

22. Monitor finger-stick blood glucose every 6 hours until maximum administration rate is reached and maintained for 24 hours.

23. Monitor intake and output every 24 hours.

24. Weigh patient daily until maximum administration rate is reached and maintained for 24 hours; then weigh patient three times per week at the same time using the same scale.

25. Observe return of normal laboratory values.

26. Inspect stoma for signs of impaired skin integrity.

27. Record amount and type of feeding, patient's response to tube feeding, patency of tube, condition of skin at tube site for tubes placed in abdominal wall, and any side effects.

28. Report patient's tolerance and adverse effects.

STUDENT: _____ DATE: _____

INSTRUCTOR: _____ DATE: _____

## Skill Performance Checklist
## Skill 42-6 Inserting a Large-Bore Nasoenteric or Orogastric Tube for Gastric Suctioning

| | S | U | NP | Comments |
|---|---|---|---|---|
| 1. Assess patient for the need for large-bore tube (i.e., for gastric suctioning or lavage). | ___ | ___ | ___ | _____ |
| A. Review physician's order for type of tube and enteral feeding schedule. | ___ | ___ | ___ | _____ |
| 2. Perform hand hygiene. Assess patency of nares. Have patient close each nostril alternately and breathe. Examine each naris for patency and skin breakdown. | ___ | ___ | ___ | _____ |
| 3. Assess the gag reflex. Place tongue blade in patient's mouth, touching uvula to induce a gag response. | ___ | ___ | ___ | _____ |
| 4. Review patient's medical history for nasal problems (e.g., nosebleeds, oral or facial surgery, anticoagulation therapy, history of aspiration). | ___ | ___ | ___ | _____ |
| 5. Stand on same side of bed as naris for insertion, and assist patient to high-Fowler's position unless that position is contraindicated. Place pillow behind patient's head and shoulders. | ___ | ___ | ___ | _____ |
| 6. Place absorbent pad over patient's chest. Keep facial tissues within reach. | ___ | ___ | ___ | _____ |
| 7. Determine length of tube to be inserted, and mark with tape. Traditional method: Measure distance from tip of nose to earlobe to xiphoid process of sternum. | ___ | ___ | ___ | _____ |
| 8. Prepare nasogastric or nasointestinal tube for intubation. | ___ | ___ | ___ | _____ |
| 9. Perform hand hygiene, and put on gloves. | ___ | ___ | ___ | _____ |
| 10. Cut tape 10 cm long, or prepare tube fixation device. Split one end of tape lengthwise 5 cm. | ___ | ___ | ___ | _____ |
| 11. Dip tube with surface lubricant into glass of water. If tube is not self-lubricating, then water-soluble lubricant should be used. | ___ | ___ | ___ | _____ |
| 12. Insert tube through nostril to back of throat (posterior nasopharynx). Aim back and down toward ear. | ___ | ___ | ___ | _____ |
| 13. Emphasize the need to mouth-breathe and swallow during the procedure (when possible). | ___ | ___ | ___ | _____ |
| 14. When tip of tube reaches the carina (about 25 cm in an adult), stop insertion, hold end of tube near your ear, and listen for air exchange from the distal portion of the tube. | ___ | ___ | ___ | _____ |
| 15. Check for position of tube in back of throat with penlight and tongue blade. | ___ | ___ | ___ | _____ |
| 16. Perform measures to verify placement of tube, by measuring pH. | ___ | ___ | ___ | _____ |
| A. Examine gastric contents and yield. | ___ | ___ | ___ | _____ |
| 17. After gastric aspirates are obtained, anchor tube to patient's nose, and avoid pressure on nares. Mark exit site on tube with indelible ink. Select one of the following options to secure tube: | | | | |
| A. Apply tape. | | | | |
| (1) Apply tincture of benzoin or other skin adhesive on tip of patient's nose and tube, and allow it to become "tacky." | ___ | ___ | ___ | _____ |
| (2) Place intact end of tape over bridge of patient's nose. Wrap each of the 5-cm strips around tube as it exits nose. | ___ | ___ | ___ | _____ |
| B. Apply tube fixation device, using shaped adhesive patch. | ___ | ___ | ___ | _____ |
| (1) Apply wide end of patch to bridge of patient's nose. | ___ | ___ | ___ | _____ |
| 18. Fasten end of nasogastric tube to patient's gown with a piece of tape (not safety pin). | ___ | ___ | ___ | _____ |
| 19. Remove gloves. Perform hand hygiene, then apply clean gloves and administer oral hygiene. Cleanse tubing at nostril. | ___ | ___ | ___ | _____ |
| 20. Remove gloves, dispose of equipment, and perform hand hygiene. | ___ | ___ | ___ | _____ |
| 21. Inspect naris and oropharynx for any irritation after insertion. | ___ | ___ | ___ | _____ |
| 22. Ask patient whether he or she feels comfortable. | ___ | ___ | ___ | _____ |
| 23. Observe patient for any difficulty breathing, for coughing, or for gagging. | ___ | ___ | ___ | _____ |
| 24. Auscultate lung sounds. | ___ | ___ | ___ | _____ |
| 25. Connect tube to suction device as ordered. | ___ | ___ | ___ | _____ |
| 26. Record the procedure. Identify the make and size of tube inserted, patient's response to procedure, and method used to confirm placement. | ___ | ___ | ___ | _____ |

STUDENT: _____ DATE: _____

INSTRUCTOR: _____ DATE: _____

## Skill Performance Checklist
## Skill 43-1 Collecting a Midstream (Clean-Voided) Urine Specimen

| | S | U | NP | Comments |
|---|---|---|---|---|
| 1. Assess the patient's voiding status. | | | | |
|   A. When patient last voided | ___ | ___ | ___ | _____ |
|   B. Level of awareness or developmental stage | ___ | ___ | ___ | _____ |
|   C. Mobility, balance, and physical limitations | ___ | ___ | ___ | _____ |
| 2. Assess the patient's understanding of the purpose of the test and method of collection. | ___ | ___ | ___ | _____ |
| 3. Explain the procedure to the patient. | | | | |
|   A. Reason why midstream specimen is needed | ___ | ___ | ___ | _____ |
|   B. Ways in which the patient and family can assist | ___ | ___ | ___ | _____ |
|   C. Ways to obtain a specimen free of feces | ___ | ___ | ___ | _____ |
| 4. Provide fluids to drink 30 minutes before collecting the specimen, unless contraindicated (i.e., fluid restriction) if the patient does not feel the urge to void. | ___ | ___ | ___ | _____ |
| 5. Provide privacy for the patient by closing the door or bed curtain. | | | | |
| 6. Give the patient or family members soap, washcloth, and towel to cleanse the perineal area. | ___ | ___ | ___ | _____ |
| 7. Perform hand hygiene, put on nonsterile gloves, and assist nonambulatory patients with perineal care. Assist female patient onto bedpan. | ___ | ___ | ___ | _____ |
| 8. Using surgical aseptic technique, open the sterile kit or prepare sterile supplies. Put on sterile gloves after opening the sterile specimen cup, placing the cap with sterile inside surface up; do not touch the inside of the container or cap. | ___ | ___ | ___ | _____ |
| 9. Pour antiseptic solution over cotton balls or gauze pads unless kit contains prepared gauze pads in antiseptic solution. | ___ | ___ | ___ | _____ |
| 10. Assist or allow the patient to cleanse perineal area and collect specimen. | ___ | ___ | ___ | _____ |
|   A. Female patient | | | | |
|     (1) Spread the patient's labia with the thumb and forefinger of your nondominant hand. | ___ | ___ | ___ | _____ |
|     (2) Cleanse the area with a cotton ball or gauze, moving from front (above urethral orifice) to back (toward anus). Using a fresh swab each time, repeat front-to-back motion three times (begin left side, then right side, then centre). | ___ | ___ | ___ | _____ |
|     (3) If employer policy indicates, rinse area with sterile water, and dry with cotton ball or gauze. | ___ | ___ | ___ | _____ |
|     (4) While you continue holding the patient's labia apart, the patient should initiate urine stream; after stream begins, pass container into stream, and collect 30 to 60 mL of urine. | ___ | ___ | ___ | _____ |
|   B. Male patient | | | | |
|     (1) Hold the patient's penis with one hand; using circular motion and antiseptic swab, cleanse the end of the penis, moving from centre to outside. In uncircumcised men, the foreskin should be retracted before cleansing. | ___ | ___ | ___ | _____ |
|     (2) If employer policy indicates, rinse the area with sterile water, and dry with a cotton ball or gauze. | ___ | ___ | ___ | _____ |
|     (3) After patient has initiated urine stream, pass specimen collection container into stream, and collect 30 to 60 mL of urine. | ___ | ___ | ___ | _____ |
| 11. Remove specimen container before urine flow stops and before you release labia or penis. The patient finishes voiding in the bedpan or toilet. If the foreskin was retracted for specimen collection, it must be replaced over the glans. | ___ | ___ | ___ | _____ |
| 12. Replace cap securely on the specimen container (touch only the outside). | ___ | ___ | ___ | _____ |
| 13. Cleanse any urine from the exterior surface of the container. Place the container in a plastic specimen bag. | ___ | ___ | ___ | _____ |
| 14. Remove the bedpan (if applicable), assist the patient to a comfortable position, and provide a handwashing basin, if needed. | ___ | ___ | ___ | _____ |

*Continued*

450

| | S | U | NP | Comments |
|---|---|---|---|---|
| 15. Label the specimen, and attach a laboratory requisition slip. | ___ | ___ | ___ | _____ |
| 16. Remove gloves, dispose of them in a proper receptacle, and perform hand hygiene. | ___ | ___ | ___ | _____ |
| 17. Transport the specimen to the laboratory within 15 minutes, or refrigerate it immediately. | ___ | ___ | ___ | _____ |
| 18. Record date and time urine specimen was obtained in nurses' notes. | ___ | ___ | ___ | _____ |
| 19. Notify physician or nurse practitioner of any significant abnormalities. | ___ | ___ | ___ | _____ |

STUDENT: _____ DATE: _____

INSTRUCTOR: _____ DATE: _____

## Skill Performance Checklist
## Skill 43-2 Inserting a Straight or In-Dwelling Catheter

| | S | U | NP | Comments |
|---|---|---|---|---|
| 1. Review the patient's medical record, including physician's order and nurses' notes. | ___ | ___ | ___ | _____ |
| 2. Close bedside curtain or door. | ___ | ___ | ___ | _____ |
| 3. Assess the status of the patient. | | | | |
| A. Urinary status: Ask the patient when he or she last voided, or check intake and output flow sheet, or palpate bladder. | ___ | ___ | ___ | _____ |
| B. Level of awareness or developmental stage | ___ | ___ | ___ | _____ |
| C. Mobility and physical limitations of the patient | ___ | ___ | ___ | _____ |
| D. The patient's gender and age | ___ | ___ | ___ | _____ |
| E. Bladder distension | ___ | ___ | ___ | _____ |
| F. Perform hand hygiene. Apply clean gloves. Inspect perineum for erythema, drainage, and odour. | ___ | ___ | ___ | _____ |
| G. Any pathological condition that may impair passage of catheter (e.g., enlarged prostate in men) | ___ | ___ | ___ | _____ |
| H. Allergies | ___ | ___ | ___ | _____ |
| 4. Assess the patient's knowledge of the purpose of catheterization. | ___ | ___ | ___ | _____ |
| 5. Explain the procedure to the patient. | ___ | ___ | ___ | _____ |
| 6. Arrange for extra nursing assistance if necessary. | ___ | ___ | ___ | _____ |
| 7. Perform hand hygiene. | ___ | ___ | ___ | _____ |
| 8. Raise the bed to an appropriate working height. | ___ | ___ | ___ | _____ |
| 9. Facing the patient, stand on the left side of the bed if you are right-handed (on the right side if you are left-handed). Clear the bedside table, and arrange equipment. | ___ | ___ | ___ | _____ |
| 10. Raise the side rail on the opposite side of the bed, and put the side rail down on the working side. | ___ | ___ | ___ | _____ |
| 11. Place a waterproof pad under the patient. | ___ | ___ | ___ | _____ |
| 12. Position the patient. | | | | |
| A. Female patient | | | | |
| (1) Assist the patient to the dorsal recumbent position. Ask the patient to relax her thighs so that the hips can be rotated externally. | ___ | ___ | ___ | _____ |
| (2) Assist the patient to a side-lying (Sims') position with the upper leg flexed at the hip if the patient is unable to assume the dorsal recumbent position. If this position is used, you must take extra precautions to cover the rectal area with a drape to reduce chance of cross-contamination. | ___ | ___ | ___ | _____ |
| B. Male patient | | | | |
| (1) Assist the patient to a supine position with thighs slightly abducted. | ___ | ___ | ___ | _____ |
| 13. Drape patient. | | | | |
| A. Female patient | | | | |
| (1) Drape with a bath blanket. Place the blanket in a diamond shape over the patient, with one corner at the patient's midsection, side corners over each thigh and the abdomen, and the last corner over the perineum. | ___ | ___ | ___ | _____ |
| B. Male patient | | | | |
| (1) Drape the patient's upper trunk with a bath blanket, and cover the lower extremities with bedsheets so that only genitalia are exposed. | ___ | ___ | ___ | _____ |
| 14. Wearing disposable gloves, wash the perineal area with soap and water as needed; dry thoroughly. Remove and discard gloves; perform hand hygiene. | ___ | ___ | ___ | _____ |
| 15. Position a lamp to illuminate the perineal area. (If you use a flashlight, have an assistant hold it.) | ___ | ___ | ___ | _____ |
| 16. Open the package containing the drainage system. Place the drainage bag over the edge of the bottom bed frame, and bring the drainage tube up between side rail and mattress. | ___ | ___ | ___ | _____ |

*Continued*

|  | S | U | NP | Comments |
|---|---|---|---|---|
| 17. Open the catheterization kit according to directions, keeping the bottom of the container sterile. | ___ | ___ | ___ | _____ |
| 18. Place the plastic bag that contained the kit within reach of the work area to use as a waterproof bag in which used supplies can be placed for disposal. | ___ | ___ | ___ | _____ |
| 19. Put on sterile gloves. | ___ | ___ | ___ | _____ |
| 20. Organize supplies on a sterile field. Open the inner sterile package containing the catheter. Pour sterile antiseptic solution into the correct compartment containing sterile cotton balls. Open the packet containing lubricant. Remove the specimen container (the lid should be placed loosely on top) and the prefilled syringe from the collection compartment of the tray, and set them aside on the sterile field. | ___ | ___ | ___ | _____ |
| 21. Lubricate 2.5 to 5 cm of the catheter for female patients and 12.5 to 17.5 cm for male patients. | ___ | ___ | ___ | _____ |
| 22. Apply the sterile drape. | | | | |
| A. Female patient | | | | |
| (1) Allow the top edge of the drape to form a cuff over both gloved hands. Place the drape on the bed between the patient's thighs. Slip the cuffed edge just under the patient's buttocks, taking care not to touch the contaminated surface with gloves. | ___ | ___ | ___ | _____ |
| (2) Pick up the fenestrated sterile drape and allow it to unfold without touching any unsterile objects. Apply the drape over the patient's perineum, exposing labia, taking care not to touch the contaminated surface with gloves. | ___ | ___ | ___ | _____ |
| B. Male patient | | | | |
| (1) Two methods are used for draping, depending on preference. | | | | |
| *First method*: Apply the drape over the thighs and under the penis without completely opening fenestrated drape. | ___ | ___ | ___ | _____ |
| *Second method*: Apply the drape over the thighs just below the penis. Pick up the fenestrated sterile drape, allow it to unfold without touching any unsterile objects, and drape it over the penis, with the fenestrated slit resting over the penis. | ___ | ___ | ___ | _____ |
| 23. Place the sterile tray and contents on the sterile drape. Open the specimen container. | ___ | ___ | ___ | _____ |
| 24. Cleanse the urethral meatus. | | | | |
| A. Female patient | | | | |
| (1) With your nondominant hand, carefully retract the labia to fully expose the urethral meatus. Maintain position of your nondominant hand throughout the procedure. | ___ | ___ | ___ | _____ |
| (2) Holding forceps in your sterile dominant hand, pick up a cotton ball saturated with antiseptic solution, and clean the patient's perineal area, wiping from clitoris toward anus (front to back). Using a new cotton ball for each area, wipe along the far labial fold, the near labial fold, and directly over the centre of the urethral meatus. | ___ | ___ | ___ | _____ |
| B. Male patient | | | | |
| (1) If the patient is not circumcised, retract the foreskin with your nondominant hand. Grasp the penis at the shaft, just below the glans. Retract the urethral meatus between your thumb and forefinger. Maintain your nondominant hand in this position throughout the procedure. | ___ | ___ | ___ | _____ |
| (2) With your sterile dominant hand, use forceps to pick up a cotton ball saturated with antiseptic solution, and clean the penis. Move the cotton ball in circular motion from the urethral meatus down to the base of the glans. Repeat cleansing three more times, using a clean cotton ball each time. | ___ | ___ | ___ | _____ |
| 25. Pick up the catheter with your gloved dominant hand, 7.5 to 10 cm from the catheter tip. Hold the end of the catheter loosely coiled in the palm of your dominant hand. (Optional: Grasp the catheter with forceps.) | ___ | ___ | ___ | _____ |

*Continued*

|  | S | U | NP | Comments |
|---|---|---|---|---|

26. Insert the catheter.
    A. Female patient
       (1) Ask the patient to bear down gently as if to void urine, and slowly insert the catheter through the urethral meatus. — — — _____
       (2) Advance the catheter a total of 5 to 7.5 cm in an adult or until urine flows out the catheter's end. When urine appears, advance the catheter another 2.5 to 5 cm. Do not use force against resistance. — — — _____
       (3) Release the labia, and hold the catheter securely with your nondominant hand. Slowly inflate the balloon if the in-dwelling catheter is being used. — — — _____
    B. Male patient
       (1) Lift the patient's penis to position perpendicular to the patient's body, and apply light traction. — — — _____
       (2) Ask the patient to bear down gently as if to void urine, and slowly insert the catheter through the urethral meatus. — — — _____
       (3) Advance the catheter 17 to 22.5 cm in an adult or until urine flows out the catheter's end. If resistance is felt, withdraw the catheter; do not force it through the urethra. When urine appears, advance the catheter another 2.5 to 5 cm. Do not use force against resistance. — — — _____
       (4) Lower the patient's penis, and hold the catheter securely in your nondominant hand. Place the end of the catheter in the urine tray. Inflate the balloon if an in-dwelling catheter is being used. — — — _____
       (5) Reduce (or reposition) the foreskin. — — — _____
27. Collect the urine specimen as needed. Fill the specimen cup or jar to the desired level (20 to 30 mL) by holding the end of the catheter over the cup with your dominant hand. — — — _____
28. Allow the patient's bladder to empty fully (about 800 to 1000 mL) unless institution policy restricts the maximal volume of urine to drain with each catheterization. Check institution policy before beginning catheterization. — — — _____
29. Inflate the balloon fully per manufacturer's recommendation, and then release the catheter with your nondominant hand, and pull gently. — — — _____
30. Attach the end of the in-dwelling catheter to the collecting tube of the drainage system. The drainage bag must be below the level of the bladder. Attach the bag to the bed frame; do not place the bag on the bed's side rails. — — — _____
31. Anchor the catheter.
    A. Female patient
       (1) Secure the catheter tubing to the patient's inner thigh or abdomen with a strip of nonallergenic tape (or multipurpose tube holders with a Velcro strap). Allow for slack so that movement of the thigh does not create tension on the catheter. — — — _____
    B. Male patient
       (1) Secure the catheter tubing to the top of the thigh or lower abdomen (with the penis directed toward the chest). Allow for slack so that movement does not create tension on the catheter. — — — _____
32. Assist the patient to a comfortable position. Wash and dry the perineal area as needed. — — — _____
33. Remove gloves, and dispose of equipment, drapes, and urine in proper receptacles. — — — _____
34. Perform hand hygiene. — — — _____
35. Palpate the patient's bladder. — — — _____
36. Ask whether the patient is comfortable. — — — _____
37. Observe the character and amount of urine in the drainage system. — — — _____
38. Ensure that no urine is leaking from the catheter or tubing connections. — — — _____
39. Record and report size of catheter inserted, amount of fluid used to inflate the balloon, characteristics and amount of urine, specimen collection (if performed), and patient's response to procedure and teaching concepts. — — — _____
40. Initiate intake and output records. — — — _____

STUDENT: _____  DATE: _____

INSTRUCTOR: _____  DATE: _____

## Skill Performance Checklist
## Skill 43-3 In-Dwelling Catheter Care

|  | S | U | NP | Comments |
|---|---|---|---|---|
| 1. Assess for episodes of bowel incontinence or patient discomfort, or provide care as per employer routine regarding hygiene measures. | ___ | ___ | ___ | _____ |
| 2. Explain the procedure to the patient. Offer the able patient an opportunity to perform self-care. | ___ | ___ | ___ | _____ |
| 3. Close the door or bedside curtain. | ___ | ___ | ___ | _____ |
| 4. Perform hand hygiene. | ___ | ___ | ___ | _____ |
| 5. Position patient. | | | | |
| A. Female patient | | | | |
| (1) Dorsal recumbent position | ___ | ___ | ___ | _____ |
| B. Male patient | | | | |
| (1) Supine or Fowler's position | ___ | ___ | ___ | _____ |
| 6. Place a waterproof pad under the patient. | ___ | ___ | ___ | _____ |
| 7. Drape a bath blanket over the patient so that only the perineal area is exposed. | ___ | ___ | ___ | _____ |
| 8. Put on disposable gloves. | ___ | ___ | ___ | _____ |
| 9. Remove the anchor device to free the catheter tubing. | ___ | ___ | ___ | _____ |
| 10. With your nondominant hand, prepare the patient for the procedure. | ___ | ___ | ___ | _____ |
| A. Female patient | | | | |
| (1) Gently retract the labia to expose the urethral meatus and the catheter insertion site fully, maintaining the position of your hand throughout the procedure. | ___ | ___ | ___ | _____ |
| B. Male patient | | | | |
| (1) Retract foreskin if the patient is not circumcised, and hold the penis at the shaft just below the glans, maintaining this position throughout the procedure. | ___ | ___ | ___ | _____ |
| 11. Assess the urethral meatus and surrounding tissue for inflammation, swelling, and discharge. Note amount, colour, odour, and consistency of discharge. Ask the patient whether any burning sensation or discomfort has been experienced. | ___ | ___ | ___ | _____ |
| 12. Cleanse the perineal tissue. | ___ | ___ | ___ | _____ |
| A. Female patient | | | | |
| (1) Use a clean cloth and perineal cleanser. Cleanse around the urethral meatus and catheter. Moving from pubis toward anus, clean the labia minora. Use a clean side of the cloth for each wipe. Clean around the anus. Dry each area well. | ___ | ___ | ___ | _____ |
| B. Male patient | | | | |
| (1) While spreading the urethral meatus, cleanse around the catheter first, and then wipe in circular motion around meatus and glans. | ___ | ___ | ___ | _____ |
| 13. Reassess the urethral meatus for discharge. | ___ | ___ | ___ | _____ |
| 14. With the towel and perineal cleanser, wipe in a circular motion along the length of the catheter for 10 cm. | ___ | ___ | ___ | _____ |
| 15. In a male patient, reduce (or reposition) the foreskin. | ___ | ___ | ___ | _____ |
| 16. Reanchor the catheter tubing. | ___ | ___ | ___ | _____ |
| 17. Place the patient in a safe, comfortable position. | ___ | ___ | ___ | _____ |
| 18. Dispose of contaminated supplies, remove gloves, and perform hand hygiene. | ___ | ___ | ___ | _____ |
| 19. Report and record the presence and characteristics of drainage, the condition of the perineal tissue, and any discomfort reported by the patient. | ___ | ___ | ___ | _____ |
| 20. If infection is suspected, report your findings to a physician. | ___ | ___ | ___ | _____ |

STUDENT: _____   DATE: _____

INSTRUCTOR: _____   DATE: _____

## Skill Performance Checklist
## Skill 43-4 Closed and Open Catheter Irrigation

| | S | U | NP | Comments |
|---|---|---|---|---|
| 1. Assess the physician's order for type of irrigation and irrigation solution to use. | ___ | ___ | ___ | _____ |
| 2. Assess the colour of urine and the presence of mucus or sediment. | ___ | ___ | ___ | _____ |
| 3. Determine the type of catheter in place. | | | | |
| A. Triple-lumen (one lumen to inflate the balloon, one to instill irrigation solution, one to allow outflow of urine) | ___ | ___ | ___ | _____ |
| B. Double-lumen (one lumen to inflate the balloon, one to allow outflow of urine) | ___ | ___ | ___ | _____ |
| 4. Determine the patency of the drainage tubing. | ___ | ___ | ___ | _____ |
| 5. Assess the amount of urine in the drainage bag (you may want to empty the drainage bag before irrigation). | ___ | ___ | ___ | _____ |
| 6. Explain the procedure and purpose to the patient. | ___ | ___ | ___ | _____ |
| 7. Perform hand hygiene, and put on clean disposable gloves for closed methods. | ___ | ___ | ___ | _____ |
| 8. Provide privacy by pulling bed curtains closed. Fold back covers so that the catheter is exposed. Cover the patient's upper torso with the bath blanket. | ___ | ___ | ___ | _____ |
| 9. Assess the lower abdomen for bladder distension. | | | | |
| 10. Position the patient in the dorsal recumbent or supine position. | ___ | ___ | ___ | _____ |
| 11. Closed intermittent irrigation (with double-lumen catheter) | | | | |
| A. Prepare prescribed solution in a sterile graduated cup. | ___ | ___ | ___ | _____ |
| B. Draw sterile solution into a syringe, using aseptic technique. | ___ | ___ | ___ | _____ |
| C. Clamp in-dwelling catheter just distal to soft injection (specimen) port. | ___ | ___ | ___ | _____ |
| D. Cleanse injection port with antiseptic swab (same port used for specimen collection). | ___ | ___ | ___ | _____ |
| E. Insert the syringe at a 30-degree angle toward the bladder. | ___ | ___ | ___ | _____ |
| F. Slowly inject fluid into the catheter and bladder. | ___ | ___ | ___ | _____ |
| G. Withdraw the syringe, remove the clamp, and allow solution to drain into the drainage bag. If ordered by the physician, keep the bag clamped to allow solution to remain in the bladder for a short time (20 to 30 minutes). | ___ | ___ | ___ | _____ |
| 12. Closed continuous irrigation (with triple-lumen catheter) | | | | |
| A. Using aseptic technique, insert the tip of the sterile irrigation tubing into the bag of sterile irrigating solution. | ___ | ___ | ___ | _____ |
| B. Close the clamp on the tubing, and hang the bag of solution on the intravenous pole. | ___ | ___ | ___ | _____ |
| C. Open the clamp, and allow solution to flow through tubing, keeping the end of tubing sterile. Close the clamp. | ___ | ___ | ___ | _____ |
| D. Wipe off the irrigation port of the triple-lumen catheter, or attach a sterile Y connector to the double-lumen catheter, and then attach to irrigation tubing. | ___ | ___ | ___ | _____ |
| E. Be sure that the drainage bag and tubing are securely connected to drainage port of the triple-lumen catheter or other arm of the Y connector. | ___ | ___ | ___ | _____ |
| F. For intermittent flow, clamp the tubing on the drainage system, open the clamp on the irrigation tubing, and allow the prescribed amount of fluid to enter the bladder (100 mL is normal for adults). Close the irrigation clamp and then open the drainage tubing clamp. (Optional: Leave the clamp closed for 20 to 30 minutes if ordered.) | ___ | ___ | ___ | _____ |
| G. For continuous drainage, calculate the drip rate, and adjust the clamp on the irrigation tubing accordingly. Ensure that the clamp on the drainage tubing is open, and check the volume of drainage in the drainage bag. Ensure that drainage tubing is patent, and avoid kinks. | ___ | ___ | ___ | _____ |

*Continued*

458

|  | S | U | NP | Comments |
|---|---|---|---|---|

13. Open irrigation (with double-lumen catheter)
    A. Open the sterile irrigation tray, establish a sterile field, pour the required volume of sterile solution into the sterile container, and replace the cap on the large container of solution. ___ ___ ___ _____
    B. Put on sterile gloves. ___ ___ ___ _____
    C. Position the sterile waterproof drape under the catheter. ___ ___ ___ _____
    D. Aspirate 30 mL of solution into the sterile irrigating syringe. ___ ___ ___ _____
    E. Move the sterile collection basin close to the patient's thighs. ___ ___ ___ _____
    F. Disconnect the catheter from the drainage tubing, allowing urine from the catheter to flow into the collection basin. Allow urine in tubing to flow into the drainage bag. Cover the end of tubing with a sterile protective cap. Position tubing in a safe place.
    G. Insert the tip of the syringe into the catheter lumen, and gently instill solution. ___ ___ ___ _____
    H. Withdraw the syringe, lower the catheter, and allow solution to drain into the basin. Repeat instillation until the prescribed solution has been used or until drainage is clear, depending on the purpose of irrigation. ___ ___ ___ _____
    I. If solution does not return, have the patient turn onto the side facing you. If changing position does not help, reinsert the syringe and gently aspirate solution. ___ ___ ___ _____
    J. After irrigation is complete, remove the protector cap from the tubing, cleanse the end with an alcohol swab (or the employer's recommended solution), and re-establish the drainage system. ___ ___ ___ _____
14. Reanchor the catheter to the patient with tape or an elastic tube holder. ___ ___ ___ _____
15. Assist the patient to a comfortable position. ___ ___ ___ _____
16. Lower the bed to the lowest position. Put the side rails up if appropriate. ___ ___ ___ _____
17. Dispose of contaminated supplies, remove gloves, and perform hand hygiene. ___ ___ ___ _____
18. Calculate the amount of fluid used to irrigate the bladder, and subtract from total output. ___ ___ ___ _____
19. Assess characteristics of output: viscosity, colour, and presence of matter (e.g., sediment, clots, blood). ___ ___ ___ _____
20. Record type and amount of irrigation solution used, amount returned as drainage, and the character of drainage. ___ ___ ___ _____
21. Record and report any findings such as complaints of bladder spasms, inability to instill fluid into bladder, or presence of blood clots. ___ ___ ___ _____

STUDENT: _____ DATE: _____

INSTRUCTOR: _____ DATE: _____

## Skill Performance Checklist
## Skill 45-1 Moving and Positioning Patients in Bed

| | S | U | NP | Comments |
|---|---|---|---|---|
| 1. Assess the patient's body alignment and comfort level while the patient is lying down. | ___ | ___ | ___ | _____ |
| 2. Assess for risk factors that may contribute to complications of immobility. | | | | |
| A. Paralysis: Hemiparesis resulting from cerebrovascular accident; decreased sensation | ___ | ___ | ___ | _____ |
| B. Impaired mobility: Traction or arthritis or other contributing disease processes | ___ | ___ | ___ | _____ |
| C. Impaired circulation | ___ | ___ | ___ | _____ |
| D. Age: Very young children, older adults | ___ | ___ | ___ | _____ |
| E. Level of consciousness and mental status | ___ | ___ | ___ | _____ |
| F. Condition of patient's skin | ___ | ___ | ___ | _____ |
| 3. Assess patient's physical ability to help with moving and positioning. | | | | |
| A. Age | ___ | ___ | ___ | _____ |
| B. Level of consciousness and mental status | ___ | ___ | ___ | _____ |
| C. Disease process | ___ | ___ | ___ | _____ |
| D. Strength, coordination | ___ | ___ | ___ | _____ |
| E. Range of motion | ___ | ___ | ___ | _____ |
| 4. Assess physician's orders. Clarify whether any positions are contraindicated because of the patient's condition (e.g., spinal cord injury; respiratory difficulties; certain neurological conditions; presence of incisions, drain, or tubing). | ___ | ___ | ___ | _____ |
| 5. Perform hand hygiene. | ___ | ___ | ___ | _____ |
| 6. Assess for the presence of tubes, incisions, and equipment (e.g., traction). | ___ | ___ | ___ | _____ |
| 7. Assess the ability and motivation of the patient, family members, and primary caregiver to participate in moving and positioning the patient in bed in anticipation of discharge to home. | ___ | ___ | ___ | _____ |
| 8. Raise the level of the bed to a comfortable working height. Get extra help if needed. | ___ | ___ | ___ | _____ |
| 9. Perform hand hygiene. | ___ | ___ | ___ | _____ |
| 10. Explain the procedure to the patient. | ___ | ___ | ___ | _____ |
| 11. Position the patient flat in bed, if this is tolerated. | ___ | ___ | ___ | _____ |
| 12. Position the patient in bed. | | | | |
| A. Assist the patient in moving up in bed (one or two nurses). *Note:* Only a young child or a lightweight patient requiring minimal assistance can be safely moved by one nurse. | ___ | ___ | ___ | _____ |
| (1) Remove the pillow from under the patient's head and shoulders, and place the pillow at the head of the bed. Ask the patient to cross arms across the chest. | ___ | ___ | ___ | _____ |
| (2) Face the head of the bed. | ___ | ___ | ___ | _____ |
| (a) Each nurse should have one arm under the patient's shoulders and one arm under the patient's thighs. | ___ | ___ | ___ | _____ |
| (d) Alternative position: Position one nurse at patient's upper body. The nurse's arm nearest the head of the bed should be under the patient's head and opposite shoulder; other arm should be under the patient's closest arm and shoulder. Position the other nurse at the patient's lower torso. The nurse's arms should be under the patient's lower back and torso. | ___ | ___ | ___ | _____ |
| (3) Place your feet apart, with the foot nearest head of bed behind the other foot (forward–backward stance). | ___ | ___ | ___ | _____ |
| (4) Ask the patient to flex knees with feet flat on the bed. | ___ | ___ | ___ | _____ |
| (5) Instruct the patient to flex the neck, tilting the chin toward the chest. | ___ | ___ | ___ | _____ |
| (6) Instruct the patient to assist moving by pushing with feet on the bed surface. | ___ | ___ | ___ | _____ |

*Continued*

|  | S | U | NP | Comments |
|---|---|---|---|---|

(7) Flex your knees and hips, bringing your forearms closer to the level of the bed.

(8) Instruct the patient to push with heels and elevate the trunk while breathing out, thus moving toward the head of the bed, on a count of three.

(9) On a count of three, rock and shift weight from back to front leg. At the same time, patient pushes with heels and elevates the trunk.

B. Move immobile patient up in bed with drawsheet or friction-reducing device (two nurses are needed).

(1) Adjust the bed to an appropriate height for the caregiver's body mechanics. Place a drawsheet or friction-reducing device under the patient by turning the patient side to side. Have the sheet extend from shoulders to thighs. Return the patient to the supine position.

(2) Position one nurse at each side of patient.

(3) Grasp the drawsheet or friction-reducing device firmly near the patient, with your palms facing up.

(4) Place your feet apart in forward–backward stance. Flex your knees and hips. Shift weight from front to back leg, and move patient and drawsheet or friction-reducing device to the desired position in bed.

(5) Realign the patient in correct body alignment.

C. Position the patient in supported Fowler's position.

(1) Elevate the head of the bed 45 to 60 degrees.

(2) Rest the patient's head against the mattress or on a small pillow.

(3) Use pillows to support the patient's arms and hands if the patient does not have voluntary control or use of them.

(4) Position the pillow at the patient's lower back.

(5) Place a small pillow or roll under the thigh.

(6) Position the patient's heel in heel boots or other heel pressure-relief device.

D. Position a hemiplegic patient in supported Fowler's position.

(1) Elevate the head of the bed 45 to 60 degrees.

(2) Position the patient in a sitting position as straight as possible.

(3) Position the patient's head on a small pillow with the chin slightly forward. If the patient is totally unable to control head movement, hyperextension of the neck must be avoided.

(4) Flex the patient's knees and hips by using a pillow or folded blanket under the knees.

(5) Support the patient's feet in dorsiflexion with a firm pillow or therapeutic boots or splints.

E. Position the patient in the supine position.

(1) Be sure the patient is comfortable on the back, with the head of the bed flat.

(2) Place a small rolled towel under the lumbar area of the back.

(3) Place a pillow under the upper shoulders, neck, or head.

(4) Place trochanter rolls or sandbags parallel to the lateral surface of the thighs.

(5) Place a small pillow or roll under the ankles to elevate the heels.

(6) Place firm pillows against the bottom of the patient's feet.

(7) Place foot boots on the patient's feet, if necessary.

(8) Place pillows under the patient's pronated forearms, and keep the patient's upper arms parallel to the patient's body.

(9) Place hand rolls in patient's hands. Consider occupational therapy referral for the use of hand splints, if necessary.

F. Position a hemiplegic patient in the supine position.

(1) Place the patient on the back, with the head of the bed flat.

(2) Place a folded towel or small pillow under the patient's shoulder or affected side.

(3) Keep the affected arm away from the patient's body, with the elbow extended and palm up. (An alternative is to place the arm out to the side, with the elbow bent and hand toward the head of the bed.)

(4) Place a folded towel under the hip of the patient's involved side.

*Continued*

| | S | U | NP | Comments |
|---|---|---|---|---|

(5) Flex the patient's affected knee 30 degrees by supporting it on a pillow or folded blanket.

(6) Support the patient's feet with soft pillows at a right angle to the leg.

G. Position the patient in prone position. Two staff members are required to position the patient safely.

    (1) With the drawsheet under the patient, move the patient toward one side of the bed. Ensure that the side rail on the opposite side is up for safety. With the patient supine, roll the patient over the arm positioned close to the body, with elbow straight, and hand under hip. Position on abdomen in the centre of the bed.

    (2) Turn the patient's head to one side, and support the head with a small pillow.

    (3) Place a small pillow under the patient's abdomen, below the level of the diaphragm.

    (4) Support the arms in flexed position, level at the shoulders.

    (5) Support the lower legs with pillows to elevate the toes.

H. Position a hemiplegic patient in prone position.

    (1) Move the patient toward the unaffected side.

    (2) Roll the patient onto that side.

    (3) Place a pillow on the patient's abdomen.

    (4) Roll the patient onto the abdomen by positioning the involved arm close to the patient's body, with the elbow straight and hand under hip. Roll the patient carefully over the arm.

    (5) Turn the patient's head toward the involved side.

    (6) Position the patient's involved arm out to the side, with elbow bent, hand toward the head of the bed, and fingers extended (if possible).

    (7) Flex the knees slightly by placing a pillow under the legs from knees to ankles.

    (8) Keep feet at right angles by using a pillow high enough to keep toes off the mattress.

I. Position the patient in lateral (side-lying) position.

    (1) Lower the head of bed completely or as low as the patient can tolerate.

    (2) Position the patient to the side of the bed.

    (3) Prepare to turn the patient onto the side. Flex the patient's knee that will not be next to the mattress. Place one of your hands on the patient's hip and your other hand on the patient's shoulder.

    (4) Roll the patient onto the side, toward you.

    (5) Place a pillow under the patient's head and neck.

    (6) Bring the shoulder blade forward.

    (7) Position both the patient's arms in slightly flexed position. The upper arm is supported by a pillow level with shoulder; other arm, by the mattress.

    (8) Place a tuck-back pillow behind the patient's back. (Make it by folding a pillow lengthwise. The smooth area is slightly tucked under the patient's back.)

    (9) Place a pillow under the semiflexed upper leg level at hip from groin to foot.

   (10) Place a sandbag parallel to the plantar surface of the dependent foot.

J. Position the patient in Sims' (semiprone) position.

    (1) Lower the head of the bed completely.

    (2) Be sure the patient is comfortable in the supine position.

    (3) Position the patient in the lateral position, with the dependent arm straight along the patient's body and with the patient lying partially on the abdomen.

    (4) Carefully lift the patient's dependent shoulder, and bring the arm back behind the patient.

    (5) Place a small pillow under the patient's head.

    (6) Place a pillow under the flexed upper arm, supporting the arm level with the shoulder.

    (7) Place pillow under flexed upper leg, supporting the leg level with the hip.

    (8) Place sandbags or pillows parallel to the plantar surface of the foot.

*Continued*

466

|  | S | U | NP | Comments |
|---|---|---|---|---|
| K. Logroll the patient (this requires three nurses). | | | | |
| (1) Place a pillow between the patient's knees. | ___ | ___ | ___ | _____ |
| (2) Cross the patient's arms on the chest. | ___ | ___ | ___ | _____ |
| (3) Position two nurses on the side of the bed to which the patient will be turned. Position the third nurse on the other side of the bed. | ___ | ___ | ___ | _____ |
| (4) Fan-fold or roll the drawsheet or pull sheet. | ___ | ___ | ___ | _____ |
| (5) Move the patient as one unit in a smooth, continuous motion on the count of three. | ___ | ___ | ___ | _____ |
| (6) The nurse on the opposite side of the bed places pillows along the length of the patient. | ___ | ___ | ___ | _____ |
| (7) Gently lean the patient as a unit back toward the pillows for support. | ___ | ___ | ___ | _____ |
| 13. Perform hand hygiene. | ___ | ___ | ___ | _____ |
| 14. Evaluate the patient's comfort level and ability to assist in position change. | ___ | ___ | ___ | _____ |
| 15. After each position change, evaluate the patient's body alignment and the presence of any pressure areas. Observe for areas of erythema or breakdown involving skin. | ___ | ___ | ___ | _____ |
| 16. Record procedure and observations (e.g., condition of skin, joint movement, patient's ability to assist with positioning). | ___ | ___ | ___ | _____ |
| 17. Report observations at change of shift, and document in nurses' notes. | ___ | ___ | ___ | _____ |

STUDENT: _____    DATE: _____

INSTRUCTOR: _____    DATE: _____

## Skill Performance Checklist
## Skill 45-2 Using Safe and Effective Transfer Techniques

| | S | U | NP | Comments |
|---|---|---|---|---|
| 1. Assess the patient for the following: | | | | |
| A. Muscle strength (legs and upper arms) | ___ | ___ | ___ | _____ |
| B. Joint mobility and contracture formation | ___ | ___ | ___ | _____ |
| C. Paralysis or paresis (spastic or flaccid) | ___ | ___ | ___ | _____ |
| D. Orthostatic hypotension | ___ | ___ | ___ | _____ |
| E. Activity tolerance | ___ | ___ | ___ | _____ |
| F. Presence of pain | ___ | ___ | ___ | _____ |
| G. Vital signs | ___ | ___ | ___ | _____ |
| 2. Assess the patient's sensory status. | | | | |
| A. Adequacy of central and peripheral vision | ___ | ___ | ___ | _____ |
| B. Adequacy of hearing | ___ | ___ | ___ | _____ |
| C. Loss of sensation | ___ | ___ | ___ | _____ |
| 3. Assess the patient's cognitive status. | ___ | ___ | ___ | _____ |
| 4. Assess the patient's level of motivation. | | | | |
| A. The patient's eagerness or unwillingness to be mobile | ___ | ___ | ___ | _____ |
| B. Whether the patient avoids activity and offers excuses | ___ | ___ | ___ | _____ |
| 5. Assess previous mode of transfer (if applicable). | ___ | ___ | ___ | _____ |
| 6. Assess patient's specific risk of falling when transferred. | ___ | ___ | ___ | _____ |
| 7. Assess special transfer equipment needed for the home setting. Assess the home environment for hazards. | ___ | ___ | ___ | _____ |
| 8. Perform hand hygiene. | ___ | ___ | ___ | _____ |
| 9. Explain the procedure to the patient. | ___ | ___ | ___ | _____ |
| 10. Transfer the patient. | | | | |
| A. Assist the patient to a sitting position (bed at waist level). | | | | |
| (1) Place the patient in supine position. | ___ | ___ | ___ | _____ |
| (2) Face the head of the bed at a 45-degree angle, and remove pillows. | ___ | ___ | ___ | _____ |
| (3) Place your feet apart, with the foot nearer the bed behind the other foot, continuing at a 45-degree angle to the head of the bed. | ___ | ___ | ___ | _____ |
| (4) Place your hand farther from the patient under the patient's shoulders, supporting the patient's head and cervical vertebrae. | ___ | ___ | ___ | _____ |
| (5) Place your other hand on the bed surface. | ___ | ___ | ___ | _____ |
| (6) Raise the patient to a sitting position by shifting weight from your front to back leg. Pivot your feet as weight is shifted from your front to back leg so that your upper body does not twist. | ___ | ___ | ___ | _____ |
| (7) Push against the bed, using your arm that is placed on the bed surface. | ___ | ___ | ___ | _____ |
| B. Assist the patient to sitting position on the side of the bed with the bed in low position. | | | | |
| (1) Turn the patient to the side, facing you on the side of the bed on which the patient will be sitting. | ___ | ___ | ___ | _____ |
| (2) With the patient supine, raise the head of the bed 30 degrees. | ___ | ___ | ___ | _____ |
| (3) Stand opposite the patient's hips. Turn diagonally so that you face the patient and the far corner of the foot of the bed. | ___ | ___ | ___ | _____ |
| (4) Place your feet apart, with the foot closer to the head of the bed in front of the other foot. | ___ | ___ | ___ | _____ |
| (5) Place your arm nearer the head of the bed under the patient's shoulder, supporting the patient's head and neck. | ___ | ___ | ___ | _____ |
| (6) Place your other arm over the patient's thighs. | ___ | ___ | ___ | _____ |
| (7) Move the patient's lower legs and feet over the side of the bed. Pivot toward your rear leg, allowing the patient's upper legs to swing downward. | ___ | ___ | ___ | _____ |
| (8) At the same time, shift weight to your rear leg, and elevate the patient. Pivot your feet in the direction of movement to avoid twisting your upper body. | ___ | ___ | ___ | _____ |

*Continued*

|  | S | U | NP | Comments |
|---|---|---|---|---|

C. Transfer the patient from bed to chair with the bed in low position.

  (1) Assist the patient to a sitting position on the side of the bed. Position the chair at a 45-degree angle to the bed. If the patient has hemiparesis or hemiplegia, place the chair on the patient's unaffected side. ___ ___ ___ _____

  (2) Apply a transfer belt or other transfer aids. ___ ___ ___ _____

  (3) Ensure that the patient has stable, nonskid shoes. The patient's weight-bearing or unaffected (strong) leg is placed back, and the affected (weak) knee is slightly forward or parallel. ___ ___ ___ _____

  (4) Place your feet shoulder-width apart. ___ ___ ___ _____

  (5) Flex your hips and knees, supporting the patient's weaker knee or leg with your knees. ___ ___ ___ _____

  (6) Grasp the transfer belt from underneath. ___ ___ ___ _____

  (7) Rock the patient up to a standing position on a count of three while straightening your hips and legs and keeping your knees slightly flexed. Unless it is contraindicated, the patient may be instructed to use hands to push up, if applicable. ___ ___ ___ _____

  (8) Maintain stability of the patient's weak or paralyzed leg between your knees. ___ ___ ___ _____

  (9) Pivot on your foot farther from the chair. Instruct the patient to stand straight. Pivot your body in the direction of the chair, instructing the patient to take small steps toward the chair. Ask the patient to tell you when the chair touches the back of his or her knees. ___ ___ ___ _____

  (10) Instruct the patient to use armrests on the chair for support, and ease the patient into the chair. ___ ___ ___ _____

  (11) Flex your hips and knees while lowering the patient into the chair. ___ ___ ___ _____

  (12) Assess the patient for proper alignment for the sitting position. Provide support for paralyzed extremities. Use a lapboard or sling to support a flaccid arm. Stabilize the patient's legs with a bath blanket or pillow. ___ ___ ___ _____

  (13) Praise the patient's progress, effort, and performance. ___ ___ ___ _____

D. Transfer the patient from bed to stretcher or another bed, using a drawsheet or friction-reducing device.

  (1) Place the bed flat, and position at the same level as the stretcher. Ensure that bed brakes are locked. ___ ___ ___ _____

  (2) Lower the side rails. Have two caregivers stand on the side where the stretcher will be, while the third caregiver stands on the other side. ___ ___ ___ _____

  (3) Two caregivers help the patient roll onto the side toward one caregiver. ___ ___ ___ _____

  (4) Work together to position the friction-reducing device properly under the patient's back. ___ ___ ___ _____

  (5) Roll the stretcher alongside the bed. Lock the wheels of the stretcher once it is in place. Instruct the patient to place his or her arms across the chest and not to move. ___ ___ ___ _____

  (6) All three caregivers place feet widely apart with one foot slightly in front of the other, and grasp the friction-reducing device. ___ ___ ___ _____

  (7) On the count of three, caregivers pull the patient from the bed onto the stretcher, using the friction-reducing device and shifting weight appropriately. ___ ___ ___ _____

  (8) Put up the side rail of the stretcher on the side where caregivers are, and then roll the stretcher away from the side of the bed, and put side rails up on that side. ___ ___ ___ _____

E. Use mechanical or hydraulic lift to transfer the patient from bed to chair. Before using the lift, be thoroughly familiar with its operation. Gather all necessary equipment and caregivers.

  (1) Choose the appropriate-size sling for the patient's weight and height. Position lift properly at the bedside. ___ ___ ___ _____

  (2) Position a chair near the bed, and allow adequate space to manoeuvre the lift. ___ ___ ___ _____

  (3) Raise the bed to a high position, with the mattress flat. Lower the side rail. ___ ___ ___ _____

  (4) Keep the bed side rail up on the side opposite you. ___ ___ ___ _____

*Continued*

| | S | U | NP | Comments |
|---|---|---|---|---|
| (5) Roll the patient on the side away from you. | ___ | ___ | ___ | _____ |
| (6) Place the sling under the patient. Place the lower edge under the patient's knees (wide piece) and the upper edge under the patient's shoulders (narrow piece). | ___ | ___ | ___ | _____ |
| (7) Roll the patient to the opposite side, and pull the sling through. | ___ | ___ | ___ | _____ |
| (8) Roll the patient supine onto the sling. | ___ | ___ | ___ | _____ |
| (9) Remove the patient's glasses, if present. | ___ | ___ | ___ | _____ |
| (10) If you are using a transportable Hoyer lift, place the lift's horseshoe bar under the side of the bed (on the side with the chair). | ___ | ___ | ___ | _____ |
| (11) Lower the horizontal bar to sling level by releasing the hydraulic valve. Lock the valve. | ___ | ___ | ___ | _____ |
| (12) Attach hooks on the strap (chain) to holes in the sling. Short straps hook to top holes of the sling; longer straps hook to bottom holes of the sling. | ___ | ___ | ___ | _____ |
| (13) Elevate the head of the bed. | ___ | ___ | ___ | _____ |
| (14) Fold the patient's arms over the chest. | ___ | ___ | ___ | _____ |
| (15) Pump hydraulic handle using long, slow, even strokes until patient is raised off bed. Use the steering handle to pull the lift from the bed and manoeuvre to the chair. | ___ | ___ | ___ | _____ |
| (16) Position the patient, and slowly lower the patient into the chair. | ___ | ___ | ___ | _____ |
| (17) Close the check valve as soon as the patient is down, and release straps. | ___ | ___ | ___ | _____ |
| (18) Remove straps and mechanical or hydraulic lift. | ___ | ___ | ___ | _____ |
| (19) Check the patient's sitting alignment. | ___ | ___ | ___ | _____ |
| 11. Perform hand hygiene. | ___ | ___ | ___ | _____ |
| 12. With each transfer, evaluate the patient's tolerance and level of fatigue and comfort. | ___ | ___ | ___ | _____ |
| 13. After each transfer, evaluate the patient's body alignment. | ___ | ___ | ___ | _____ |
| 14. Record procedure, including the following pertinent observations: patient's weakness, ability to follow directions, weight-bearing ability, balance, and ability to pivot; number of personnel needed to assist; and amount of assistance (muscle strength) required. | ___ | ___ | ___ | _____ |
| 15. Report any unusual occurrence to the nurse in charge. Report transfer ability and assistance needed to next shift or other caregivers. Report progress or remission to rehabilitation staff (physiotherapist or occupational therapist). | ___ | ___ | ___ | _____ |

STUDENT: _____   DATE: _____

INSTRUCTOR: _____   DATE: _____

## Skill Performance Checklist
## Skill 46-1 Assessment for Risk of Pressure Ulcer Development

| | S | U | NP | Comments |
|---|---|---|---|---|
| 1. Identify at-risk individuals needing prevention and the specific factors placing them at risk. | | | | |
| A. Use a validated risk assessment tool (e.g., the Braden Scale). | ___ | ___ | ___ | _____ |
| B. Assess the patient on admission to the hospital, long-term care facility, home care program, or other health care facility. | ___ | ___ | ___ | _____ |
| C. Inspect the condition of the patient's skin at least once a day, and examine all bony prominences, noting skin integrity. (Check employer policy for reassessment, and reassess at periodic intervals.) If redness or discoloration is noted, palpate area of redness for blanchable erythema. | ___ | ___ | ___ | _____ |
| D. Observe all assistive devices, such as braces or casts, and medical equipment, such as nasogastric and enteral tubes and catheters, for pressure points. | ___ | ___ | ___ | _____ |
| 2. Determine the patient's ability to respond meaningfully to pressure-related discomfort (sensory perception). | ___ | ___ | ___ | _____ |
| 3. Assess the degree to which the patient's skin is exposed to moisture. | ___ | ___ | ___ | _____ |
| 4. Evaluate the patient's activity level. | | | | |
| A. Determine the patient's ability to change and control body position (mobility). | ___ | ___ | ___ | _____ |
| B. Determine patient's preferred positions. | ___ | ___ | ___ | _____ |
| 5. Assess the patient's usual food and fluid intake pattern (nutrition and hydration). | | | | |
| A. Review weight pattern and nutritional laboratory values. | ___ | ___ | ___ | _____ |
| B. Complete a fluid intake assessment. | ___ | ___ | ___ | _____ |
| 6. Evaluate the presence of friction and shear. | ___ | ___ | ___ | _____ |
| 7. Document the risk assessment on admission, on a regular basis according to institutional policy, and if any change in status occurs. | ___ | ___ | ___ | _____ |
| A. Observe the Braden Scale scores. As they become lower, predicted risk becomes higher. Existing skin breakdown increases the risk by one level. | ___ | ___ | ___ | _____ |
| B. Link the risk assessment to preventive protocols. | ___ | ___ | ___ | _____ |
| C. Institute mild-risk interventions (score of 15 to 16). Plan of care should include frequent turning; maximum remobilization; off-loading of heel pressure; use of pressure-reducing support surface; management of moisture, nutrition, and friction and shear. | ___ | ___ | ___ | _____ |
| D. Institute moderate-risk interventions (score of 13 to 14). Plan of care should include interventions for mild risk, as well as use of foam wedges to position the patient in the 30-degree lateral position. | ___ | ___ | ___ | _____ |
| E. Institute high-risk interventions (score of 10 to 12). Plan of care should include interventions for moderate risk, as well as instructions to turn the patient with small shifts in weight. | ___ | ___ | ___ | _____ |
| F. Institute very high-risk interventions (score of 10). Plan of care should include interventions for high risk, as well as use of a pressure-relieving surface, which still requires frequent repositioning of patient. | ___ | ___ | ___ | _____ |
| 8. Provide education to the patient and family regarding pressure ulcer risk and prevention. | ___ | ___ | ___ | _____ |
| 9. Evaluate measures to reduce pressure ulcer development. | | | | |
| A. Observe the patient's skin for areas at risk. | ___ | ___ | ___ | _____ |
| B. Observe the patient's tolerance for positioning. | ___ | ___ | ___ | _____ |
| C. Monitor the success of a toileting program or other measures to reduce the frequency of incontinence of urine or stool. | ___ | ___ | ___ | _____ |
| D. Evaluate laboratory nutrition values. | ___ | ___ | ___ | _____ |
| 10. Record patient's risk score and subscores. | ___ | ___ | ___ | _____ |
| 11. Record appearance of skin (at pressure points, etc.). | ___ | ___ | ___ | _____ |
| 12. Describe position, turning intervals, pressure-relieving devices, and other prevention strategies. | ___ | ___ | ___ | _____ |
| 13. Report any need for additional consultations (e.g., wound care specialist or dietitian) for the high-risk patient. | ___ | ___ | ___ | _____ |

STUDENT: _____  DATE: _____

INSTRUCTOR: _____  DATE: _____

## Skill Performance Checklist
## Skill 46-2 Treating Pressure Ulcers

|  | S | U | NP | Comments |
|---|---|---|---|---|
| 1. Assess the patient's level of comfort, using a scale of 1 to 10, and the need for pain medication. | ___ | ___ | ___ | _____ |
| 2. Determine whether the patient has allergies to topical agents. | ___ | ___ | ___ | _____ |
| 3. Review physician's order for topical agent or dressing. | ___ | ___ | ___ | _____ |
| 4. Close the room door or bedside curtains. Position the patient to allow dressing removal. | ___ | ___ | ___ | _____ |
| 5. Perform hand hygiene, and put on clean gloves. Remove dressing and place it in a plastic bag. | ___ | ___ | ___ | _____ |
| 6. Assess pressure ulcer(s). All pressure ulcers require individual assessments. | | | | |
| A. Note colour, type, and percentage of tissue present in the wound base. | ___ | ___ | ___ | _____ |
| B. Measure width and length of the ulcer(s). Determine width by measuring the dimension from left to right and the length from top to bottom. | ___ | ___ | ___ | _____ |
| C. Measure depth of pressure ulcer by using a sterile cotton-tipped applicator. | ___ | ___ | ___ | _____ |
| D. Measure depth of undermining, using a cotton-tipped applicator to gently probe under skin edges. | ___ | ___ | ___ | _____ |
| 7. Assess the periwound skin; check for maceration, redness, and denuded areas. | ___ | ___ | ___ | _____ |
| 8. Change to sterile gloves (check employer policy). | ___ | ___ | ___ | _____ |
| 9. Cleanse ulcer thoroughly with normal saline or a cleansing agent. Use an irrigating syringe for deep ulcers. | ___ | ___ | ___ | _____ |
| 10. Apply topical agents, as prescribed. | | | | |
| A. Enzymes (where available) | | | | |
| (1) Apply a thin, even layer of ointment over only necrotic areas of the ulcer where eschar has been scored if required. Protect periwound skin. | ___ | ___ | ___ | _____ |
| (2) Apply secondary nonadherent gauze dressing directly over the ulcer. | ___ | ___ | ___ | _____ |
| (3) Tape securely in place. | ___ | ___ | ___ | _____ |
| B. Hydrogel | | | | |
| (1) Cover the surface of the ulcer with a thin layer of hydrogel, using the applicator or your gloved hand. | ___ | ___ | ___ | _____ |
| (2) Apply secondary nonadherent gauze dressing or transparent dressing over the wound, and make it adhere to intact skin. | ___ | ___ | ___ | _____ |
| C. Calcium alginate | | | | |
| (1) Lightly pack wound with alginate, using an applicator or your gloved fingers. | ___ | ___ | ___ | _____ |
| (2) Apply secondary dressing of nonadherent gauze, absorbent pad, or foam over alginate. Tape in place. | ___ | ___ | ___ | _____ |
| 11. Remove gloves, and dispose of soiled supplies. Perform hand hygiene. | ___ | ___ | ___ | _____ |
| 12. Assess the pressure ulcer at each dressing change or sooner if the wound or patient's condition deteriorates. Utilize the employer's tool for wound assessment. | ___ | ___ | ___ | _____ |
| 13. Compare wound assessment to the identified plan of care. If the wound is not progressing toward healing, it will be indicated by an increase in size, increased presence of pain, foul-smelling drainage, or increase in devitalized tissue. | ___ | ___ | ___ | _____ |
| 14. Complete wound documentation required for one of the wound assessment instruments per employer's protocol. | ___ | ___ | ___ | _____ |
| 15. Record assessment of ulcer in patient's record. | ___ | ___ | ___ | _____ |
| 16. Describe type of topical agent used, dressing applied, and patient's response. | ___ | ___ | ___ | _____ |
| 17. Report any deterioration in ulcer appearance. | ___ | ___ | ___ | _____ |

STUDENT: _____ DATE: _____

INSTRUCTOR: _____ DATE: _____

## Skill Performance Checklist
## Skill 46-3 Applying Dry and Moist Dressings

| | S | U | NP | Comments |
|---|---|---|---|---|
| 1. Perform hand hygiene. Obtain information about size and location of the wound. | ___ | ___ | ___ | _____ |
| 2. Assess the patient's level of comfort. | ___ | ___ | ___ | _____ |
| 3. Review orders for dressing change procedure. | ___ | ___ | ___ | _____ |
| 4. Explain procedure to the patient, and instruct the patient not to touch the wound area or sterile supplies. | ___ | ___ | ___ | _____ |
| 5. Close the room or cubicle curtains and windows. | ___ | ___ | ___ | _____ |
| 6. Position the patient comfortably, and drape with a bath blanket to expose only the wound site. | ___ | ___ | ___ | _____ |
| 7. Place a disposable bag within reach of the work area. Fold the top of bag to make a cuff. | ___ | ___ | ___ | _____ |
| 8. Put on a face mask and protective eyewear, if needed. | ___ | ___ | ___ | _____ |
| 9. Put on clean, disposable gloves, and remove tape, bandage, or ties. | ___ | ___ | ___ | _____ |
| 10. Remove tape. Pull parallel to skin toward dressing; remove remaining adhesive from skin. | ___ | ___ | ___ | _____ |
| 11. With your gloved hand, carefully remove gauze dressings, one layer at a time, taking care not to dislodge drains or tubes. | ___ | ___ | ___ | _____ |
|    A. If dressing sticks on a wet-to-dry dressing, do not moisten it; instead gently free the dressing, and alert the patient of potential discomfort. | ___ | ___ | ___ | _____ |
| 12. Observe the character and amount of drainage on the dressing and the appearance of wound. | ___ | ___ | ___ | _____ |
| 13. Fold dressings with drainage contained inside, and remove gloves inside out. With small dressings, remove gloves inside out over the dressing. Dispose of gloves and soiled dressings in disposable bag. Perform hand hygiene. | ___ | ___ | ___ | _____ |
| 14. Open the sterile dressing tray or individually wrapped sterile supplies. Place on the bedside table. | ___ | ___ | ___ | _____ |
| 15. If ordered, cleanse or irrigate the wound. | | | | |
|    A. Pour the ordered solution into the sterile irrigation container. | ___ | ___ | ___ | _____ |
|    B. Using a syringe, gently allow the solution to flow over the wound. | ___ | ___ | ___ | _____ |
|    C. Continue until the irrigation flow is clear. | ___ | ___ | ___ | _____ |
|    D. Dry the surrounding skin. | ___ | ___ | ___ | _____ |
| 16. Apply dressing. | | | | |
|    A. Dry dressing | | | | |
|      (1) Put on sterile gloves. | ___ | ___ | ___ | _____ |
|      (2) Inspect the wound for appearance, drains, drainage, and integrity. | ___ | ___ | ___ | _____ |
|      (3) Cleanse the wound with solution. | ___ | ___ | ___ | _____ |
|        (a) Clean from the least contaminated area to the most contaminated area. | ___ | ___ | ___ | _____ |
|      (4) Dry the area. | ___ | ___ | ___ | _____ |
|      (5) Apply sterile, dry dressing to cover the wound. | ___ | ___ | ___ | _____ |
|      (6) Apply topper dressing if indicated. | ___ | ___ | ___ | _____ |
|    B. Moist dressing | | | | |
|      (1) Put on clean gloves. | | | | |
|      (2) Remove and discard old dressings. | ___ | ___ | ___ | _____ |
|      (3) Assess the surrounding skin. Discard gloves. | ___ | ___ | ___ | _____ |
|      (4) Put on sterile gloves. | ___ | ___ | ___ | _____ |
|      (5) Cleanse the wound base with normal saline or commercially prepared wound cleanser. Assess the wound base. | ___ | ___ | ___ | _____ |
|      (6) Moisten gauze with the prescribed solution. Gently wring out excess solution. Unfold gauze. | ___ | ___ | ___ | _____ |

*Continued*

| | S | U | NP | Comments |
|---|---|---|---|---|

(7) Apply gauze as a single layer directly onto the wound surface. If the wound is deep, gently pack dressing into the wound base by hand or with forceps until all wound surfaces are in contact with the gauze. If tunnelling is present, use a cotton-tipped applicator to place gauze into the tunnelled area. Be sure gauze does not touch the surrounding skin.

(8) Cover with sterile dry gauze and topper dressing.

17. Secure dressing.

  A. Tape: Apply nonallergenic tape to secure dressing in place.

  B. Montgomery ties

    (1) Expose adhesive surface of tape on the end of each tie.

    (2) Place ties on opposite sides of the dressing.

    (3) Place adhesive directly on the skin, or use a skin barrier.

  C. For dressings on an extremity, secure dressing with rolled gauze or an elastic net.

18. Remove gloves, and dispose of them in the bag. Remove any mask or eyewear.

19. Dispose of supplies, and perform hand hygiene.

20. Assist the patient to a comfortable position.

21. Report brisk, bright-red bleeding or evidence of wound dehiscence or evisceration to health care provider immediately.

22. Report wound and periwound tissue appearance, colour, and tissue type and presence and characteristics of exudate, type and amount of dressings used, and tolerance of patient to procedure.

23. Record patient's level of comfort.

24. Write date and time dressing applied on tape in ink (not marker).

STUDENT: _____   DATE: _____

INSTRUCTOR: _____   DATE: _____

## Skill Performance Checklist
## Skill 46-4 Performing Wound Irrigation

| | S | U | NP | Comments |
|---|---|---|---|---|
| 1. Assess the patient's level of pain. Administer prescribed analgesic 30 to 45 minutes before starting wound irrigation procedure. | ___ | ___ | ___ | _____ |
| 2. Review the medical record for physician's prescription for irrigation of open wound and type of solution to be used. | ___ | ___ | ___ | _____ |
| 3. Assess recent recording of signs and symptoms related to patient's open wound. | | | | |
| A. Condition of skin and wound | ___ | ___ | ___ | _____ |
| B. Elevation of body temperature | ___ | ___ | ___ | _____ |
| C. Drainage from wound (amount, colour) | ___ | ___ | ___ | _____ |
| D. Odour | ___ | ___ | ___ | _____ |
| E. Consistency of drainage | ___ | ___ | ___ | _____ |
| F. Size of wound, including depth, length, and width | ___ | ___ | ___ | _____ |
| 4. Explain the procedure of wound irrigation and cleansing to the patient. | ___ | ___ | ___ | _____ |
| 5. Perform hand hygiene. | ___ | ___ | ___ | _____ |
| 6. Position the patient comfortably to permit gravitational flow of irrigating solution through the wound and into the collection receptacle. Position the patient so that the wound is vertical to the collection basin. | ___ | ___ | ___ | _____ |
| 7. Warm irrigation solution to approximately body temperature. | ___ | ___ | ___ | _____ |
| 8. Form a cuff on the waterproof bag, and place the bag near the bed. | ___ | ___ | ___ | _____ |
| 9. Close the room door or bed curtains. | ___ | ___ | ___ | _____ |
| 10. Put on gown and goggles, if needed. | ___ | ___ | ___ | _____ |
| 11. Put on disposable gloves, remove soiled dressing, and discard in waterproof bag. Discard gloves. | ___ | ___ | ___ | _____ |
| 12. Prepare equipment; open sterile supplies. | ___ | ___ | ___ | _____ |
| 13. Put on sterile gloves (check employer policy). | ___ | ___ | ___ | _____ |
| 14. Irrigating a wound with a wide opening: | | | | |
| A. Fill a 35-mL syringe with irrigation solution. | ___ | ___ | ___ | _____ |
| B. Attach a 19-gauge needle or angiocatheter. | ___ | ___ | ___ | _____ |
| C. Hold the syringe tip 2.5 cm above the upper end of the wound and over the area being cleansed. | ___ | ___ | ___ | _____ |
| D. Using continuous pressure, flush the wound; repeat steps 14A, B, and C until the solution draining into the basin is clear. | ___ | ___ | ___ | _____ |
| 15. Irrigating a deep wound with a very small opening: | | | | |
| A. Attach a soft angiocatheter to the filled irrigating syringe. | ___ | ___ | ___ | _____ |
| B. Lubricate the tip of the catheter with irrigating solution; then gently insert the tip of the catheter, and pull out about 1 cm. | ___ | ___ | ___ | _____ |
| C. Using slow, continuous pressure, flush wound. | ___ | ___ | ___ | _____ |
| D. Pinch off the catheter just below the syringe while keeping the catheter in place. | ___ | ___ | ___ | _____ |
| E. Remove and refill the syringe. Reconnect it to the catheter, and repeat steps 15A to D until solution draining into basin is clear. | ___ | ___ | ___ | _____ |
| 16. Cleanse the wound with a hand-held shower. | | | | |
| A. With the patient seated comfortably in the shower chair, adjust the spray to gentle flow; water temperature should be warm. | ___ | ___ | ___ | _____ |
| B. Cover the showerhead with a clean washcloth, if needed. | ___ | ___ | ___ | _____ |
| C. Have the patient shower for 5 to 10 minutes with the showerhead 30 cm from the wound. | ___ | ___ | ___ | _____ |
| 17. Obtain cultures, if needed, after cleansing with nonbacteriostatic saline. | ___ | ___ | ___ | _____ |
| 18. Dry the wound edges with gauze; dry the patient, if a shower or whirlpool is used. | ___ | ___ | ___ | _____ |
| 19. Apply appropriate dressing. | ___ | ___ | ___ | _____ |
| 20. Remove gloves and, if worn, mask, goggles, and gown. | ___ | ___ | ___ | _____ |
| 21. Dispose of equipment and soiled supplies. Perform hand hygiene. | ___ | ___ | ___ | _____ |
| 22. Assist the patient to a comfortable position. | ___ | ___ | ___ | _____ |

*Continued*

478

| | S | U | NP | Comments |
|---|---|---|---|---|
| 23. Assess the type of tissue in the wound bed. | ___ | ___ | ___ | _____ |
| 24. Inspect the dressing periodically. | ___ | ___ | ___ | _____ |
| 25. Evaluate skin integrity. | ___ | ___ | ___ | _____ |
| 26. Observe the patient for signs of discomfort. | ___ | ___ | ___ | _____ |
| 27. Observe for presence of retained irrigant. | ___ | ___ | ___ | _____ |
| 28. Record wound irrigation and patient response on progress notes. | ___ | ___ | ___ | _____ |
| 29. Immediately report to attending physician any evidence of fresh bleeding, sharp increase in pain, retention of irrigant, or signs of shock. | ___ | ___ | ___ | _____ |

STUDENT: _____   DATE: _____

INSTRUCTOR: _____   DATE: _____

## Skill Performance Checklist
## Skill 46-5 Applying an Abdominal or Breast Binder

|  | S | U | NP | Comments |
|---|---|---|---|---|
| 1. Observe the patient with a need for support of the thorax or abdomen. Observe ability to breathe deeply and cough effectively. | ___ | ___ | ___ | _____ |
| 2. Review the medical record for whether a medical prescription for a particular binder is required and reasons for application. | ___ | ___ | ___ | _____ |
| 3. Inspect the skin for actual or potential alterations in integrity. Observe for irritation, abrasion, skin surfaces that rub against each other, or allergic response to adhesive tape used to secure dressing. | ___ | ___ | ___ | _____ |
| 4. Inspect any surgical dressing. | ___ | ___ | ___ | _____ |
| 5. Assess the patient's comfort level, using an analogue scale of 0 to 10, noting any objective signs and symptoms of pain. | ___ | ___ | ___ | _____ |
| 6. Gather necessary data regarding the size of patient and appropriate binder. | ___ | ___ | ___ | _____ |
| 7. Explain the procedure to the patient. | ___ | ___ | ___ | _____ |
| 8. Teach the skill to the patient or significant other. | ___ | ___ | ___ | _____ |
| 9. Perform hand hygiene and put on gloves (if you are likely to contact wound drainage). | ___ | ___ | ___ | _____ |
| 10. Close the curtains or room door. | ___ | ___ | ___ | _____ |
| 11. Apply the binder. | | | | |
| A. Abdominal binder | | | | |
| (1) Position the patient in the supine position with the head slightly elevated and knees slightly flexed. | ___ | ___ | ___ | _____ |
| (2) Fan-fold the far side of the binder toward the midline of the binder. | ___ | ___ | ___ | _____ |
| (3) Instruct and help the patient to roll away from you toward the raised side rail while firmly supporting the abdominal incision and dressing with hands. | ___ | ___ | ___ | _____ |
| (4) Place the fan-folded ends of the binder under the patient. | ___ | ___ | ___ | _____ |
| (5) Instruct or assist patient to roll over the folded ends. | ___ | ___ | ___ | _____ |
| (6) Unfold and stretch the ends out smoothly on the far side of the bed. | ___ | ___ | ___ | _____ |
| (7) Instruct the patient to roll back into the supine position. | ___ | ___ | ___ | _____ |
| (8) Adjust the binder so that the supine patient is centred over the binder; use the symphysis pubis and costal margins as lower and upper landmarks. | ___ | ___ | ___ | _____ |
| (9) Close the binder. Pull one end of the binder over the centre of the patient's abdomen. While maintaining tension on that end of the binder, pull the opposite end of binder over the centre, and secure with Velcro closure tabs, metal fasteners, or horizontally placed safety pins. | ___ | ___ | ___ | _____ |
| B. Breast binder | | | | |
| (1) Assist the patient in placing arms through the binder's armholes. | ___ | ___ | ___ | _____ |
| (2) Assist the patient to the supine position in bed. | ___ | ___ | ___ | _____ |
| (3) Pad the area under the breasts, if necessary. | ___ | ___ | ___ | _____ |
| (4) Using Velcro closure tabs or horizontally placed safety pins, secure the binder at nipple level first. Continue closure process above and then below the nipple line until the entire binder is closed. | ___ | ___ | ___ | _____ |
| (5) Make appropriate adjustments, including individualizing fit of shoulder straps and pinning waistline darts to reduce binder size. | ___ | ___ | ___ | _____ |
| (6) Instruct the patient in self-care related to reapplying breast binder, and observe skill development. | ___ | ___ | ___ | _____ |
| 12. Remove gloves, and perform hand hygiene. | ___ | ___ | ___ | _____ |
| 13. Assess the patient's comfort level, using an analogue scale of 0 to 10, noting any objective signs and symptoms. | ___ | ___ | ___ | _____ |
| 14. Adjust the binder, as necessary. | ___ | ___ | ___ | _____ |
| 15. Observe the site for skin integrity, circulation, and characteristics of the wound. (Periodically remove binder and surgical dressing to assess wound characteristics.) | ___ | ___ | ___ | _____ |

*Continued*

|  | S | U | NP | Comments |
|---|---|---|---|---|
| 16. Assess the patient's ability to breathe properly. | ___ | ___ | ___ | _____ |
| 17. Identify the patient's need for assistance with activities such as hair combing. | ___ | ___ | ___ | _____ |
| 18. Report any skin irritation at between-shift report. | ___ | ___ | ___ | _____ |
| 19. Record application of binder, condition of skin, circulation, integrity of dressing, and patient's comfort level. | ___ | ___ | ___ | _____ |
| 20. Report ineffective lung expansion to physician immediately. | ___ | ___ | ___ | _____ |

STUDENT: _____     DATE: _____

INSTRUCTOR: _____     DATE: _____

## Skill Performance Checklist
## Skill 46-6 Applying an Elastic Bandage

|  | S | U | NP | Comments |
|---|---|---|---|---|
| 1. Perform hand hygiene and put on gloves, if needed. Inspect the patient's skin for alterations in integrity as indicated by abrasions, discoloration, chafing, or edema. (Look carefully at bony prominences.) | ___ | ___ | ___ | _____ |
| 2. Inspect surgical dressing. Remove gloves and perform hand hygiene. | ___ | ___ | ___ | _____ |
| 3. Observe adequacy of circulation (distal to bandage) by noting surface temperature, skin colour, and sensation of body parts to be wrapped. | ___ | ___ | ___ | _____ |
| 4. Review the medical record for specific orders related to application of elastic bandage. Note the area to be covered, the type of bandage required, the frequency of change, and previous response to treatment. | ___ | ___ | ___ | _____ |
| 5. Identify patient's and primary caregiver's current knowledge level of skill, if bandaging will be continued at home. | ___ | ___ | ___ | _____ |
| 6. Explain the procedure to the patient. | ___ | ___ | ___ | _____ |
| 7. Teach the skill to the patient or primary caregiver. | ___ | ___ | ___ | _____ |
| 8. Perform hand hygiene and put on gloves if drainage is present. | ___ | ___ | ___ | _____ |
| 9. Close the room door or curtains. | ___ | ___ | ___ | _____ |
| 10. Help the patient assume a comfortable, anatomically correct position. | ___ | ___ | ___ | _____ |
| 11. Hold a roll of elastic bandage in your dominant hand, and use your other hand to lightly hold beginning of bandage at the distal body part. Continue transferring roll to dominant hand as bandage is wrapped. | ___ | ___ | ___ | _____ |
| 12. Apply bandage from the distal point toward the proximal boundary, using a variety of turns to cover various shapes of body parts. | ___ | ___ | ___ | _____ |
| 13. Unroll and very slightly stretch bandage. | ___ | ___ | ___ | _____ |
| 14. Overlap turns by one-half to two-thirds' width of the bandage roll. | ___ | ___ | ___ | _____ |
| 15. Secure the first bandage with a clip or tape before applying additional rolls. | ___ | ___ | ___ | _____ |
| 16. Apply additional rolls without leaving any skin surface uncovered. Secure the last bandage applied. | ___ | ___ | ___ | _____ |
| 17. Remove gloves, if worn, and perform hand hygiene. | | | | |
| A. Assess distal circulation when the bandage application is complete and at least twice during the next eight-hour period. | ___ | ___ | ___ | _____ |
| B. Observe skin colour for pallor or cyanosis. | ___ | ___ | ___ | _____ |
| C. Palpate skin for warmth. | ___ | ___ | ___ | _____ |
| D. Palpate pulses, and compare them bilaterally. | ___ | ___ | ___ | _____ |
| E. Ask whether the patient is aware of pain, numbness, tingling, or other discomfort. | ___ | ___ | ___ | _____ |
| F. Observe mobility of the extremity. | ___ | ___ | ___ | _____ |
| 18. Have the patient demonstrate bandage application. | ___ | ___ | ___ | _____ |
| 19. Document condition of the wound, integrity of dressing, application of bandage, circulation, and patient's comfort level. | ___ | ___ | ___ | _____ |
| 20. Report any changes in neurological or circulatory status to the nurse in charge or physician. | ___ | ___ | ___ | _____ |

STUDENT: _____  DATE: _____

INSTRUCTOR: _____  DATE: _____

## Skill Performance Checklist
## Skill 48-1 Demonstrating Postoperative Exercises

| | S | U | NP | Comments |
|---|---|---|---|---|
| 1. Assess the patient for risk of postoperative respiratory complications. Review the medical history to identify the presence of chronic pulmonary conditions (e.g., emphysema, chronic bronchitis, asthma), any condition that affects chest wall movement, history of smoking, and presence of reduced hemoglobin. | ___ | ___ | ___ | _____ |
| 2. Assess the patient's ability to cough and breathe deeply by having the patient take a deep breath and observing movement of shoulders and chest wall. Measure chest excursion during deep breath. Ask the patient to cough after taking a deep breath. | ___ | ___ | ___ | _____ |
| 3. Assess risk for postoperative thrombus formation. (Older patients, those with active cancer, and those immobilized for more than three days are most at risk.) Observe for localized tenderness along the distribution of the venous system, swollen calf or thigh, calf swelling more than 3 cm in comparison with asymptomatic leg, pitting edema in symptomatic leg, and collateral superficial veins. If any of these signs are present, notify the physician. | ___ | ___ | ___ | _____ |
| 4. Assess the patient's ability to move independently while in bed. | ___ | ___ | ___ | _____ |
| 5. Explain postoperative exercises to the patient, including their importance to recovery and physiological benefits. | ___ | ___ | ___ | _____ |
| 6. Demonstrate exercises. | | | | |
| A. Diaphragmatic breathing | | | | |
| (1) Assist the patient to a comfortable sitting position on the side of the bed or in a chair or to standing position. | ___ | ___ | ___ | _____ |
| (2) Stand or sit facing the patient. | ___ | ___ | ___ | _____ |
| (3) Instruct the patient to place the palms of the hands across from each other, down and along the lower borders of the anterior rib cage. Place the tips of the third fingers lightly together. Demonstrate for the patient. | ___ | ___ | ___ | _____ |
| (4) Have the patient take slow, deep breaths, inhaling through the nose and pushing the abdomen against the hands. Tell the patient to feel the middle fingers separate during inhalation. Demonstrate. | ___ | ___ | ___ | _____ |
| (5) Explain that the patient will feel normal downward movement of the diaphragm during inspiration. Explain that abdominal organs descend and the chest wall expands. | ___ | ___ | ___ | _____ |
| (6) Avoid using auxiliary chest and shoulder muscles while inhaling, and instruct patient in the same manner. | ___ | ___ | ___ | _____ |
| (7) Have the patient hold a slow, deep breath for count of three, and then slowly exhale through the mouth as if blowing out a candle (with pursed lips). Tell the patient that the middle fingertips will touch as the chest wall contracts. | ___ | ___ | ___ | _____ |
| (8) Repeat breathing exercise three to five times. | ___ | ___ | ___ | _____ |
| (9) Have the patient practise the exercise. Instruct the patient to take ten slow, deep breaths every hour while awake during postoperative period until mobile. | ___ | ___ | ___ | _____ |
| B. Incentive spirometry | | | | |
| (1) Perform hand hygiene. | ___ | ___ | ___ | _____ |
| (2) Instruct the patient to assume semi-Fowler's or high-Fowler's position. | ___ | ___ | ___ | _____ |
| (3) Either set or indicate to the patient on the device scale the volume level to be attained with each breath. | ___ | ___ | ___ | _____ |
| (4) Demonstrate to the patient how to place the mouthpiece of the spirometer so that the lips completely cover it. | ___ | ___ | ___ | _____ |

*Continued*

| | S | U | NP | Comments |
|---|---|---|---|---|

(5) Instruct patient to inhale slowly and maintain constant flow through the unit, attempting to reach goal volume. When maximal inspiration is reached, the patient should hold breath for two or three seconds and then exhale slowly. Number of breaths should not exceed 10 to 12 per minute in each session.

(6) Instruct the patient to breathe normally for a short period.

(7) Have the patient repeat the manoeuvre until goals are achieved.

(8) Perform hand hygiene.

C. Positive expiratory pressure therapy and "huff" coughing

  (1) Perform hand hygiene.

  (2) Set positive expiratory pressure device to the setting ordered.

  (3) Instruct the patient to assume semi-Fowler's or high-Fowler's position, and place nose clip on the patient's nose.

  (4) Have the patient place lips around the mouthpiece. The patient should take a full breath and then exhale two to three times longer than inhalation. This pattern should be repeated for 10 to 20 breaths.

  (5) Remove device from the patient's mouth, and have the patient take a slow, deep breath and hold for three seconds.

  (6) Instruct the patient to exhale in quick, short, forced inhalations, or "huffs."

D. Controlled coughing

  (1) Explain the importance of maintaining an upright position.

  (2) Demonstrate coughing. Take two slow, deep breaths, inhaling through the nose and exhaling through the mouth.

  (3) Inhale deeply a third time, and hold breath to a count of three. Cough fully for two or three consecutive coughs without inhaling between coughs. (Tell the patient to push all air out of lungs.)

  (4) Caution the patient against simply clearing the throat instead of coughing. Explain that coughing will not cause injury to the incision when done correctly.

  (5) If the surgical incision will be abdominal or thoracic, teach the patient to place one hand over the incisional area and the other hand on top of it. During breathing and coughing exercises, the patient presses gently against incisional area to splint or support it. A pillow over the incision is optional.

  (6) The patient continues to practise coughing exercises, splinting the imaginary incision. Instruct the patient to cough two to three times every two hours while awake.

  (7) Instruct the patient to examine any sputum for consistency, odour, amount, and colour changes.

E. Turning

  (1) Instruct the patient to assume the supine position and move to the side of the bed if permitted by surgery. Have the patient move by bending knees and pressing heels against the mattress to raise and move buttocks. Top side rails on both sides of the bed should be raised.

  (2) Instruct the patient to place the right hand over the incisional area to splint it.

  (3) Instruct the patient to keep the right leg straight and flex the left knee up. If back or vascular surgery is being performed, the patient will need to logroll or will require assistance with turning.

  (4) Have the patient grab the right side rail with the left hand, pull toward the right, and roll onto the right side.

  (5) Instruct the patient to turn every two hours while awake.

F. Leg exercises

  (1) Have the patient assume the supine position in bed. Demonstrate leg exercises by performing passive range-of-motion exercises and simultaneously explaining exercise.

  (2) Rotate each ankle in a complete circle. Instruct the patient to draw imaginary circles with the big toe. Repeat five times.

  (3) Alternate dorsiflexion and plantar flexion of both feet. Direct the patient to feel calf muscles contract and relax alternately. Repeat five times.

*Continued*

|  | S | U | NP | Comments |
|---|---|---|---|---|

(4) Perform quadriceps setting by tightening thigh muscles and bringing the knee down toward the mattress, then relaxing. Repeat five times.

(5) Have the patient alternately raise each leg straight up from the bed surface, keeping legs straight, and then have the patient bend the leg at the hip and knee. Repeat five times.

7. Have the patient practise exercises at least every two hours while awake. Instruct the patient to coordinate turning and leg exercises with diaphragmatic breathing, incentive spirometry, and coughing exercises.

8. Observe the patient's ability to perform all five exercises independently.

9. Record the exercises demonstrated and whether the patient can perform them independently.

10. Report any problems the patient has in practising exercises to the nurse assigned to the patient on the next shift for follow-up.